Disalienation

CHICAGO STUDIES IN PRACTICES OF MEANING

A series edited by Andreas Glaeser, William Mazzarella, William Sewell Jr., Kaushik Sunder Rajan, and Lisa Wedeen

Published in collaboration with the Chicago Center for Contemporary Theory
http://ccct.uchicago.edu

Recent books in the series

Capitalism and the Emergence of Civic Equality in Eighteenth-Century France
by William H. Sewell Jr.

Routine Crisis: An Ethnography of Disillusion
by Sarah Muir

Justice Is an Option: A Democratic Theory of Finance for the Twenty-First Century
by Robert Meister

Authoritarian Apprehensions: Ideology, Judgment, and Mourning in Syria
by Lisa Wedeen

Deadline: Populism and the Press in Venezuela
by Robert Samet

Guerrilla Marketing: Counterinsurgency and Capitalism in Colombia
by Alexander L. Fattal

What Nostalgia Was: War, Empire, and the Time of a Deadly Emotion
by Thomas Dodman

The Mana of Mass Society
by William Mazzarella

The Sins of the Fathers: Germany, Memory, Method
by Jeffrey K. Olick

The Politics of Dialogic Imagination: Power and Popular Culture in Early Modern Japan
by Katsuya Hirano

Disalienation

POLITICS, PHILOSOPHY,
AND RADICAL PSYCHIATRY
IN POSTWAR FRANCE

Camille Robcis

The University of Chicago Press   Chicago and London

The University of Chicago Press, Chicago 60637
The University of Chicago Press, Ltd., London
© 2021 by The University of Chicago
All rights reserved. No part of this book may be used or reproduced
in any manner whatsoever without written permission, except in
the case of brief quotations in critical articles and reviews.
For more information, contact the University of Chicago Press,
1427 E. 60th St., Chicago, IL 60637.
Published 2021
Printed and bound by CPI Group (UK) Ltd,
Croydon, CR0 4YY

30 29 28 27 26 25 24 23 22 21   1 2 3 4 5

ISBN-13: 978-0-226-77760-3 (cloth)
ISBN-13: 978-0-226-77774-0 (paper)
ISBN-13: 978-0-226-77788-7 (e-book)
DOI: https://doi.org/10.7208/chicago/9780226777887.001.0001

Library of Congress Cataloging-in-Publication Data

Names: Robcis, Camille, author.
Title: Disalienation : politics, philosophy, and radical psychiatry in
postwar France / Camille Robcis.
Other titles: Politics, philosophy, and radical psychiatry in postwar
France | Chicago studies in practices of meaning.
Description: Chicago ; London : The University of Chicago Press,
2021. | Series: Chicago studies in practices of meaning | Includes
bibliographical references and index.
Identifiers: LCCN 2020046180 | ISBN 9780226777603 (cloth) |
ISBN 9780226777740 (paperback) | ISBN 9780226777887 (ebook)
Subjects: LCSH: Psychotherapy—France—History—20th century. |
Psychiatry—Political aspects—France. | Psychiatry—Philosophy—
History—20th century. | France—Intellectual life—20th century.
Classification: LCC RC450.F7 R63 2021 | DDC 616.89/140944—dc23
LC record available at https://lccn.loc.gov/2020046180

♾ This paper meets the requirements of ANSI/NISO Z39.48-1992
(Permanence of Paper).

For Cate

CONTENTS

List of Illustrations ix
List of Abbreviations xi

INTRODUCTION: A POLITICS OF MADNESS *1*

1: FRANÇOIS TOSQUELLES, SAINT-ALBAN,
AND THE INVENTION OF
INSTITUTIONAL PSYCHOTHERAPY *15*

2: FRANTZ FANON, THE PATHOLOGIES OF FREEDOM,
AND THE DECOLONIZATION OF
INSTITUTIONAL PSYCHOTHERAPY *48*

3: FÉLIX GUATTARI, LA BORDE,
AND THE SEARCH FOR ANTI-OEDIPAL POLITICS *74*

4: MICHEL FOUCAULT, PSYCHIATRY,
ANTIPSYCHIATRY, AND POWER *107*

EPILOGUE: THE HOSPITAL AS A LABORATORY OF
POLITICAL INVENTION *143*

Acknowledgments 151
Notes 157
Bibliography 195
Index 209

ILLUSTRATIONS

Chapter 1

1.1 Postcard of the Saint-Alban Hospital before the war 16
1.2 Institut Pere Mata in Reus, Catalonia, Spain 20
1.3 Postcard of the Camp de Judes in Septfonds 28
1.4 Map of the Camp de Septfonds 29
1.5 François Tosquelles with his assistants at the Septfonds Camp infirmary 30
1.6 Portrait of François Tosquelles painted by one of the prisoners at Septfonds 31
1.7 Transfer order of Tosquelles from Septfonds to Saint-Alban on December 14, 1939 32
1.8 Tosquelles with co-workers at Saint-Alban 38
1.9 Poster of a theater performance at Saint-Alban in 1977 42
1.10 Editorial by Frantz Fanon in *Trait d'union* during his residency at Saint-Alban in March 1953 43
1.11 Tosquelles with a sculpture by Auguste Forestier 45

Chapter 2

2.1 The Psychiatric Hospital of Blida-Joinville 62
2.2 Frantz Fanon and his medical team in Blida 65
2.3 The kitchen of the Blida hospital 65

Chapter 3

3.1 Félix Guattari 76
3.2 Postcard of the Château de La Borde 76

ILLUSTRATIONS

3.3 Map of La Borde 77
3.4 The "Grid" (la "Grille") at La Borde 80
3.5 A CERFI meeting in the 1970s 102

Chapter 4

4.1 Michel Foucault in Münsterlingen with Roland Kuhn and Georges Verdeaux 114
4.2 May '68 Poster: "Bourgeois Medicine Does Not Heal, It Repairs Workers" 126
4.3 *Tankonalasanté*, November 1974 134
4.4 *Psychiatrisés en lutte*, May–August 1975 135

ABBREVIATIONS

AERLIP Association pour l'étude et la rédaction du livre des institutions psychiatriques
BOC Bloque Obrero y Campesino
CERFI Centre d'étude, de recherche et de formation institutionnelles
CNT Confederación Nacional del Trabajo
ERC Esquerra Republicana de Catalunya
FFI Forces françaises de l'intérieur
FFL Forces françaises libres
FGERI Fédération des groupes d'études et de recherches institutionnelles
FLN Front de libération nationale
GIA Groupe information asiles
GIP Groupe d'information sur les prisons
GIS Groupe information santé
GTPSI Groupe de travail de psychothérapie et sociothérapie institutionnelle
ICE Izquierda Comunista de España
IPA International Psychoanalytic Association
PCE Partido Comunista Español
PCF Parti communiste français
POUM Partido Obrero de Unificación Marxista
UEC Union des étudiants communistes

INTRODUCTION

A Politics of Madness

From 1940 to 1945, during the German Occupation of France, forty thousand patients died in French psychiatric hospitals. Like much of the French territory during these years, hospitals suffered greatly from the war, from the chronic shortage of food, medicine, and heat. These deaths, however, were due not simply to scarcity and strenuous living conditions, as official authorities contended, but as several historians have suggested, to a specific policy of extermination of the cognitively disabled that the Nazi state promoted and the Vichy regime silently endorsed.[1] Unlike the Third Reich, which actively embraced eugenics and the forced euthanasia of the "incurably sick," the Vichy regime opted for a "soft extermination" that would let patients die of cold, starvation, or lack of care within the confines of the hospitals themselves. In Saint-Alban-sur-Limagnole, a small and isolated village in the Lozère, in central France, one psychiatric hospital attempted to resist and feed its patients by hoarding extra food with the help of the local population.

Alongside these efforts to provide sustenance and basic care, the doctors and the staff that worked at Saint-Alban began to rethink the practical and theoretical bases of psychiatric care. Fascism and the war had made clear the extent to which the political and the psychic were interconnected. Not only was the murder of the physically and mentally disabled central to the Nazi project of social regeneration, but fascism, authoritarianism, and collaboration were clearly not simple political choices: they required a particular state of mind. For the doctors at Saint-Alban, psychiatry needed to take into account this connection between the political and the psychic and fight on both fronts if it wanted to avoid being complicit with genocidal practices. This movement, which began in Saint-Alban and which had a significant influence on the world of psychiatry and in postwar French thought, came to be known as institutional psychotherapy.[2]

This book traces the history of institutional psychotherapy from its inception at Saint-Alban to its various transformations between 1945 and 1975. It begins with an analysis of Saint-Alban during the war, focusing on one of the most important theorizers and practitioners of institutional psychotherapy, François Tosquelles. Tosquelles was a Catalan psychiatrist and one of the founders of the POUM (Partido Obrero de Unificación Marxista), the anarchist-inspired and anti-Stalinist leftist movement that flourished in the Republican Spain of the 1930s. After fighting against Franco's army during the Spanish Civil War, Tosquelles fled to France where he was placed in a refugee camp close to the Pyrenees before he made his way to the Saint-Alban Hospital. At the front and within the camp, Tosquelles set up therapeutic communities where, with the help of other soldiers and prisoners, he treated combatants and refugees who had been severely affected psychologically by the violence of the war. These improvised psychiatric experiments convinced Tosquelles that psychiatry could be practiced anywhere.

Tosquelles liked to repeat that in the course of his life he had been exposed to multiple forms of physical and ideological "occupations": as a Catalan citizen fighting Spanish imperialism; as a leftist activist struggling against Stalinist domination; as an opponent to fascism, first in Spain and later in the Resistance in Vichy France; and as a refugee detained in the dire setting of a French concentration camp. These various forms of encampment, colonization, or incarceration had rendered him particularly sensitive to the dangers of "concentrationism"—or as he called it, le-tout-pouvoir (the-all-power). As he observed, "concentrationism" was not simply a mode of social and political organization: it also resulted from a particular psychic disposition, and it always had a specifically psychic outcome. In this context, psychiatry could play a key role: it could offer the necessary tools to recognize the traces of this "concentrationism" in the mind, but it could also combat its alienating effects. As Tosquelles's colleague Jean Oury put it, the main goal of institutional psychotherapy was to set up "mechanisms to fight, every day, against all that could turn the whole collective toward a concentrationist or segregationist structure."[3] Institutional psychotherapy was, in the words of Tosquelles, an attempt to cure not only the patients, not only the doctors, but an "attempt to cure life itself."

During the war and the immediate postwar years, institutional psychotherapy drew the attention of several psychiatrists who traveled to Saint-Alban as visitors, residents, or interns. Saint-Alban also became a haven for Surrealist poets such as Paul Éluard and visual artists interested in *art brut* such as Jean Dubuffet who had long been fascinated by madness, which, they believed, represented a more authentic form of existence. The doctors at Saint-Alban came from various social backgrounds, but they all shared a vision of psychiatry as a deeply political practice. Some of these doctors had been involved in communist or anarchist politics prior to the war, and most had joined the Resistance against the Vichy regime. Others arrived at Saint-Alban because they were frustrated with the biological essentialism of mainstream psychiatry, its exclusively neurological approach to the brain, and its hostility to most psychoanalytic, philosophical, or sociological insights. Still others, horrified by the humanitarian disaster taking place in psychiatric hospitals, hoped to find in Saint-Alban a more compassionate form of medical care. In all cases, the inhabitants of the hospital called for a "politics of madness" that would bring together neurology, psychology, psychoanalysis, phenomenology, aesthetics, and social and political theory. The point of institutional psychotherapy was never to devise a fixed dogma or model that could be applied indiscriminately, but rather to offer an "ethics" in Michel Foucault's sense of the term — a practice of everyday life.

One of the essential premises of institutional psychotherapy was the belief that theory and practice were inextricably linked — including in the treatment of psychosis. According to the practitioners of institutional psychotherapy, the two fields that had most studied madness, psychiatry and psychoanalysis, were both fundamentally hindered by their erroneous understanding of psychosis, from a conceptual and from a therapeutic point of view. Mainstream psychiatry, as these doctors had concluded after their medical training, remained hopelessly enamored with the ideal of neutrality and rigid objectivism. Its focus on brain localization (hoping to find the cause of specific behaviors in the brain) left little space for the patients' self-accounts or for the study of how social, familial, and cultural factors came into play in the genesis of mental processes.[4] Furthermore, for institutional psychotherapy, psychiatry still refused to recognize the explicitly political nature of all medical practice and, more generally, of all scientific research, its historical entanglement with structures of power, and its responsibility in the stigmatization of madness. In this sense, the work of the historian of science Georges Canguilhem, who spent some time at Saint-Alban in 1944 while he was in the Resistance, was crucial for the theorists of institutional psychotherapy. Instead of treating psychosis as an aberration, institutional psychotherapy, following Canguilhem, considered it a variation of the normal, another form of life.

Given these limitations of mainstream psychiatry, many of the practitioners of institutional psychotherapy turned to psychoanalysis as a framework that could take into better consideration the various factors that intervened in the causality of mental developments. In fact, Sigmund Freud himself shared many of these apprehensions concerning psychiatry, and we could say that Freud invented psychoanalysis at the end of the nineteenth century as a way to bypass the rigid determinism of psychiatry. In particular, Freud devised two concepts that became absolutely central to institutional psychotherapy: the existence of an unconscious and the importance of transference in all clinical work. The unconscious allowed Freud to posit a model of causality that went beyond culture and biology. Indeed, as he observed, his first patients—primarily hysterics—exhibited a series of spectacular symptoms without displaying any specific neurological signs on their brains. If these symptoms were not natural, that is, biological or neurological in their origin, they were also not entirely culturally determined: rather, their origin was psychic. Psychoanalysis thus emerged as an alternative to conventional psychiatry, which focused primarily on the brain, but also to sociological explanations that assumed that if all behavior was learned, it could also be unlearned. His patients' symptoms, Freud was noticing, were not disappearing simply because they wanted them to. The fantasmatic was just as "real" as the empirical: what his patients remembered or had come to believe was just as important as what had really happened. Freud thus invented the "talking cure" as a way to gain access to this other reality, psychic reality.

Freud's talking cure relied on a second concept that became a cornerstone for institutional psychotherapy: transference. This was the term that Freud coined to designate the patient's affective bond with his or her analyst. This unconscious bond functioned as a conduit to study the structure of the patient's other intersubjective relationships, social or familial for example. Freud, however, was forced to reconsider his understanding of transference when he was presented with psychotic patients who had a relation to language that was radically different from his and for whom intersubjective interactions operated quite differently. As Jacques Lacan would later put it, psychosis was characterized by the foreclosure of the symbolic order, the domain of alterity and of the signifier in language. The difficulty of relying on the psychoanalytic talking cure to treat psychotic patients was especially clear to Freud after his case study of Daniel Paul Schreber, the German judge who suffered from paranoid delusions and who, in 1903, published a memoir that provided the groundwork for Freud's inquiry. Schreber, whom we would most likely categorize today as a paranoid schizophrenic, had lost his sense of social reality as his fantasies became autonomous. Freud concluded that psychoanalysis was primarily a theory geared toward neurotics (who suffered from obsessive behavior, anxiety, hysteria, phobias ...) rather than psychotics whose delusions and hallucinations had taken over.

Many of Freud's followers remained unhappy with this observation and continued to study psychosis through a psychoanalytic lens. Jacques Lacan, for example, devoted his 1932 medical thesis to the question of paranoid psychosis and its relation to the personality. Lacan's point was not simply that psychoanalysis could be compatible with psychiatry but, more provocatively, that psychiatry needed to be anchored in a Freudian understanding of subjectivity. As Lacan insisted, psychosis was the product of a complex interaction of neurological, biological, psychological, and social factors, and psychiatry's obsession with locating a single cause in the brain was simply absurd. Lacan's work, and his attention to language especially, provided foundational references for the practitioners of institutional psychotherapy. As psychoanalysis throughout the world began moving toward ego psychology and behaviorism after the Second World War, Lacan remained an unconditional advocate of the Freudian unconscious and of transference, the two pillars that, as he argued, marked the specificity of psychoanalysis as a method.[5]

The intention of institutional psychotherapy was to take Lacan's "return to Freud" one step further and to explore how psychoanalysis could be useful for psychotic patients within the confines of the hospital, and not just in one-on-one sessions. Indeed, as the doctors associated with institutional psychotherapy had witnessed in their clinical work, psychotic patients did have transferential relations, but they were not intersubjective, person-to-person, as they were in the case of neurosis: they were collective. Tosquelles referred to the psychotic transference as a "burst transference" (*transfert éclaté*); Oury as a "transferential constellation"; Félix Guattari as a "transversality." In all cases, the social remained the most significant space to observe the operations of the psychotic unconscious, to analyze the projection of desires and fantasies, to study identifications, and to eventually try to work with them.

These were the theoretical premises that guided Tosquelles and his colleagues at Saint-Alban as they set up a series of concrete practices that would favor this transferential constellation, reconfigure the social, and, they hoped, attenuate their patients' suffering: group therapies, general meetings, self-managed unions, ergotherapy workshops (printing, binding, woodwork, pottery ...), libraries, publications, and a wide range of cultural activities (movies, concerts, theater ...). The idea was to constantly imagine and reimagine institutions that would produce

6 INTRODUCTION

new vectors of transference, different forms of identifications, and alternative, less hierarchical, and less oppressive social relations. Every hands-on experiment also had a therapeutic purpose, and every therapeutic intervention was always grounded in the practice.

Their theoretical reliance on Freudian and especially on Lacanian psychoanalysis was one of the factors that distinguished institutional psychotherapists from other practitioners of radical psychiatry who emerged in the postwar years, such as Franco Basaglia in Italy, Ronald Laing and David Cooper in Great Britain, or Thomas Szasz in the United States.[6] Laing and Basaglia, for instance, were much more interested in phenomenology and existentialism than in Lacan's turn to structural linguistics. Even though the second generation of institutional psychotherapists—especially Félix Guattari—had a more critical relationship to Lacanian orthodoxy, psychoanalysis remained a constant source of reference for institutional psychotherapy. The idea was not to choose psychiatry *or* psychoanalysis but to reform and integrate the two together.

This was another important point of difference between institutional psychotherapy and many of these other currents that came to be known in the 1960s as "antipsychiatry": institutional psychotherapy insisted on the medical specificity of psychosis. Psychosis was not simply an angry (and, according to much of antipsychiatry, justified) reaction to social or familial oppression. It was neither a cultural construction nor an effect of bourgeois power, but an illness that required medication and could benefit from a hospital setting. To be sure, like antipsychiatry, institutional psychotherapy was eminently conscious of the power structures undergirding psychiatry, but it never rejected drugs, neuroleptics, or even insulin cures and electroshocks. Similarly, institutional psychotherapy never advocated closing down hospitals, unlike much of antipsychiatry, perhaps most famously in Italy with Basaglia's *psichiatria democratica*. Again, the hospital needed to be profoundly rethought— and this was the goal of institutional psychotherapy—but institutions still retained great therapeutic potential for the treatment of psychosis. In other words, according to institutional psychotherapy, it was possible to remain institutional while critical at the same time.

From its birth at Saint-Alban, institutional psychotherapy had many admirers, including Frantz Fanon, who was a resident at Saint-Alban from 1952 to 1953 after he completed medical school in Lyon. When he arrived at the hospital, Fanon was already the author of several important works including "The North African Syndrome" and *Black Skin, White Masks*.

The kinds of experiments that Tosquelles and his colleagues had set up at Saint-Alban, and the results they were getting, confirmed many of the philosophical hypotheses that Fanon had put forth in his early work on race and racism. In particular, Fanon had argued that the psyche and the social were structurally linked, that colonialism and racism had crucial psychological effects, and that psychiatry could—and should—be political. As Fanon later put it, "all political leaders should be psychiatrists as well."[7]

At Saint-Alban, Tosquelles had a profound influence on Fanon. Fanon brought the insights of institutional psychotherapy to North Africa, first at the psychiatric hospital of Blida-Joinville in Algeria, where he lived from 1953 to 1957, and later at the Charles-Nicolle day center in Tunisia where he worked until his death in 1961. Throughout these years, Fanon treated psychotic patients as well as war combatants and wrote about institutional psychotherapy, its benefits and limits within a colonial context. At the same time, he got increasingly involved with the FLN (Front de libération nationale) and with anticolonial struggles more generally, and he wrote his most important political texts, including *The Wretched of the Earth*, during those years. In this sense, institutional psychotherapy was literally interwoven, from a theoretical standpoint but also at the very concrete level of production, with Fanon's political work.

Another early advocate of institutional psychotherapy was Jean Oury, who was a resident at Saint-Alban in 1947 and who, in 1953, founded the Clinic of La Borde in Cour-Cheverny, in the Loire region. Throughout the 1960s, La Borde became a mythical pilgrimage site for the French intellectual world, as it welcomed philosophers, artists, writers, and filmmakers, in addition to medical personnel. Fernand Deligny, the educator and film director who worked with autistic children, for example, spent several months at La Borde before moving to the Cévennes where he tried to implement a new form of living in which autistic children could thrive outside of the pathologizing gaze of medicine and society.[8]

La Borde also provided a home for the philosopher, psychoanalyst, and political activist Félix Guattari, who worked at the clinic—and lived there on and off—from 1955 until his death in 1992. Oury, Guattari, and their colleagues at La Borde borrowed and adapted many of the Saint-Alban techniques to reorganize the life of the clinic and to imagine new vectors of transference for the psychotic unconscious. Their clinical practice also evolved alongside Lacanian psychoanalysis, and many of the doctors of La Borde attended Lacan's seminars in Paris each week. For Guattari, the type of psychiatry performed at La Borde was in perfect continuity with his political and philosophical activity, what

8   INTRODUCTION

he would eventually call "institutional analysis." All provided different terrains to think through the role of the institution as a social and subjective anchor and to envision radically horizontal, anti-authoritarian, and "deterritorialized" spaces, to use his term.

Guattari brought together his clinical experience at La Borde with his political and philosophical interests in the FGERI (Fédération des groupes d'études et de recherches institutionnelles), a working group that he founded in 1964 and that in 1967 merged into the CERFI (Centre d'étude, de recherche et de formation institutionnelles). In 1966, the CERFI began publishing a journal, *Recherches*, to which various intellectuals of the time, including Gilles Deleuze, Maud Mannoni, Michel Foucault, Guy Hocquenghem, and Antonio Negri, contributed. Guattari also explored the intersections of the psychiatric and the philosophical in his magnum opus co-written with Gilles Deleuze, *Capitalism and Schizophrenia*, whose first volume, *Anti-Oedipus*, was published in 1972, followed by the second, *A Thousand Plateaus*, in 1977.

Both of these works—*Anti-Oedipus* in particular—were premised on the idea that alienation was always social and psychic at once, a lesson that Guattari and Oury had learned from Tosquelles. "Oedipalization"—the concept that Deleuze and Guattari invented to describe the entrapment of desire and its channeling into the "safe" route of the heterosexual family—did not simply configure social relations: it was also a state of being, a form of psychic renunciation of the plenitude of desire. It is in this sense that Michel Foucault referred to *Anti-Oedipus* as a "book of ethics": its goal was to convince its readers to give up their attachment to authority, domination, and power, to renounce the "fascisms in their heads." As Foucault put it: "How does one keep from being fascist, even (especially) when one believes oneself to be a revolutionary militant? How do we rid our speech and our acts, our hearts and our pleasures, of fascism? How do we ferret out the fascism that is ingrained in our behavior?"[9] Being anti-oedipal was, like institutional psychotherapy, a way to excavate the traces of "concentrationism" in our psyche and our social existence, and in this sense, a lifestyle, a mode of thinking and living.

Each chapter of this book is organized around a case study of individuals who either practiced, theorized, or engaged extensively with institutional psychotherapy. The first chapter recounts the beginnings of institutional psychotherapy at Saint-Alban, highlighting the crucial presence of Tosquelles. The second chapter focuses on Fanon, his encounter with institutional psychotherapy, and his psychiatric and political work in North Africa. The third chapter shifts to La Borde, to what was often called the second generation of institutional psychotherapy, with Oury and Guattari. The fourth and final chapter centers on Michel Foucault, who was neither a psychiatrist nor a psychoanalyst, but who thought and wrote about institutional psychotherapy. Even though Foucault considered becoming a psychiatrist as a student, he ultimately rejected the premises of institutional psychotherapy and of psychiatry more generally. Instead, he gravitated toward antipsychiatry and relied on it to formulate a new theory of power—which he called "disciplinary power"—during the 1970s. My aim is to trace the intersections of psychiatry, philosophy, and politics in the work of each of these figures. In each case, I examine how the psyche has figured as a lens to think through the political, to understand alienation and offer perspectives for "disalienation."

Much of what has been written on institutional psychotherapy has tended to be in the mode of either dismissal ("it clearly did not work") or hagiography ("it was wonderful and psychiatry needs to return to this model"). My own interest in institutional psychotherapy is somewhat different. Institutional psychotherapy was a complex and diverse movement with some incredibly visionary and progressive analyses and other remarkably conservative and retrograde positions. Despite its explicit commitment to anti-authoritarianism, it is worth noting that the doctors associated with institutional psychotherapy were mostly male and mostly white and that they often failed to question some obvious hierarchies around gender and race. Fanon's exceptionality—which I comment on extensively in chapter 2—is, in this sense, worth pausing on. I am interested in the possibilities of using certain insights of institutional psychotherapy in psychological, psychoanalytic, and psychiatric clinical work, but as a historian, I find the therapeutic potential of these experiments difficult to assess. Rather, through my study of institutional psychotherapy, I hope to contribute to three broader historiographical and theoretical discussions.

First, I want to suggest that institutional psychotherapy can add to the conversation around the history of the self.[10] Indeed, one of the clearest goals of institutional psychotherapy was to question the idea that psychic manifestations, in psychosis but also in subjectivity more generally, resulted from a single cause. As the practitioners of institutional psychotherapy maintained, neurological, unconscious, familial, and social factors constantly interacted in the construction of the self. This is why psychiatry needed to remain open to literature, philosophy, anthropology, art, and social and political theory and to draw from the various tools that these disciplines offered. In this sense, this book is an attempt to put intellectual history and the history of science in dialogue. It is also an effort to bring together the neurosciences, the social sciences, and the humanities and to recall this moment in history in which brain and psyche were perceived not as mutually exclusive but as complementary in the understanding of the self.

Second, I want to revisit the relationship between the psychic and the political through this cast of characters who maintained not only that psychiatry was political but also that politics needed to take the unconscious seriously. One of my goals in this book is to read institutional psychotherapy as a political theory, as an attempt to envision a different political imaginary that can still be useful today. More specifically, the founders of institutional psychotherapy conceived of their project against the two dominant political frameworks of their time: liberalism and State Marxism in its bureaucratic Cold War version. By foregrounding the decisive role of drives, affect, and desire, institutional psychotherapy challenged the liberal ideal—inherited from the Enlightenment—of a bound, individualized, and rational self. However, it also refused the crude Marxist vision according to which the libidinal and the fantasmatic were simply displacements of a more accurate material reality, whether it be class interest, capitalist hegemony, or social structure. For institutional psychotherapy, the unconscious was not simply important to politics. It was not a supplement to a political analysis. Rather, the unconscious was constitutive of the political. Institutional psychotherapy developed this point extensively in relation to three questions: its theory of alienation, its understanding of fantasy, and its analysis of institutions.

The problem of alienation and disalienation was at the heart of institutional psychotherapy. Psychosis was first and foremost a form of alienation, or rather, a double alienation as the French term *aliéné* denotes. Alienation was a psychic state—being mad, insane—but also a social condition that left patients feeling estranged, trapped, isolated from others. This theory of "double alienation" was what led Tosquelles to regularly refer to Marx and Freud as the "two legs" of institutional psychotherapy. Marxism was necessary to understand and address social alienation, but it needed to be complemented by psychoanalysis, indispensable to grasp its psychic dimension. As Tosquelles liked to say throughout his life, when one leg walked, the other needed to follow. Alienation more broadly, however, was not specific to psychosis: it was coextensive with the human condition, and this is why psychosis could be helpful in formulating a more general theory of subjectivity.

The question of alienation seemed especially pressing in the aftermath of the Second World War. First and foremost, institutional psychotherapy sought to come to terms with fascism. How was fascism able to succeed in Europe, and, in the context of their particular discipline, how did psychiatry close its eyes to the mass murder of the physically and mentally disabled? As Dagmar Herzog has recently put it, "unlearning eugenics" in post-Nazi Europe required a particular intellectual shift.[11] But more generally, for many of the practitioners of institutional psychotherapy, the turn to the psyche was necessary to overcome the impasses which, they believed, had paralyzed the left in the postwar period. Indeed, by 1950, it was clear that ideology was not the exclusive weapon of a ruling class seeking to oppress another. It was also clear that alienation was unlikely to disappear, even when the proletariat managed to acquire the means of production as in the Soviet Union and other socialist nations. In other words, if alienation would not end with a Marxist revolution, another framework to understand politics was necessary. This is where the unconscious could be useful.

As Deleuze and Guattari argued in *Anti-Oedipus*, if workers continued to vote against their interest and to sabotage their potential emancipation, it was because they had been conditioned—unconsciously—to think and act in particular ways. As these authors saw it, by the 1970s, the most important obstacle for any leftist or progressive political action was not so much the fascism of Hitler and Mussolini that was easily recognizable, but the "fascisms in our heads," the fascisms that caused us to "love power, to desire the thing that dominates and exploits us," as Foucault would claim.[12] To be sure, Deleuze, Guattari, and Foucault used the term "fascism" hyperbolically and metaphorically—and, we could say, quite problematically from a historical point of view—to refer to authoritarianism more broadly.[13] Still, their more general point was that any political analysis required a notion of the unconscious just as any study of the unconscious needed to include a social perspective.

Institutional psychotherapy was not the only attempt to bring together Marx and Freud in the twentieth century. Several thinkers associated with the Frankfurt School (especially Herbert Marcuse and Erich Fromm) or with Marxist existentialism (Jean-Paul Sartre for example) had already tried.[14] Many of these authors, however, remained committed to a revolutionary horizon, to "disalienation" as a possible and reachable goal, rather than constructing alienation as the very condition of human existence. This is why fantasy—and the psychoanalytic understanding of fantasy—was so important for institutional psychotherapy. At the level of the self, taking fantasy seriously meant that identity was never unified or whole but discontinuous and often contradictory. At the level of the group, fantasy was equally central, and most of the group work of institutional psychotherapy sought to create various stages for these fantasies and these conflicts to play out in a clinical setting. At the level of society, fantasy could help us understand a phenomenon such as fascism but also authoritarianism, racism, xenophobia, misogyny, and the extreme right more generally. From this perspective, fascism was neither a "failure of rationality" or a political pathology as liberalism maintained, nor a "false consciousness," a displacement of social reality, as Marxism suggested. According to institutional psychotherapy, both of these accounts failed to understand the actual *desire* expressed in these mass movements, the collective fantasy of a cleansing violence and a regenerated social body.

If alienation and fantasy were constitutive of the self and of all social processes, institutional psychotherapy proposed to work with them through the framework of institutions. Indeed, as its name indicates, institutional psychotherapy argued that institutions were necessary for the construction of subjectivity and for social organization. This was another way in which it differed significantly from Italian, British, or American antipsychiatry, which blamed institutions (including the asylum) for human unhappiness and often fought for their destruction. It is also, as we will see, one of the ways in which institutional psychotherapy departed most considerably from Foucault, who depicted institutions as sites of power, knowledge, and subjectification—and certainly not as vectors of emancipation.

According to the theorizers of institutional psychotherapy, the problem with institutions was not that they existed or that they generated conflicts but that they all had the potential to become "concentrationist"— authoritarian, hierarchical, oppressive, and stagnant. Institutional psychotherapy strove not to eliminate institutions or to suppress conflicts but rather to imagine a philosophy, a social theory, and a clinical practice that would prevent the reappearance of these political and psychic "concentrationisms"—to imagine institutions that could be constantly rethought, reworked, and remapped. This was the principle that guided all therapeutic activities within the hospital. And in this sense, the hospital could offer a template to rethink the community at large, what Oury called the Collective. From this perspective, psychiatry could also function as a form of systematic critique, suspicious of doctrinal purity and theoretical a prioris. As I develop in the epilogue, institutional psychotherapy sought to convert the hospital into a laboratory of political invention to conceive a new "common," a radically horizontal social space committed to the renewed destabilization of centers and authorities—a conduit to a permanent revolution of the political and the psychic at once.

The third broader ambition of this book is more specific to intellectual history. Indeed, this project is engaged in a historiographical dis-

A Politics of Madness 13

cussion as it strives to be both a microhistory of particular hospitals and a transnational study that extends beyond France, to Algeria, Tunisia, and Spain. My aim is not to claim that Saint-Alban, La Borde, or Blida was the sole origin of this diverse intellectual production but rather to explore the role that a particular setting or context can have in fostering ideas. The book interweaves archival research and oral interviews, historical analysis, and philosophical and theoretical close readings in order to map out various overlapping networks of professional collaboration, intellectual exchange, and personal friendships. Each chapter attempts to set up a dialogue between texts and their various contexts, following Dominick LaCapra's valuable notion of a "dialogic" approach to reading and interpretation.[15] Instead of opting for a model of causality ("this person was influenced by this person"), I would like to think of the figures in this book as a *constellation* in Walter Benjamin's sense, as a spatial arrangement without an origin or an end point in which certain links and connections can come to light or be obscured, depending on the viewer's perspective.[16]

How, for instance, can we rethink the supposedly European parameters of the history of medicine and what is generally referred to as "French theory" if we highlight the importance of Tosquelles and Catalonia for Fanon, Oury, and Guattari? How do we rewrite the history of "Western" psychiatry if we consider Fanon the strictest interpreter of institutional psychotherapy who was forced to revise the Saint-Alban lessons—to "deterritorialize" them—for the colonial context of Blida? How does intellectual history shift if we regard Lacan as a psychiatrist rather than a philosopher and if we take into account the role that the Saint-Alban doctors played in popularizing his work in medical spheres? How are our commonly held ideas on Foucault challenged if we treat him as a close interlocutor of psychiatry rather than an unconditional critic? How were anticolonialism and radical psychiatry brought together by certain journals such as *Esprit* and certain publishers, most notably François Maspero? Why was the psychiatric field so foundational for postwar French thought? Finally, how can the central notions of institutional psychotherapy—the unconscious as individual and social at once; desire and fantasy as foundational and always already conflictual; collective transference; institutional praxis—still help us today to apprehend the permanence of extreme-right movements, fascisms real and "in our heads," still spreading and gaining force throughout the world?

CHAPTER 1

François Tosquelles, Saint-Alban, and the Invention of Institutional Psychotherapy

Institutional psychotherapy was born during the Second World War in a small and remote village in central France called Saint-Alban-sur-Limagnole. Since 1821, the castle of Saint-Alban had served as an asylum for the Lozère region, housing approximately six hundred patients by the turn of the century (fig. 1.1). Managed by administrators who were, according to the testimony of Marius Bonnet, a nurse who arrived at Saint-Alban in 1931, more interested in "minimizing costs and troubles" than in the welfare of the patients, the asylum slowly deteriorated.[1] Without heat, drugs, and basic sanitation, the inhabitants of the Saint-Alban asylum lived in miserable conditions.[2] As Bonnet recalls, the patients slept in haystacks that also served as their toilets, amongst screams, foul smells, chronic illness, and death. They were "constantly locked up, day and night, without electricity, in complete inactivity, without ever seeing the doctor" or anyone else from the outside world, since visits were forbidden.[3] In 1914 a fire destroyed much of the building, and in 1936 a typhoid epidemic ravaged the institution. Both crises highlighted the pressing need to modernize the insalubrious facilities and to implement serious hygienic measures.[4] This was the context in which Paul Balvet assumed the directorship of the asylum, which, in 1937, was declared a psychiatric hospital. It was also the context in which François Tosquelles, one of the most important theorizers and practitioners of institutional psychotherapy, arrived at Saint-Alban, where he worked from 1940 to 1962.

This chapter focuses on the life, the ideas, and the work of François Tosquelles, who had a decisive influence on various of the other figures who appear in this book, including Jean Oury, Félix Guattari, Lucien Bonnafé, Frantz Fanon, and Georges Canguilhem. More specifically, this chapter makes two arguments. First, I want to suggest that

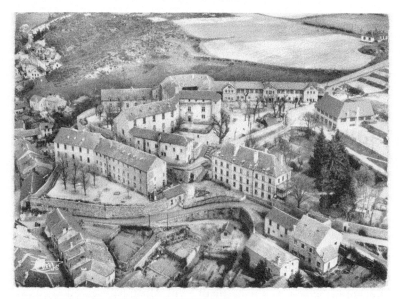

1.1 Postcard of the Saint-Alban Hospital before the war
© Association Culturelle SACPI

Tosquelles played a key role in the dialogue between psychoanalysis and psychiatry in twentieth-century France. Tosquelles brought many of the insights of Freud and especially of Lacan to the domain of psychiatry, both in his theoretical writings and in his medical practice. Tosquelles's reliance on psychoanalysis revealed the constraints of biological and neurological essentialism in psychiatry. It also exposed the theoretical limits of Freud's own understanding of psychoanalysis as a departure from psychiatry and as a treatment geared primarily toward neurotics as opposed to psychotics for whom repression, symptoms, language—and hence transference—operated quite differently.[5]

The second argument that I wish to develop in this chapter is that Tosquelles's psychiatric work was fundamentally shaped by his activism in radical politics in Catalonia and by his experience during the Spanish Civil War, first as a doctor for the Republican army at the front and later as a refugee in a French concentration camp. This experience of physical occupation—whether this occupation came in the form of Spanish nationalism, Stalinism, Fascism, Vichy, or World War II—convinced Tosquelles of the intimate link between political and psychic oppression, between political and psychic freedom. Consequently, politics and psychiatry needed to work together to "disalienate" subjects and "disoccupy" their minds. Marx and Freud were thus complementary figures for Tosquelles, the two sides of one same struggle in what he called a "politics of madness" (*une politique de la folie*). Whereas Marx was necessary to grasp social alienation, Freud was essential for diagnosing psychic disaffection.[6] As Tosquelles explained in a 1984 interview: "From age ten, I already knew what I wanted to do: bring Freud to the asylum, and bring psychoanalysis to the patients. Later, I understood that without Marx, a psychiatrist is nothing. Marx talks about the problems of man as a social being and Freud talks about the psychopathology of man, why he is condemned to suffer. Without them, we cannot understand anything about man, let alone about the mad. This is what all these biological psychiatrists refuse to understand when they think that they can cure the world with a pill."[7] It is this process of bringing together the theories of Freud and Marx and applying them to the asylum that I explore in this chapter.

Marx and Freud in Catalonia

Marx and Freud were indeed the two most important references for Tosquelles before he left Spain and sought refuge in France in 1939. Born in 1912 in Reus, a city south of Barcelona, Tosquelles was deeply marked by the Catalan political and cultural effervescence of the turn of the century. With the electoral victory of the ERC (Esquerra Republicana de Catalunya), which advocated socialism and Catalan independence, Catalonia became the first region of Spain to proclaim itself a republic in 1931. These were vibrant years for the labor movement, which was marked by strong anarchist and syndicalist currents.[8] The CNT (Confederación Nacional del Trabajo), founded in Barcelona in 1910, anchored itself in the important neighborhood-based sociability and reciprocity networks that had emerged in the last decades of the nineteenth century. Significant philosophical and tactical disagreements divided the myriad workers' collectives during these years, but many on the left bonded over their disillusion with the PCE (Partido Comunista Español), the official communist party, which they perceived as too subservient to Moscow, too eager to accept integration and centralization. Instead, the CNT and many groups on the radical left advocated federalism and decentralization, worker solidarity and self-management, and consciousness-raising, particularly through culture.[9]

In 1935, activists from two of these subgroups, the ICE (Izquierda Comunista de España) and the BOC (Bloque Obrero y Campesino) under the leadership of Andreu Nin and Joaquín Maurín, founded the POUM (Partido Obrero de Unificación Marxista). Nin and Maurín, who had both begun their political activism within the CNT, embraced its vision of society as federated communes. Having traveled to Russia, both were also very much attracted to the thought of Leon Trotsky and his idea of permanent revolution. Most important, the POUM supporters were adamant about their opposition to Stalinism and to the centralized, antidemocratic, authoritarian, and bureaucratic turn that the Soviet Union had taken.[10] As its leaders stated in a 1936 manifesto "Who Is the POUM and What Does It Want?," the POUM fought for "a revolution committed to democratic-socialist ideals, workers' alliances, the recognition of regional nationalisms and the creation of an Iberian Union of Socialist Republics that would replace the centralized nation, and the right to criticize the policies of the leaders of the USSR when they were counterproductive for the march of the world revolution."[11]

The POUM's advocacy of federalism, regionalism, and anti-authoritarianism clashed with the Comintern's directives for socialist movements throughout Europe and with Stalin's foreign policy, which had become increasingly obsessed with the notion of sabotage and treachery after successive defeats in Germany, Estonia, Bulgaria, and China throughout the 1920s. As the POUM's leaders reiterated, Stalin's Comintern was a perfect example of ideological colonialism, a "grotesque attempt to impose the map of Russia over that of Spain."[12] Although Stalin immediately denounced the POUM as a "Trotskyite organization" filled with "fascist spies," the POUM eventually broke with Trotsky who, in their eyes, also sought to force a Russian framework onto Spain. The POUM thus refused to adhere to Trotsky's Fourth International, preferring to remain politically independent. It is this spirit of critique that pushed the POUM to stand alone amongst international leftist organizations in denouncing the Moscow show trials, and in particular the execution of Lev Kamenev and Grigori Zinoviev in 1936.[13]

Tosquelles was among the founding members of the POUM, which, by 1936, had grown larger than the official Communist Party of Spain (PCE).[14] Fiercely loyal to Stalin and the Comintern, the PCE quickly began calling for the extermination of the POUM. Although the POUM was apprehensive about the strategy of "popular fronts" advocated by Stalin, it chose to participate in the Spanish Popular Front of Manuel Azaña, which gathered republicans, communists, and socialists. The Spanish Popular Front eventually won the elections of February 1936, five months before Francisco Franco's coup d'état in July 1936 and the beginning of the Spanish Civil War. As Tosquelles recalled in an interview, it was his activism in the POUM that taught him to refuse the "all-power" (le tout-pouvoir). As he put it, "Stalin wanted the POUM to join Madrid and to spread Spanish propaganda—with the monarchy, the military in power—and say 'all-power-to-the Soviets.' No republicans, no anarchists, no socialists, nothing." To accept centralization was to accept to speak *castellano* "when the Castilians are our oppressors."[15] It was through his activism in the POUM and through his exposure to Catalan anarchism that Tosquelles became especially interested in promoting decentralization, self-management, and solidarity within the confines of the psychiatric hospital, as mechanisms to prevent authoritarianism, reification, and stagnation.

Parallel to his political activism, Tosquelles began medical school in 1927 and chose to specialize in psychiatry, a booming field in the Catalonia of the early twentieth century. As the historian of psychiatry Josep Comelles has suggested, psychiatric reform was central to the Catalanist political project during these years, especially once the nationalists were able to gain control of the four provincial governments of Catalonia between 1914 and 1925. Catalan "psychiatric nationalism," to use Comelles's expression, was premised on the idea that individual subjectivity and social communities were conceptually analogous, and thus, that psychiatric care needed to be adapted to the Catalan regional specificity.[16] Between 1911 and 1925, one of the government's main structural initiatives was to decentralize psychiatric care through the implementation of district divisions known as *comarcas*. The idea behind these *comarcas* was to allow patients who did not require hospitalization to continue living with their families, in their usual surroundings.[17] As Félix Martí Ibáñez, an anarchist psychiatrist who became director of the health and social services of Catalonia after the 1936 Revolution, put it:

> In view of the special structure of Catalonia, we chose the *comarca*, which in this region possesses well-defined geographic and economic characteristics and, because it represents an unheard-of abundance of creative energy and new vitality, it could renew so much of the archaic health care system. We were persuaded that the form of the future revolutionary social organization would be the *comarca*. In the new Catalan anatomy, it will enjoy a new flowering of life, it will be a palpitating organ in the regional whole, and its warmth will expand the great *comarcal* capitals which will become the cultural and economic mirrors of the *comarca* reflected in them, instead of the way things were in the past, when these cities were socioeconomic deserts of little vitality in which, from time to time, an oasis bloomed with false splendor.[18]

In many ways, the *comarca* system laid the foundations for what would later be called in France *psychiatrie de secteur*, a movement that

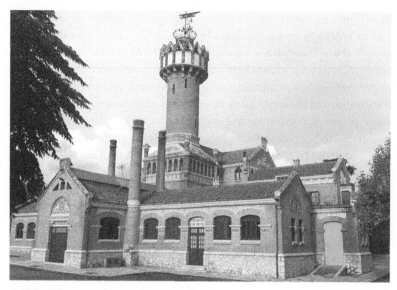

1.2 Institut Pere Mata in Reus, Catalonia, Spain
© Camille Robcis

Tosquelles and his associates first developed at Saint-Alban and that was eventually adopted by the French Ministry of Health and generalized to the rest of the national territory after 1960.

Among the most important actors in this Catalan psychiatric reform movement of the early twentieth century was Tosquelles's mentor, Emilio Mira y López.[19] Like Tosquelles, Mira was actively involved in leftist politics, and he was one of the founders of the Catalan-Balearic Communist Federation. But Mira was also a psychiatrist who worked at the Institut Pere Mata in Tosquelles's hometown, Reus (fig. 1.2). Tosquelles, who was already well acquainted with the Pere Mata clinic through his uncle, who was also a doctor there, joined the medical team soon after finishing medical school. Mira, who was a prolific writer and who held the first chair of psychiatry at the University of Barcelona in 1933, was also one of the main popularizers of Freud's thought in Catalonia. An avid reader of phenomenology, Surrealism, and psychoanalysis, Mira incorporated many of these insights into his teaching, his writings, and his medical practice.[20] As Tosquelles recalls, it was Mira who, during their clinical briefings at the Pere Mata, taught him to question the idea of a detached and objective psychiatrist—the positivist ideal throughout the nineteenth century—and to take into consideration the doctor's own transference with his patients and with the hospital.[21]

Throughout these years, Mira was in close contact with Maurice

Dide, a psychiatrist based in Toulouse who eventually played a key role in bringing Tosquelles to Saint-Alban, and who regularly visited Mira in Barcelona and in Reus.[22] Mira—and Tosquelles—admired Dide's clinical approach, which emphasized the patient's humanity and which called for a psychiatric practice tolerant and accepting of madness. This new approach to madness also appealed to many Surrealist writers and artists—including those based in Toulouse—who saw in madness the key to a more genuine form of human existence. After he had come to terms with what he perceived as the obvious failure of "moral treatment" as preached by Philippe Pinel and the other founding fathers of psychiatry in the nineteenth century, Dide's philosophy was to "leave the mad alone."[23] It was through Mira, finally, that Tosquelles first encountered the work of Jacques Lacan, who, as we will see, remained a constant source of inspiration throughout his life.[24] Mira's teaching and the reading of Lacan convinced Tosquelles that there was no necessary conflict between psychiatry and psychoanalysis, as many psychiatrists maintained. To deepen his understanding of psychoanalysis, Tosquelles began in 1933 an analysis with Sandor Eiminder, a Hungarian-Jewish doctor who had belonged to the Aichhorn group in Vienna and one of the many Eastern European exiles who had landed in Barcelona—often described as a "small Vienna" throughout the early thirties.[25]

Theoretical Bases: Simon and Lacan

Aside from Mira, whom he described as his "master," Tosquelles was deeply indebted to two books that, as he recalled in various interviews, he brought with him into France, "across the Pyrenees," in 1939, when he escaped the Spanish fascist regime: Jacques Lacan's 1932 thesis on paranoia and Hermann Simon's 1929 account of his psychiatric work at the Gütersloh asylum in Germany. These texts, which Tosquelles translated, photocopied, and distributed at Saint-Alban before they were readily available to the French public, were foundational for the development of the theory and practice of institutional psychotherapy.[26] Tosquelles became acquainted with the work of Simon through Ramón Sarró, a Catalan psychiatrist, an expert on schizophrenia, and a colleague of Mira's, who, after living in Vienna and in close contact with Freud and his circle for two years, played a central role in the diffusion of psychoanalysis in interwar Spain. More generally, Simon became well-known in psychiatric milieus of the early twentieth century for introducing the notion of a "more active therapy" in the hospital. After noticing that patients became "calm and lucid when they could undertake a small task, no matter how small," he began to set up various activities for his patients so that by 1919, 90 percent of the residents were working.[27] As he explained, the three main problems undermining psychiatric work were the "patient's lack of activity, an unfavorable environment in the asylum, and a fundamental belief in the unaccountability [*irresponsabilité*] of the mentally ill."[28] To address these issues, Simon advocated building libraries, setting up workshops, and promoting a system of "open doors."[29] Similarly, he advised nurses to avoid using a "harsh and imperative military tone."[30] The goal of his "more active therapy" was to lead to freedom, a true freedom that was not equivalent to laissez-faire but one that would allow patients to lead a life as independent as possible, "free of doctors and immediate assistance."[31] Rather than focusing on the particular symptoms of individuals, it was important to address "the whole": the institution, the team, the group. It is in this sense that Tosquelles referred to Simon's work as a "practical application, banal in fact, but often forgotten, of Gestalt theory."[32]

To be sure, Simon was not the first psychiatrist to recommend physical work as a cure for mental illness. As Tosquelles reminds us, by the end of the nineteenth century, Philippe Pinel was already insisting on the importance of keeping patients busy to "soothe the mind" (*adoucir les moeurs*).[33] Similarly, the goal of occupational therapy as it was developed in Great Britain and in the United States was to reintroduce war veterans into the workplace.[34] According to Tosquelles, however, Simon's greatest contribution was to change the attitudes of doctors and nurses vis-à-vis the patients.[35] Work was not simply a distraction for the patients, and it certainly was not a "moral treatment" in the way that Pinel had intended it. Rather, work was a way to hold the patients accountable (*responsables*): "holding the patients accountable for Simon meant trusting them and trusting the existence of a general law of all living beings, a 'logos' that regulated and ordered everything."[36] This general law was not a moral code, Tosquelles insisted, but more like an ethics, a way of life. As Tosquelles put it, "the point was not to 'make the patients work' to alleviate this or that symptom but to make the patients and the staff work to cure the institution."[37] It is this ethical—and fundamentally social—understanding of psychiatry that Tosquelles brought to Saint-Alban and that was particularly influential for thinkers such as Jean Oury and Félix Guattari.

This idea of a "general law" anchored in language was also articulated—although differently—in Lacan's work, especially in his notion of the symbolic. As Lacan suggested throughout his life, madness (or psychosis) was founded and expressed in a form of linguistic alienation—what Lacan later called a foreclosure from the symbolic order. Like Simon's, Lacan's work played a foundational role for Tosquelles because of its theoretical weight but also because of its institutional impact within the world of early twentieth-century European psychiatry. Indeed, before he was known as a psychoanalyst, Lacan was a psychiatrist in a time and in a context in which adhering to Freud's theses was not an obvious or an easy choice.[38] After a classical training in neurology and psychiatry (*clinique des maladies mentales et de l'encéphale* under the direction of Doctor Henri Claude), Lacan spent the summer of 1930 as a resident in the famous Swiss clinic of Burghölzli, where doctors were developing a new approach to madness. In addition to the typical nosographic evaluations, the doctors at Burghölzli insisted on the importance of listening to the patients' narration of their lives and ailments. Back in Sainte-Anne, one of the most important psychiatric institutions in France, Lacan discussed these ideas with several other young psychiatrists including Henri Ey, who also became an important reference for Tosquelles. Immersed in philosophy, phenomenology, and Surrealism, Lacan and Ey were eager to distinguish themselves from the old organicism that prevailed at Sainte-Anne, especially under Édouard Toulouse, a strong believer in the power of heredity and a proponent of the degeneration thesis.[39]

Lacan's early theoretical observations culminated in two works that were regularly cited by Tosquelles and his colleagues at Saint-Alban: a doctoral thesis titled *On Paranoid Psychosis and Its Relations to the Personality* published in 1932 and an article, "Beyond the 'Reality Principle,'" that appeared in 1936 in the journal *L'Évolution psychiatrique* and that was eventually republished in *Écrits*. For Tosquelles, Lacan's work was pioneering not only for the concepts it put forth but also for its methodological and institutional consequences. Indeed, given the reluctance of the French medical and psychological profession to accept Freudian psychoanalysis—for complicated reasons that had to do with chauvinism, anti-Semitism, and Germanophobia—Lacan's early work appeared quite revolutionary. As Lacan made clear in his thesis, which he defended in 1932 in front of a committee of psychiatrists chaired by Henri Claude, his goal was twofold: to radically reform psychiatry with the help of psychoanalysis and to rethink psychoanalysis through the lens of paranoia—that is, through the lens of psychosis. Through his case study of Aimée, a thirty-eight-year-old railway clerk who had inexplicably tried to kill a famous actress in Paris, Lacan was especially interested in putting forth a methodological point. As he put it, he sought to deepen not only the "description" of Aimée's illness but its very "conception."[40]

Was paranoid psychosis, Lacan asked, the result of the "development of a personality, and thus, did it come about from a constitutive anomaly or a reactionary deformation? Or was psychosis an autonomous illness, that reshaped the personality by breaking the course of its development?"[41] In other words, did madness originate in the brain as many neuroscientists believed, in the body as an acquired disease, or in the social and familial worlds? Lacan's answer was clear: "It is absurd to attribute these phenomena to a specifically neurological *automatism*."[42] Rather than focusing on a single origin, Lacan argued, researchers needed to study psychosis in relation to the formation of a specific "personality." If psychosis also had a social "origin, exercise, and meaning,"[43] it was important to consider three factors: "the childhood history of the patient, the conceptual structures of his delirium, and the drives and intentions behind his social behavior."[44] Psychiatric clinical work thus needed to remain open to sociological inquiry, medical exams, and, most important, psychoanalytic treatment. Indeed, psychoanalysis was, according to Lacan, the only discipline able to provide a coherent theory of subjectivity: a subject resulted from conscious and unconscious representations constructed in relation to an Other and to others more generally.[45] Lacan had already come to understand the fundamental role of others in the elaboration of the self after attending Alexandre Kojève's seminar on Hegel.[46] For Lacan, this philosophical insight could fundamentally help psychiatry, which should no longer focus exclusively on the brain or on the will (as Pinel's "moral treatment" required) but rather on the unconscious. As Elisabeth Roudinesco suggests, Lacan's argument was not simply that psychiatry should incorporate psychoanalytic concepts in its practice, but rather that psychiatry needed to be anchored in a Freudian understanding of the unconscious and in a Freudian understanding of the subject.[47]

Lacan's thesis was not exactly rejected by the psychiatric community, but it was essentially ignored. Rather, its early champions were the Surrealists, who welcomed Lacan's innovative approach to madness and discussed him in various of their journals. A few years after the publication of his thesis, Lacan pursued his defense of Freudian subjectivity in his article "Beyond the 'Reality Principle,'" published in 1936 in *L'Évolution psychiatrique*. This journal, founded in 1925 by the avant-garde of French psychiatry, had, under the influence of Henri Ey amongst others, become more receptive to Freudian ideas. As a 1936 editorial stated: "the study of Freudian theories and the observation of clinical cases through a psychoanalytic technique have emerged as important aspects of scientific psychiatry."[48] A few months later, Lacan pushed this statement further as he proclaimed in his opening paragraph: "The new psychology not only fully accepts psychoanalysis; by constantly corroborating it by research in disciplines that begin from other starting points, it demonstrates the value of psychoanalysis' pioneering work."[49] Lacan's text began with a strong attack against nineteenth-century psychiatry and psychology. Despite their claim to scientificity, these disciplines clung to an "associationist conception of the psyche" (derived from neurobiology) that was neither objective nor materialist. The rest of the text can be read as a preliminary or companion text to Lacan's more well-known 1949 essay "The Mirror Stage as Formative of the I Function," in which Lacan set forth his understanding of subjectivity and of language.[50]

Indeed, in "Beyond the 'Reality Principle,'" Lacan introduced many of the techniques and concepts that distinguished him later in his career. He defended, for instance, "Freud's revolutionary method" grounded in "the subject's own account [*témoignage*]"—grounded, in other words, in language. Similarly, Lacan praised Freud's "law of free association" during the analytic session, a method that encouraged the patients' "nonomission" and "nonsystematization" of their thoughts.[51] In opposition to the biological notion of *association*, Lacan put forth the concept of *identification*. The configuration of various identifications would eventually lead to the construction of a particular *personality*. Within the process of identification, Lacan also singled out the notion of the *complex*, which he distinguished from the *instinct*. Whereas the instinct belonged to the realm of nature and biology, the complex could be social or cultural while still operating at the level of the body: "It is through the pathway of the *complex* that the images that inform the broadest units of behavior are instated in the psyche, images with which the subject identifies one after the other in order to act out, as sole actor, the drama of their conflicts."[52]

Tosquelles and his colleagues at Saint-Alban were among the first doctors to celebrate Lacan's structural understanding of the personality, the complex, and psychic identification.[53] As Tosquelles explained in an article co-written with Lucien Bonnafé and André Chaurand for the *Annales médico-psychologiques* in 1946: "It is in Lacan's work that we find the theses that best reveal the structural aspects of pathological existence, as a psychoanalytic perspective highlights."[54] This was especially true of Lacan's notion of the complex, "which shap[ed] the ways in which patients perceive their own morbid experience and their situation as sick people within society."[55] "This understanding of the complex," they continued, "has allowed Lacan to clarify his concept of identification. It goes beyond the global assimilation of an imago viewed statically and includes the potential implied by the development through the imago."[56] As we will see, the founders of institutional psychotherapy were especially interested in thinking about the role of the doctors, the medical staff, and the hospital itself in the process of identification of psychotic patients. Lacan's early work provided Tosquelles and his colleagues a model of madness as "a phenomenal totality, already manifested in the personality," which they could study through various means.[57]

War Psychiatry

In July 1936, a few months after the election of a left-wing Popular Front government, which included the POUM, a group of army officers led by General Francisco Franco staged a military coup that marked the beginning of the Spanish Civil War. Tosquelles joined the resistance through the POUM, which, by this point, was persecuted by both the military and the Communist Party under Stalin's directives. As the war developed, Mira became an advisor to the republican army. From that position, he recommended that Tosquelles be appointed head of military psychiatric services and sent to the southern front. The Catalan government's plan to decentralize mental health care through the *comarcas* was obviously interrupted by the war, but Mira believed that it could still be carried out within the structure of the army. Tosquelles, who possessed a thorough knowledge of Catalan health policies and who was committed to this new modern and reformed psychiatry, seemed like an ideal candidate to carry this mission through.

It was in this context that Tosquelles set up his first therapeutic community, in the middle of the war, in Almodovar del Campo. There, he tested many of the theories and practices that he later developed at Saint-Alban, in particular, a *politique de secteur* inspired by the *comarcas*. Tosquelles's idea was to treat the patients close to their homes and families so as not to uproot them further. As he recalled in an interview: "I avoided having patients sent two hundred kilometers away from the front. I treated them there, where things had started, less than fifteen kilometers away, along a principle that could be compared to that of the *politique de secteur*. If you send a war neurotic one hundred and fifty kilometers away from the front, you make his illness chronic. You have to cure him close to his family where the problems had started."[58] A few years later, the Second World War popularized the practice of therapeutic communities in other countries. In Great Britain for example, the Tavistock Clinic worked in close association with the Army Psychiatric Services, and Maxwell Jones ran the Effort Syndrome Unit in the Mill Hill public school.[59] Interestingly enough, many of the policies adopted by these therapeutic communities (which were often run by people with no formal training in psychiatry or psychology) resembled those implemented in Saint-Alban around the same time: "hospital clubs" run by the patients designed to give them a sense of purpose, identity, and autonomy; less paternalistic doctors; group therapies; and a general commitment to a more democratic and open vision of the psychiatric hospital.

Mira and Tosquelles also brought to the front some of the discoveries of German psychiatry during World War I, in particular the treatment of panic attacks, shell shock, and war neurosis. They advised the chiefs of staff on questions of leave rotation, on combat units going back and forth between the front line and the rearguard, on possible psychological support for the troops, and much more.[60] Both insisted on the importance of providing psychiatric care not only for civilians and combatants but also for the doctors themselves. This holistic approach to psychiatry remained consistent in all of Tosquelles's work—from his endorsement of Lacan's "total" vision of madness, to his interest in Simon's work on the hospital as a total institution that needed to be treated and cured. Psychiatry, he believed, could be practiced anywhere. As Tosquelles recounted his experience during the war:

> I learned from Mira that someone called Bartz had proposed and organized a series of non-hospital-based services that . . . allowed for many different forms of treatment according to a staggered series of interventions. A practice known as *geopsychiatry* could take place outside the hospital and consisted of breaking bread with the mentally ill in their homes. . . . I brought to Saint Alban this notion of active involvement, this plan for working at the comarcal level . . . by sector. Of course, the war helped it to take root there: working with peasants, the local police . . . not to speak of the schoolteachers, some priests, the notaries. We worked with the local doctors, the moviehouses, with families in their homes. . . . Cooperation between social classes . . . why not? . . . an institution is a space of exchange, a place where exchanges are possible. In other words, singularity doesn't exist outside the context of a group, or an institution.[61]

This experience at the front was crucial for Tosquelles's work at Saint-Alban but also for what would later be known as "social psychiatry."

In June 1937, the POUM was dissolved after the assassination of its political leader by agents of Stalin's secret intelligence services. In January 1939, Barcelona fell to Franco's army, and in March of that year, the fascist final military victory put a tragic end to the Spanish Republic and to the Civil War.[62] In the months that followed, Tosquelles, like many other republicans, fled Spain and crossed the Pyrenees into France as part of the massive exodus that came to be known as the *Retirada*. France had followed the Spanish Civil War closely as left and right projected many of their political hopes and fears into their southern neigh-

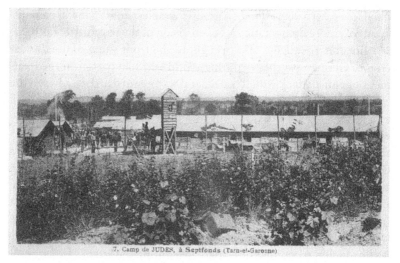

1.3 Postcard of the Camp de Judes in Septfonds
© Jean-Marc Labarta

bor. Despite the fact that the French government had officially committed to welcome Spanish refugees, the defeat of the Popular Front in April 1938, the growing economic crisis, the rise of xenophobia and anti-Semitism, and the looming war with Germany significantly complicated this promise. As the government headed by Édouard Daladier made clear, France would serve primarily as a place of transit rather than as a permanent home for these Spanish refugees often described in official documents as "undesirable" (*indésirables*). To that effect, the French government built a series of camps or "special centers," as they were called, to manage the 450,000 refugees who had reached French soil. Furthermore, seeking to appease the campaign of fear launched by the extreme right, which immediately condemned the "anarchist scum" (*racaille*) that was invading France, the minister of the interior, Albert Sarraut, made national security a priority. He imposed a strict military discipline within the camps and worked closely with the police to weed out potential "subversives."[63]

When he arrived in France, Tosquelles was placed in one of these camps, the Camp de Judes, in the town of Septfonds in the southwest, not far from Montauban.[64] As historians have documented and as the archives confirm, living conditions in these camps were especially harsh, causing many to die from hunger, disease, or exhaustion and driving others to suicide. The refugees were amassed in overcrowded barracks surrounded by barbed wire, electrical projectors, and surveillance posts (figs. 1.3 and 1.4). They slept in haystacks with only a little wood available

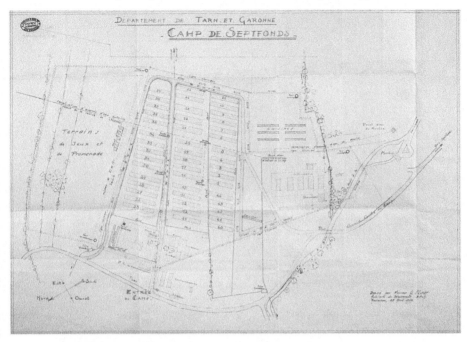

1.4 Map of the Camp de Septfonds
©Archives Départementales de Tarn-et-Garonne, 4M1

for heat and in deplorable hygienic and sanitary conditions. Many of the testimonies from Septfonds also recall the brutal treatment from the guards and the system of surveillance and classification to which the refugees were subjected. According to one account, the walk to the camp from the train station was so long and tiring that French soldiers had to poke the Spaniards with their rifles to urge them to walk faster: "treat us like humans," this refugee pleaded. Another witness described these walks as making him feel like "cattle."[65] Upon their arrival, the refugees were "thrown like rags, *piltrajas*, abandoned by the whole world."[66] After passing through shower stations, where they were washed and where their clothes were disinfected, they were sent to their barracks and eventually thrown some bread, "like animals."[67] As many reports suggest, the camp looked and felt, more than anything, like a prison.

Furthermore, the noxious effects of the camp were not simply physical; they were also psychic. As the historian Scott Soo has suggested, "there was agreement on one basic premise: internment caused psychological harm."[68] The "war neuroses" of the Spanish camps took several names, including "barbed-wire disease" and *arentitis* or "sanditis" because of the sandy and windy conditions in which the refugees lived.

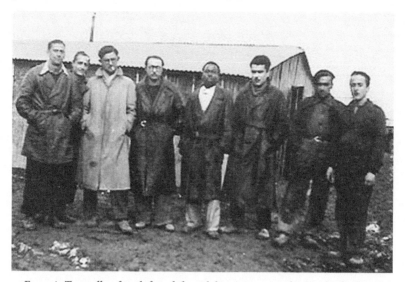

1.5 François Tosquelles, fourth from left, with his assistants at the Septfonds Camp infirmary
© Marie-Rose Ourabah

As one detainee put it: "the sand has entered my soul and body. And I feel like crying to dry the ink with which I am writing, for my tears have turned to sand."[69] According to another testimony, "neurasthenia ravaged us. There were many obsessives and maniacs. The lack of food weakened our heads, desperation capsized our reason."[70] As he recalled in various interviews, Tosquelles was deeply marked by his experience at Septfonds and what he described as its "concentrationist" and "carceral" environment. Tosquelles claimed that the camp reminded him of a "badly organized" psychiatric hospital.

The camp's commander, Lieutenant Colonel Vigouroux, happened to come from a family of psychiatrists that included Raymond Vigouroux, a close colleague of Jean-Martin Charcot, with whom he had practiced hypnotism at the end of the nineteenth century. Worried by the rampant psychic disarray in the camp and by the growing number of suicides, Vigouroux welcomed the arrival of Tosquelles, along with his colleague Jaime Sauret.[71] Vigouroux thus allowed Tosquelles and Sauret to set up a psychiatric service within the camp where Tosquelles tested many of his theoretical insights (fig. 1.5). Septfonds had the reputation of being the most "intellectual" camp since many of its prisoners happened to be political activists, artists, and musicians. Tosquelles thus relied on these prisoners to help him organize activities—concerts, art, theater productions, publications, but also group therapies—that would temper some of the effects of this "camp psychosis" (fig. 1.6). As

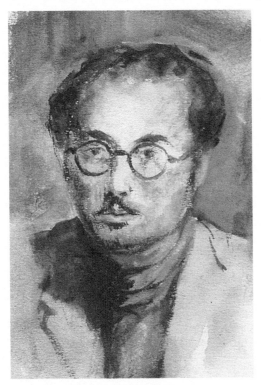

1.6 Portrait of François Tosquelles painted by one of the prisoners at Septfonds
© Marie-Rose Ourabah

Tosquelles remembered, at Septfonds, "There was only one psychiatric nurse; the rest were normal people. I think it is one of the places where I conducted very good psychiatry, in this concentration camp, in the mud."[72] This account is confirmed by other prisoner testimonies who recall that Tosquelles and Sauret treated the refugees, especially those traumatized by the war. As one observer put it, being a doctor did not prevent Tosquelles from doing the "heavy work" (*corvées*) like everybody else.[73]

News of Tosquelles's work in the camp and at the front traveled in medical circles and eventually came to the attention of Paul Balvet, who had taken over the administration of the Saint-Alban Hospital in 1937. Both André Chaurand and Maurice Dide recommended Tosquelles to Balvet, who was concerned with staffing the hospital during the war and with modernizing its decaying facilities. Balvet thus contacted the local state representative (*préfet de la Lozère*) to release Tosquelles, and on January 6, 1940, he arrived at Saint-Alban (fig. 1.7).[74] At first

1.7 Transfer order of Tosquelles from Septfonds to Saint-Alban on December 14, 1939
© Archives Départementales de Tarn-et-Garonne, 4M1

sight, Tosquelles was an odd choice for Balvet, a fervently Catholic supporter of Philippe Pétain's rule, who was, in addition, vehemently anticommunist. Balvet, however, admired Tosquelles's extensive knowledge of phenomenology and psychoanalysis. He had written a medical thesis on the "Cotard delusion," a type of psychosis in which a patient believed that he or she was dead. Tosquelles knew this illness well, and he impressed Balvet by recommending several potential therapeutic treatments. What was important was to "go beyond the general passivity of psychiatrists, which is frequent, and beyond the aesthetic fascination

François Tosquelles, Saint-Alban, and Institutional Psychotherapy   33

with which most psychiatrists have welcomed these fabulous delirious manifestations."[75] From that point on, Tosquelles and Balvet formed a close friendship and established a particularly productive working relationship at the Saint-Alban Hospital, first trying to survive the war, and second seeking to revolutionize the practical and theoretical underpinnings of psychiatric care.[76]

Political and Psychic Resistances

Tosquelles's first years at Saint-Alban coincided with the Second World War and, after Stalinism and fascism, yet another form of political "occupation." Even though Saint-Alban was located in the free zone, Germany worked closely with the Vichy regime in various administrative matters, including the management of hospitals. The Third Reich's policy regarding mental illness has been well documented. Eugenics and the forced euthanasia of the "incurably sick" were integral to Hitler's program of racial purification. "Action T4," as this policy was later called, resulted in 70,000 official deaths, but according to some historians, the number was closer to 200,000.[77] Although the Vichy regime never had an explicit policy of extermination, between 1940 and 1945, 40,000 patients died in French psychiatric hospitals. Most of these deaths were due to the food shortage, the system of rationing, and the harsh living conditions that all of France experienced during these years. However, several historians have suggested that these deaths, in fact, resulted from a policy of "soft extermination" of the mentally ill that the Nazi state promoted and the Vichy regime silently endorsed—a true biopolitics in Michel Foucault's sense of the term that let some live and let others die.[78]

Balvet, Tosquelles, and the other doctors at Saint-Alban were acutely aware of the humanitarian disaster occurring in French psychiatric institutions during the war. Patients from the psychiatric hospitals of Rouffach in Alsace and of Ville-Evrard on the outskirts of Paris were evacuated to Saint-Alban at the beginning of the war.[79] By 1940, Saint-Alban housed 852 patients, many more than it could accommodate, and doctors and staff were forced to improvise. The first priority was to hoard enough food to feed the patients with the help of the local villagers but also by encouraging the patients to work in the fields and produce their own meats and vegetables. The second was to continue to operate the hospital without attracting the attention of the German or Vichy authorities. Saint-Alban's geographic isolation was, most likely, one of the factors that helped explain its relative independence during the war.[80] Other sources, however, including Tosquelles and Bonnafé, mentioned Balvet's *pétainiste* sympathies (which Balvet strongly repudiated by the end of the war) that afforded the doctors a certain degree of freedom.[81] This hypothesis is confirmed by a letter from the Vichy intelligence services (Renseignements Généraux) dated April 29, 1942, warning the local agents about the "most harmful influence" of Tosquelles and some of his colleagues on the hospital's personnel: "Clearly revolutionary and antinationalist tendencies . . . sympathies are pro-CGT [France's largest union] and even possibly communist." The letter, however, also specified that Tosquelles was "a good doctor who has the full confidence and appreciation of Doctor Balvet, the director of the asylum."[82]

The experience of living through and surviving the war was a major catalyst in the genesis of institutional psychotherapy. The war was especially crucial in convincing Tosquelles and his colleagues of the need to radically rethink the practical and theoretical bases of psychiatry so as not to be complicit in the biopolitical assault against the mentally ill. Finally, it was the war that brought together at Saint-Alban the particular cast of characters who eventually put in place institutional psychotherapy: Balvet and Tosquelles, but also Lucien Bonnafé, Georges Canguilhem, Georges Daumézon, Marius Bonnet, Paul Éluard, and others. Saint-Alban during the war became a center of psychiatric innovation and intellectual effervescence, but also of political resistance against Vichy and fascism. As Bonnafé recalled this period: "the occupation played an extremely important role in this initiation of the *I* towards the *Us* of the medical team. The occupation produced an experience of fraternity which was essential at Saint-Alban."[83]

Within this constellation of doctors, artists, philosophers, and writers who gathered at Saint-Alban, Lucien Bonnafé played a key role. Born in 1912 in Figeac in the Lot region, Bonnafé spent his student years in Toulouse, where he was immersed in Surrealist circles including the group Chaos, through which he first discovered psychoanalysis alongside avant-garde poetry and cinema. During these years, Bonnafé also joined the Union fédérale des étudiants and eventually the Communist Party. Like Tosquelles, Bonnafé pursued his political activism throughout his medical studies, especially during the French Popular Front and the Spanish Civil War. Self-identified as an "activist doctor," Bonnafé followed closely the Popular Front's initiatives to reform psychiatric hospitals under the impulse of the health minister, Henri Sellier—initiatives that they were unable to implement until the end of the war.[84] After the German Occupation of France, Bonnafé joined the Resistance and participated in the formation of the clandestine Health Services. This was the context in which Bonnafé arrived at Saint-Alban, in 1942, under the auspices of Balvet, who allowed him to continue his work in the Resistance, in hiding, from the hospital. After fighting in the famous battle of Mont Mouchet in 1944, Bonnafé was named chief commander of Health Services for the Forces françaises de l'intérieur (FFI) and the Forces françaises libres (FFL) in the southern zone.[85]

Bonnafé remained at Saint-Alban until 1946, and he was instrumental in the early theorization and promotion of institutional psychotherapy. During the war and the immediate postwar, he co-authored a series of articles with Tosquelles and Chaurand in which they exposed the bases of institutional psychotherapy. They presented these papers at various medical congresses and published extensively in the *Annales médico-psychologiques*. It was through Bonnafé that in November 1943, the poet Paul Éluard—whom Bonnafé knew from Surrealist circles—found refuge at Saint-Alban, where he continued to think and write about madness and freedom.[86] As Bonnafé recalled, he would travel with Éluard to a nearby village where a member of the Resistance had a printing press that they could borrow.[87] According to Bonnafé, Éluard was the "most consistent spokesperson" for the Surrealist commitment to "treat subjects who suffered from relational troubles as human subjects," and to resist "the proscriptions of difference." Surrealism, Bonnafé continued, "fought to minimize the differences that exist amongst men and as such, it refused to serve an absurd order. . . . Significantly, when poetry was called to the Resistance, it chose to share its life with a psychiatric hospital where the love of differences and the denunciation of an absurd order came together."[88] Surrealism and psychiatry, in other words, shared similar goals of rehumanizing madness and fighting against the "absurd order" of the world.

Finally, it was thanks to Bonnafé that Georges Canguilhem hid at Saint-Alban for a few weeks during the war, between June and July 1944.[89] Bonnafé had met Canguilhem in medical school in Toulouse, and they traveled in similar intellectual networks. They were both, for instance, regulars at the bookstore of Silvio Trentin, an Italian antifascist intellectual exiled in Toulouse, who had an important collection of Surrealism, psychoanalysis, and philosophy—including the work of Gaston Bachelard, who remained a foundational figure for both Canguilhem and Bonnafé.[90] During the Occupation, the bookstore served as a gathering place for the nascent Resistance movement. Bonnafé reconnected with Canguilhem in the *maquis* and more specifically during the battle of Mont Mouchet. Bonnafé offered to treat some of the wounded combatants at Saint-Alban, and Canguilhem arrived in this context.[91] Bonnafé described the meeting between Tosquelles and Canguilhem as "one of the most memorable if unexpected [*imprévus*] events in my life."[92] And indeed, many of the themes central to Canguilhem's first book, the thesis that he defended in 1943, which eventually became

The Normal and the Pathological, closely resonated with Tosquelles's reflections: the problem of objectivity in science, the relativity of norms, the social construction of diagnoses, and much more. After his stay at Saint-Alban, Canguilhem's work was routinely cited by the founding fathers of institutional psychotherapy as a theoretical framework that was complementary to their own. For instance, in a 1945 text co-authored by Bonnafé, Chaurand, and Tosquelles for the *Annales médico-psychologiques*, the doctors of Saint-Alban criticized mainstream psychiatry for assuming that patients had a fundamentally different "form of life": "As Canguilhem has recently shown in a study on the normal and the pathological . . . the morbid event is not simply a quantitatively varied prolongation of the physiological state: it is another 'form of life.'"[93]

As Bonnafé explained in a 1995 conference, the practice that developed at Saint-Alban needed to be understood as the coming together of two contexts, one medical and one political: "the resistance to the inhumanity of the psychiatric world" and the "Resistance to the Nazi occupation and collaboration." For Bonnafé, both Éluard and Canguilhem played a key role in generating this "philosophy of the no," this imperative of rupture that eventually led to psychiatric reform. In his words, the war years at Saint-Alban were characterized by "our fraternity with Éluard and the Surrealist vision of madness" and by "our participation in the work of a 'new scientific spirit' that sought to correct misconceptions and propose new conceptions, and to break with scientific narrowness, as exemplified by our friendship with Georges Canguilhem."[94] Bonnafé's point here guided much of the Saint-Alban experiment: the political and the psychic were two sides of one same project of resistance. As Bonnafé defined it, resistance meant fighting against "everything that tries to submit the subject to a power foreign to himself, to intoxicate him by convincing him that 'it is stronger than himself,' to direct his conscience and prevent him from thinking."[95]

This form of political and psychic oppression was also described in the writings of this period as "totalitarianism" or "concentrationism." Whichever name it took, this experience was foundational for the political and psychiatric work that was undertaken at Saint-Alban. Marius Bonnet, for instance, described his return from the work camps in Germany (in the Service du travail obligatoire [STO]) as a moment of awareness: "That is where I changed. In this concentration camp, I remembered the asylum and I compared my condition as prisoner to that of the mentally ill."[96] The goal of institutional psychotherapy was thus to provide a model of psychic and political resistance to this form of confinement, not only within the walls of the hospital but within the social world at large. In the words of Jean Oury: "institutional psychotherapy was the act of setting up all kinds of mechanisms to fight, every day, against all that could turn the whole collective toward a concentrationist or segregationist structure."[97] It was, as Tosquelles put it, an effort to "cure life."

The Saint-Alban Experiment

In July 1941, Tosquelles, Bonnafé, Balvet, Chaurand, and others decided to systematize this "work of tracking the perversions of totalitarian thought" and to write down some of the practices that they had put in place in the hospital during the war. This became the first manifesto of the "Société du Gévaudan," the name they chose for their group, in reference to a mythical dog-wolf monster from the region of Saint-Alban in the Lozère. According to Bonnafé, the Société du Gévaudan was "a society with multiple aims":

> there was the incessant search, anchored in a daily practice, for a new clinic founded on the nonsubmission to the dominant "clinoid" model, which clearly entailed the erasure of the subject behind the symptom. There was the constant deepening of the constructive critique of the institution instituted as the site of segregation. There was also, along similar lines, the work to institute disalienating relations in this site dedicated to the production of a system of overalienating relations, and at the same time, the development of open practices, outside the walls [of the hospital], modeled on a "geopsychiatry."[98]

The members of the Société du Gévaudan thus drew upon their experiences as doctors, activists, and resisters to lay out the principles of what would later be called institutional psychotherapy or, sometimes, socialtherapy (*socialthérapie*) (fig. 1.8).

In the founding manifesto and during the subsequent meetings of the group, Tosquelles, Bonnafé, and their colleagues insisted on three points. First, they argued, theory and practice were inexorably linked. As Bonnafé put it, "psychological and psychopathological speculation must have practical truth as its goal."[99] Or as Tosquelles explained, if doctors "sacrifice[d] the individual because of considerations that were too philosophical," they would end up with a practice that was useless. Unless they treated the hospital as an organism that participated in the social conditioning of illness, they would never understand the multiple facets of madness. Second—and this was a point that Canguilhem also emphasized in his early work—all medical diagnoses presupposed a normative ideal of health or morality. Consequently, it was fundamen-

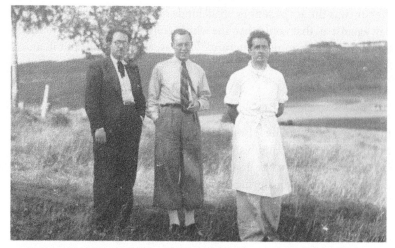

1.8 Tosquelles (left) with co-workers at Saint-Alban
© Marie-Rose Ourabah

tal for psychiatry to take into account the social aspect of illness. As Tosquelles formulated the problem: "was it possible to leave behind the mass of classifications in order to prove to clinicians and scientists that much of their research lacked a biological foundation?" To go further, doctors ought to ask, "Are these people sick? Does this notion of 'sickness' encompass all of the meanings of mental alienation?"[100]

Third, and related to this, "madness was never a personal affair." Psychosis, in other words, was individual and social at the same time. It is in this context that the members of the Société du Gévaudan turned to Lacan's work to complicate the premises of mainstream psychiatry, which, as they saw it, remained obsessed with localization—finding the sole origin of madness in a part of the brain: "We can say that madness does not have a beginning. The study of generative troubles is important but as Lacan's thesis suggests, we must consider the phenomenon of madness in its phenomenal totality, already manifested in the personality."[101] As the doctors of the Société du Gévaudan stated in the conclusion to their text: "madness never begins with a generative disorder; it is a historical and dialectical phenomenon. Genetic investigations of the patient's personality are unilateral investigations; they cannot grasp the entirety of its historical existence."[102]

Emphasizing the social and normative dimension of madness was not simply an abstract theoretical position for the doctors of Saint-Alban. It was also a conclusion that had become obvious after World War II. At the Congress of Psychiatry and Neurology held in Montpellier in 1942,

Balvet denounced the unacceptable conditions of psychiatric hospitals during the war, which he described as a "genocide." Everybody was suffering from hunger, Balvet exclaimed, but their patients were actually dying from it: "It begins with the inflation of the feet and it ends with what we call 'edematous-cachexia' [*cachexia œudémateuse*]."[103] According to Balvet, psychiatry could no longer be satisfied by praising "individual initiatives." It needed to consider the problems of mental illness and of psychiatric treatment from a structural point of view: "We do not have in psychiatry a general doctrine of care. . . . The insane asylum has changed names [to 'hospital'] but the reality is the same."[104] Much of the problem, Balvet suggested, stemmed from the fact that the medical and the administrative bodies remained separate, distanced, thus breaking the hospital's "unity of life." To fight against the alienating effects of the psychiatric hospital, Balvet called for a new model: the "asylum-village."[105] Inspired by the organic vision of the hospital put forth by Simon, the "asylum-village" could operate as a site of transference for the psychotic patient who suffered from an internal division.

The "disalienation" of the hospital—and of the psychiatric profession—thus required a series of very practical measures as well as a complete theoretical reconsideration. It needed to begin at the level of architecture. At Saint-Alban, the first step was to demolish the walls of the asylum and later the walls that separated each cell. As Marius Bonnet recalls, "one day, we tore down the walls of the compound. There was no longer a border between the hospital and the village of Saint-Alban. . . . After the war, the Liberation of the territory was also the liberation of the asylum."[106] Along similar lines, and again in accordance with Simon's teaching, the administration eliminated uniforms and medical blouses so that doctors, nurses, and patients were indistinguishable from one another. The goal was to explode fixed roles, to do away with the "look of an idle barrack or concentration camp," but also to force the medical staff to think through the singularity of the patient and his illness.[107] As Bonnafé put it: "when you cannot put a patient in a uniform or when you cannot simply lock him up, you are forced to anticipate his reactions and thus to penetrate the mechanisms of his illness."[108] This effort to respect the individuality of each patient began the minute he entered the hospital, where he was welcomed by a committee composed of doctors, nurses, and patients that would show him around the castle and explain the logistics of the treatment and of daily life.

In 1952, in a special issue of the journal *Esprit* titled "The Misery of Psychiatry," the founding fathers of institutional psychotherapy articulated these points for a more general audience. Georges Daumézon insisted on the social nature of alienation and concluded that while "the doctor could fight illness, only society could fight alienation."[109] Louis Le Guillant and Bonnafé asserted the continuity between madness and normality in an article that took to task the "myths and taboos" that have haunted psychiatry since the time of Pinel. As they concluded: "the mad were (in the eyes of the dominant class) the blacks, the *indigènes*, the Jews, the proletarians of the sick."[110] Only a new practice could bring about the much-needed transformation of psychiatric care and a new conception of mental illness in society. Because normality and pathology existed in a continuum, this new practice could ultimately help illuminate human behavior in general.

One of the pillars of this "new practice," which was eventually baptized "institutional psychotherapy" in 1952, was the hospital. In his contribution to *Esprit*, Tosquelles described the hospital as a field invested with social significance: "for most of our patients, the acts, the delusions, and the confessions often refer to intimate conflicts that are always intersocial, and more specifically familial. We can sometimes bring to light the chain of associations linked to these conflicts that tends to lead us back to typical childhood situations similar to the ones described by psychoanalysts." In this context, Tosquelles continued, "the hospital can play a role analogous to that of the psychoanalyst. It can be the object of consecutive projections of these conflicts. The dialectic of the cure would go through this mill [*laminoir*] of transferences and projections facilitated by the structure of the hospital."[111] As Tosquelles suggested, the hospital could circumvent some of the theoretical and practical difficulties that Freud had encountered in his treatment of psychotics by providing a different model of transference.

And indeed, as Tosquelles repeated throughout his life, the hospital— its architecture, its activities, its staff—represented a *collectif soignant*, a "healing collective": "It is in these collectives that emerges, within concrete social exchanges, an entirely different dynamic of 'psychic elements' that we need to understand. I am talking about collectives of 'wholes' [*collectifs des 'ensembles'*] that always function as open systems, incisions in time and space."[112] Tosquelles insisted that his point was not simply to modify the spatial organization or the laws that governed the hospital but rather to capitalize on its psychic potential. The hospital could no longer be treated as a "passive instrument" or as "a stable geographic site." Rather, it was important to grasp "its internal life as the social environment of the cure: the patient population, its groups, its relations with the staff, with the administration, and with the doctors also."[113] If madness was a social problem, then it also required a social solution, and the hospital offered a space to think these questions through.

One of the most important innovations at Saint-Alban, designed to enact this new social, this alternative transferential space, was the Club Paul Balvet. Founded in 1947, the Club was a patient-run cooperative structure, a sort of self-financed union in charge of organizing all activities within the hospital. The Club, Tosquelles claimed, was to operate as "the automatic expression of the whole hospital."[114] Elected and composed of various subcommittees, the Club planned meals, theater and music performances, sports, parties, and field trips—social activities deemed integral to the cure (fig. 1.9). It also ran the library and the different ergotherapy and work stations and elected the committee that welcomed new patients. The atmosphere at the Club Paul Balvet reminded one observer of a lively café where everyone conversed all the time. The constant discussions and the decentralization were mechanisms to provide a "permanent guarantee against the reappearance of oppressive behaviors."[115] In many ways, the Club resembled the kinds of political structures that Tosquelles had fought for during his time in the POUM throughout the 1930s: both sought to promote self-managed, organic, radically democratic, and anti-authoritarian structures. As Marius Bonnet remembered:

> When the Club's administration met, it analyzed the various proposals put forth by the committees. And when a patient, without prior warning, would begin to talk about his problems, we would drop the meeting's agenda and everybody listened. Thus began the psychotherapeutic dialogue. Or here is another example: when one patient declared, concerning the library purchases, "we should never have bought this or that book," the doctor would ask him if he had read the book, what passage bothered him. And again, we talked. You see, at Saint-Alban, everything was a pretext for dialogue and not only in these meetings. Elsewhere, also, in daily life. The gardener, the cook, the secretary, the nurse, the electrician . . . all employees intervened in the system of psychotherapy. If a gardener proposed an idea, a patient could answer that it was a bad one. Basically, when I think back to this period, I often wonder: in Saint-Alban, who cured who?[116]

This concern for the collective guided all of the Club's initiatives, and in particular two of its most important tasks: the publication of a weekly newsletter called *Trait d'union* (hyphen) and the organization of work stations for the patients. *Trait d'union* was a collection of texts (theoretical, literary, and poetic), drawings, recipes, advertisements, and letters that ran from 1950 to 1981.[117] The editorial board was composed of patients who were helped by a few staff members, and the journal was

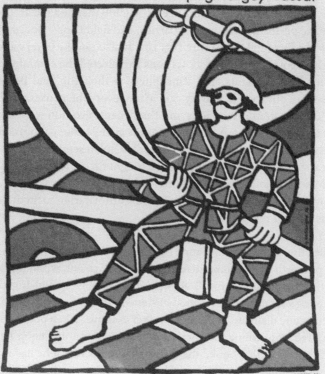

1.9 Poster of a theater performance at Saint-Alban in 1977
© Archives de Saint-Alban

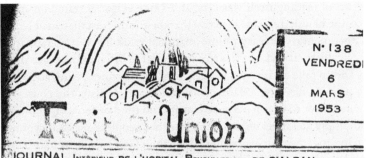

1.10 Editorial by Frantz Fanon in *Trait d'union* during his residency at Saint-Alban in March 1953
© Archives de Saint-Alban

published in the hospital itself by the printing and binding committee. Tosquelles, Bonnafé, and Fanon all contributed several editorials to the early issues of the journal (fig. 1.10). Once again, *Trait d'union* had both a theoretical and a practical mission. The content was meant to be informational but also philosophically stimulating. Most important perhaps,

44   CHAPTER ONE

the act of reading itself was crucial. As one editorial stated on July 15, 1950, the newsletter had "an active therapeutic interest that went beyond its documentary, literary, or informational value. To read a newspaper is a typically social act. . . . It is to exit oneself to listen to the voice of others and to take an interest in their joys and sorrows." And, addressing the patients directly: "Many of you have lost the taste, the courage, or the incentive to do so, because you are too tired or too sad, or because you simply no longer enjoy talking to other people. You isolate yourself; you live together but everyone stays in their little bubble. A *trait-d'union* [hyphen] between you, between you and the world, between your pavilions, between you and the staff."[118] Reading was a way to link the patients to the world, to offer them a "hyphen," literally a "line of union," to reach this broader "whole."

The Club Paul Balvet also coordinated the different work activities for the patients, activities that Tosquelles, following Simon, considered fundamental to the cure. The work was divided into three categories: agricultural (picking fruits, working on the land, overseeing animals in the field . . .), hospital-related (masonry, carpentry, painting, cooking . . .), and ergotherapy stations (art, pottery, book printing and binding, woodwork . . .).[119] For their manual labor, patients were paid a minimal amount that they could deposit in the hospital bank and possibly use later at the café or the bar. Ergotherapy was also a way to secure more regular access to food (growing vegetables, picking fruits, hunting for mushrooms . . .) especially during the wartime difficulties. As Tosquelles made clear, in ergotherapy, the object that was fabricated "did not have a therapeutic value in itself, but it was invested with affective, economic, and social values" that the staff needed to help the patient discover. This form of "consciousness-raising or of discovery of the other" was according to Tosquelles the true goal of ergotherapy.[120] Ergotherapy was a way to introduce patients to the "general law" that Tosquelles addressed in his discussion of Simon, a way to revive the symbolic dimension of life.

Within ergotherapy, art played an especially important role as a vector of symbolic expression for the patients. Many of the patients' drawings and paintings were published in *Trait d'union*, and some of the sculptures, ceramics, and wood carvings were sold, exchanged, or given to others outside of the hospital.[121] Saint-Alban thus participated quite directly in the production of the modern art current known as *art brut* that developed in the postwar years. In fact, the French artist Jean Dubuffet, who first coined the term *art brut* in 1945, traveled to Saint-Alban in the late 1940s as part of his tour of psychiatric hospitals to search for new artforms produced outside of the professional artworld (hence the En-

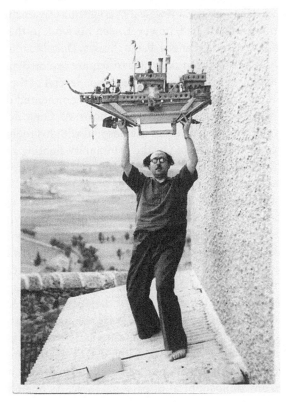

1.11 Tosquelles with a sculpture by Auguste Forestier
© Marie-Rose Ourabah

glish term, "outsider art").[122] Dubuffet had long shared the Surrealist fascination with madness, but he became especially aware of the specificity of the hospital setting after paying regular visits to his friend, the poet and playwright Antonin Artaud, who spent the last years of his life in the psychiatric hospital of Rodez. In 1948, Dubuffet traveled to several clinics in Switzerland to meet psychiatrists and acquire new works (including that of Adolf Wölfli) for his growing collection that would eventually become the Compagnie de l'art brut (first held in Paris at the Galerie René Drouin, then in New York in 1951, back in Paris in 1962, and finally in Lausanne in 1975, where it still lives today).[123]

Dubuffet was especially interested in the work of one of the patients at Saint-Alban, Auguste Forestier, a local from the Lozère region who was committed at age twenty-seven and who stayed at Saint-Alban until he died in 1958 (fig. 1.11). In a letter dated February 17, 1949, Dubuffet wrote to Jean Oury at Saint-Alban to inquire about the possibility of buying several pieces by Forestier. As Dubuffet explained, he had traveled to Saint-Alban by car a few years earlier but was unable to meet Forestier in person. He had, however, seen his work in the homes of Paul Éluard, Raymond Queneau, Pablo Picasso, Dora Maar, and Tristan Tzara.[124] Dubuffet was eventually able to acquire several pieces that are still exhibited in his collection in Switzerland. Several of the doctors at Saint-Alban, including Tosquelles and Oury, commented directly on Forestier's work in their writings on psychosis. As Oury described it, Forestier would sit in a hallway of the hospital with his tools and work there, alone but also protected by the community, fighting against "disintegration" (*l'émiettement*), against "permanent destruction," and reconstructing the world "permanently."[125]

The Club, the journal, and the activities at Saint-Alban were all designed to facilitate the emergence of a horizontal "collectivity": a new space of transference—a "transferential constellation," as Tosquelles called it—that could serve as the basis for a different treatment of psychosis. Even though the patients received one-on-one psychoanalytic sessions with the doctors, they also were invited to participate in the general meetings, which had an explicit therapeutic goal. Inspired by the "psychodramas" of Jacob Moreno, these meetings allowed patients to role-play and explore particular fantasies and behaviors in a clinical setting.[126] The meetings, which were attended by doctors, nurses, staff, and patients, were strictly anti-authoritarian, and everyone was invited to speak on any philosophical or personal topic. As one observer recounted, within the space of one month, there were 177 meetings held at Saint-Alban.[127] As Tosquelles explained, holding regular meetings was crucial: "to fight against the authorities, the hierarchies, the habits, the local feudalisms, the corporatisms. Nothing should ever be obvious, everything is subject to discussion. Everybody must be consulted, everybody can decide. Not just for the sake of democracy, but in order to facilitate the progressive conquest of speech, to learn mutual respect. The patients must be able to have a say on the conditions of their stay and their care, their rights of exchanges, expression, and circulation."[128]

The Club and the meetings were thus two very practical mechanisms designed to fight stagnation and to promote a new form of common. Once again, Tosquelles's medical reflections resonated with his political engagements prior to the war. Institutional psychotherapy was also a form of permanent critique, what he called a "permanent revolution": "the work that transforms an establishment of care into an institution, a healing team into a collective, is never finished. It requires the elaboration of material and social means, the conscious and unconscious conditions of psychotherapy." And this, Tosquelles continued, was not simply in the hands of "doctors and specialists." Rather, "it was the result of a complex assemblage [*agencement*] in which the patients themselves play a primordial role."[129]

As Tosquelles and his colleagues at Saint-Alban made clear in their written work and in their psychiatric practice, the social question was also fundamentally a psychic question and vice versa. While they never denied the reality of mental illness—in contrast to much of what would later become British antipsychiatry—the doctors at Saint-Alban insisted on the importance of social conditions in the emergence and in the treatment of psychosis. As I have suggested here, Tosquelles's experience of occupation, in Catalonia, within the POUM, in the concentration camp, and during the Second World War, shaped in crucial ways his psychiatric work. When he laid down the foundations for institutional psychotherapy, he insisted on the importance of performing a systematic "disalienation" of the medical staff, the hospital, the patients, and the theories that guided them. During the 1940s and 1950s, the medical staff at Saint-Alban worked to develop a "politics of madness" anchored in psychoanalysis, anarchism, and Surrealism. The goal of institutional psychotherapy was not to develop a rigid and all-encompassing model that could be exported to other settings but rather to offer an ethics, a way of thinking and living. Constantly evolving, adapting, and always revisable, institutional psychotherapy was meant as a permanent revolution of politics, society, and psychic life, all at once. It is precisely this ethical commitment that inspired the figures in the following chapters.

CHAPTER 2

Frantz Fanon, the Pathologies of Freedom, and the Decolonization of Institutional Psychotherapy

In December 1956, Frantz Fanon resigned from his position as medical director of the psychiatric hospital of Blida-Joinville in Algeria. In a letter addressed to Resident Minister and Governor General Robert Lacoste, Fanon explained that after three years of arduous work to improve the mental health of the local population, the reality of colonialism, its "tissue of lies, cowardice, [and] contempt for man" had finally convinced him to leave: "Madness is one of the means man has of losing his freedom. And I can say, on the basis of what I have been able to observe from this point of vantage, that the degree of alienation of the inhabitants of this country appears to me frightening. If psychiatry is the medical technique that aims to enable man no longer to be a stranger to his environment, I owe it to myself to affirm that the Arab, permanently alien [*aliéné permanent*] in his own country, lives in a state of absolute depersonalization."[1] By choosing the adjective *aliéné* to describe the colonized Algerians, Fanon was playing with the double meaning of the term in French: estranged and foreign—even in their own land—but also mentally unstable, crazy, insane. More broadly, Fanon was articulating a point that he reiterated throughout his life: colonialism had a direct psychic effect. Colonialism was not simply an economic doctrine that encouraged the pillage of natural resources, a political justification for confiscating the rights of certain groups, or the social transformation of all preexisting structures: it could literally render someone mad by hijacking their person, their being, and their sense of self. The confiscation of freedom and the alienation brought about by colonialism and by racism were always simultaneously political and psychic.

By the time Fanon wrote this letter in 1956, the war in Algeria, which had officially begun in November 1954, had turned increasingly violent. Like many other partisans of decolonization, Fanon had welcomed the

Frantz Fanon and the Decolonization of Institutional Psychotherapy   49

return of the left in the French legislative elections earlier that year. This hope, however, was short-lived as the new prime minister, Guy Mollet, was greeted by tomatoes and furious crowds in Algiers on February 6, 1956. The following month, the French legislature voted to grant the government "special powers," giving the army free rein to reestablish order in Algeria. Fanon had followed the acceleration of the war closely. By 1956, he was already involved with the Front de libération nationale (FLN), which had reached out to him in his capacity as a doctor to provide drugs and medical advice—including psychiatric help—for the combatants.[2] Fanon had been a harsh critic of the 1946 departmentalization law, a law fostered by his former mentor Aimé Césaire, which had converted Guadeloupe, Réunion, French Guyana, and his native island of Martinique into French overseas departments (*départements d'outre-mer*). As he consistently argued, decolonization had to be total. Consequently, he was sympathetic to the FLN's goal to put a decisive end to the French occupation and restore Algerian sovereignty.

As Fanon explained in his letter to Lacoste, he had finally come to realize that his "absurd gamble" to promote progressive psychiatric reforms while serving the French State was hopeless. The "lawlessness [*non-droit*], the inequality, and the multi-daily murder of man . . . raised to the status of legislative principles" had ultimately convinced him to leave. Certainly, the war had made the daily violence and web of discriminations particularly obvious, but as Fanon suggested, the state of exception was actually coexistent with colonialism. As he put it, it had become increasingly obvious that "the social structure existing in Algeria was hostile to any attempt to put the individual back where he belonged." And, as he continued: "the present-day events that are steeping Algeria in blood do not constitute a scandal for the observer. What is happening is the result neither of an accident nor of a breakdown [*panne*] in the mechanism. The events in Algeria are the logical consequence of an abortive attempt to decerebralize a people."[3] In other words, neither the intensification of the conflict after 1955 nor the "special powers" granted to the army and the widespread use of torture that ensued were anomalies or deregulations in a system that was otherwise anchored in liberalism, equality, and human rights. Instead, violence—political, social, and psychic—was *constitutive* of colonialism: it was the structure of the land, a structure that had come to condition individuals in their very psyche.

I pause on Fanon's letter because it gives us a particularly good insight into his conception of psychiatry and colonialism. More precisely, I wish to expand on two of the hypotheses that Fanon formulated in his letter: first, that the political and the psychic are intimately linked; and second, that colonial violence and racism take on a structural form that affects the psyche in a specific, structural, manner. The colony, like the asylum, was premised on a form of enclosure and segregation, a "concentrationist logic," as Tosquelles would put it, that led to political and social violence but also to mental agitation. In this sense, occupation and liberation, freedom and unfreedom, alienation and disalienation should be analyzed—and combatted—together. This is probably what Fanon meant when he told Simone de Beauvoir that "all political leaders should be psychiatrists as well."[4] Mental illness, as he put it in a 1959 medical text, was a "true pathology of freedom."[5]

In order to discern Fanon's understanding of the relationship between the psychic and the political, this chapter proceeds in three parts. It begins with Fanon's theory of the subject, which was shaped, I show, by his critiques of French mainstream psychiatry, of colonial medicine, and of various other theories of race and racism that were circulating at the time. In a second step, I discuss Fanon's encounter with François Tosquelles during his residency at Saint-Alban in 1952–53. I argue that the experience of institutional psychotherapy played a key role in Fanon's thought and medical practice. Institutional psychotherapy not only confirmed on an empirical level that alienation was always social and psychic at once but also offered a potential example of what freedom and emancipation could look like. Finally, I examine how Fanon tried to enact these forms of "freedom improvisations" both in his clinical work in Algeria and Tunisia and in his later political writings. I suggest that Fanon neither applied nor adapted a model of Western psychiatry to the colonial settings of Algeria and Tunisia. Rather, he revised the very foundations of this framework in order to promote what he considered a truly disalienated and disalienating psychiatry, a psychiatry close to the notion of "national culture" that Fanon theorized in his last and best-known book, *The Wretched of the Earth*.

To be sure, the fact that Fanon practiced psychiatry throughout his life is not new. Several rich biographies have highlighted his medical background, and many of his unpublished works, including his psychiatric writings, are now available in the excellent collection *Alienation and Freedom*.[6] Still, most scholarship on Fanon tends to consider his commitment to institutional psychotherapy as a biographical detail. David Macey, for instance, refers to Fanon as an ultimately "very conventional" psychiatrist.[7] In other words, we know that Fanon was a psychiatrist, a theorist, and an activist at the same time. We know much less about the extent to which Fanon's psychiatric work shaped his theoretical writing. My aim here is thus not to underscore once again the impor-

Frantz Fanon and the Decolonization of Institutional Psychotherapy   51

tance of psychiatry in Fanon's work. Rather, I wish to argue that the evolution of Fanon's thought across institutional and political/decolonial contexts explains as much about the history, promise, and achievements of institutional psychotherapy as it does about his political thinking. My point is not simply to restate the significance of the psyche for Fanon but rather to restate the significance of Fanon in the genealogy of what is generally called "Western radical psychiatry."

Fanon's Theory of the Subject

Before arriving at Saint-Alban in March 1952, Fanon had already been thinking about the relationship between the social and the psychic for quite some time. His early reflections on the construction of the subject culminated in three texts that he wrote as a medical student in Lyon: his thesis, defended in November 1951 and titled "Mental Alterations, Character Modifications, Psychic Disorders, and Intellectual Deficit in Spino-Cerebral Heredo-Degeneration: On a Case of Friedreich's Ataxia with Delusions of Possession"; an essay, "The North African Syndrome," printed in the journal *Esprit* in February 1952; and *Black Skin, White Masks* published in June 1952 by the Éditions du Seuil. In these three works, which all addressed the issue of causality in mental illness, Fanon elaborated a theory of subjectivity that drew on psychiatry, psychoanalysis, phenomenology, and politics. Fanon's subject was defined by a *structure* of conscious and unconscious relations rather than by biological essentialism or brain chemistry. The structural allowed Fanon to highlight the importance of the social, of others, and of alterity in the construction of the self. The structural also enabled him to go beyond three other models of subjectivity that he found inadequate: the rational individualism of liberalism; the biological determinism of nineteenth-century psychiatry; and the racism of colonial ethnopsychiatry. Psychoanalysis and philosophy, which Fanon saw as not in conflict but in continuity with psychiatry, helped him to define human reality as a construction, as the product of signifying activity always rooted in specific bodies and specific contexts.

Fanon traveled to France to study medicine in Lyon in 1946. He chose to specialize in psychiatry in 1949 under the supervision of Jean Dechaume, an expert in psychosurgery, neuropsychiatry, and neurology. As we saw in the previous chapter, French university training in the domain of psychiatry was dominated by an organicist and neuropsychiatric approach to mental illness, and this was especially true of Lyon. As one of Fanon's contemporaries put it, the Lyon medical school was a "psychiatric desert" hostile to any input from social psychology or psychoanalysis.[8] In the words of Tosquelles, Lyon was a "caricature of analytical Cartesianism, the flagship of efficiency over the anatomo-physiopathological matter at the root of medicine. . . . Lyon had produced two volumes on psychiatry and on the professional formation of psychiatrists. One chapter per illness. The sequence is well-known: diagnostic, prognostic, treatment," with treatment usually limited to confinement.[9]

Fanon admired Dechaume's scientific rigor, and he retained a certain inclination for this type of empiricism throughout his life. However, he quickly felt constrained by the theoretical narrowness of psychiatry and turned to other fields, including literature, anthropology, philosophy, and psychoanalysis. While at Lyon, he attended the lectures of the anthropologist André Leroi-Gouran and of the philosopher Maurice Merleau-Ponty. He read extensively and engaged the main intellectual theories of his period, from Claude Lévi-Strauss, Marcel Mauss, Karl Marx, Vladimir Lenin, Hegel mediated through Alexandre Kojève and Jean Hyppolite, Martin Heidegger, to Jean-Paul Sartre. During these years, Fanon also immersed himself in psychoanalysis through Freud and Lacan, and in Gestalt theory through Kurt Goldstein. Finally, he wrestled with the theses of Henri Ey and other French psychiatrists associated with the journal *L'Évolution psychiatrique* who had been seeking to reconcile psychiatry and psychoanalysis since 1925.[10] From existentialism and anthropology, Fanon learned the importance of relationality in the construction of the self. Through Marxism, he came to appreciate the decisive effect of politics on the human condition. Psychoanalysis and phenomenology offered him a model of embodiment that could complement social constructionism. Bringing together these different currents and disciplines, Fanon spent much of his time in medical school thinking about the question of psychic causation, trying to untangle the biological from the psychological, and separating the roles of ontogeny (the study of the development of organisms), phylogeny (the study of evolution), and sociogeny (Fanon's term to designate social phenomena) in the constitution of the self.

Fanon's medical thesis centered on Friedreich's ataxia, a hereditary disease that caused progressive damage to the nervous system. As he explained in his introduction, this illness was of particular interest to him because despite the fact that the state of general paralysis was "eminently neurological," it was usually accompanied by "a cluster of specifically psychiatric symptoms."[11] The close study of Friedreich's ataxia was thus a way to ponder this fundamental medical—but also philosophical—

quandary: "At what point can a neurological disease be suspected of triggering psychic alterations? At what point can it be said that the thought processes are disturbed?"[12] This was also a way to delimit neurology and psychiatry, to reflect on the issue of specialization and disciplinary borders.[13] In order to think through these questions, Fanon turned to the works of Henri Ey, Jacques Lacan, and Kurt Goldstein—three of his contemporaries who were also, as we saw, crucial for the founding fathers of institutional psychotherapy at Saint-Alban. In his thesis, Fanon mapped out the substantial differences between their respective approaches before suggesting that the three figures were linked by their desire to undercut the dichotomy between the neurological and the physiological. Ey, Fanon wrote, remained committed to a neurological framework despite the fact that he underscored the psychic nature of pathogenesis.[14] For Goldstein, "every organic manifestation . . . is the fruit of global mechanisms. For him, the organism acts as a whole."[15] In both cases, Fanon observed, neurological and psychiatric troubles went hand in hand.

Significantly, Fanon ended his thesis with an extended discussion of Lacan's theory of subject formation, which appeared closest to his own position. Referring to Lacan as an "eminently controversial figure," Fanon highlighted two concepts in Lacan's early work that he found especially helpful.[16] The first was his understanding of desire, which provided a link between on the one hand the biographical development of the subject and, on the other, his lived experience (his *Erlebnis*—a term that Fanon would take up in *Black Skin, White Masks*), his ego ideal, and his relationships (and tensions) with others.[17] The second was Lacan's notion of personality, especially important in his 1932 thesis on paranoia, which Lacan defined phenomenologically, as grounded in genetics and yet able to integrate human relations with the social order.[18] According to Fanon, through his concepts of desire and of personality, Lacan stressed the fact that madness always had something to do with the social.

Fanon's wish to complicate the classic—but by then much-contested—medical dictate that "every symptom required a lesion" was not, however, simply motivated by his wide range of readings.[19] It was also inspired by his first "hands-on" experiences in the medical field even before he chose to specialize in psychiatry. Indeed, throughout medical school, Fanon regularly accompanied doctors attending to emergencies in a predominantly Muslim neighborhood of Lyon. Fanon described finding patients in dirty beds, sordid rooms, with friends and family weeping and screaming because they were convinced that the patient was on the brink of death. Fanon and the supervising doctors would proceed with an examination that would generally reveal no significant illness. Eventually, and in response to further complaints by the patient, the doctor would recommend further testing. Three days later, the same person would show up completely cured and the French doctors would conclude that "the North African's pain, for which we can find no lesional basis, is judged to have no consistency, no reality."[20] This verdict confirmed what colonial psychiatry, especially the Algiers School, had argued for years and what much of French racism corroborated: "when you come down to it, the North African is a simulator, a liar, a malingerer, a sluggard, a thief."[21] For Fanon, however, the pain described by these patients was not imaginary but all too real. As he contended, this illness did have symptoms, but they were not necessarily physiological. He called it "the North African Syndrome."

Fanon's essay "The North African Syndrome" provided yet another confirmation of the interdependence of psyche and soma, of medicine and politics. As Fanon put it: "it so happens that there is a connection" between "the North African on the threshold of the French Nation" and "the North African in a hospital setting": "Threatened in his affectivity, threatened in his social activity, threatened in his membership in the community [*appartenance à la cité*]—the North African combines all the conditions that make a sick man. Without a family, without love, without human relations, without communion with the group, the first encounter with himself will occur in a neurotic mode, in a pathological mode; he will feel himself emptied, without life, in a bodily struggle with death, a death on this side of death, a death in life."[22] As this passage makes clear, the existence of these real-yet-imaginary illnesses displayed by North African immigrants confirmed with striking clarity the structural effects of racism and discrimination on the psyche. "Why don't they stay where they belong?" Fanon asked, provocatively: well, "the trouble is, they have been told they were French. They learned it in school. In the street. In the barracks . . . On the battlefields. They have had France squeezed into them wherever, in their bodies and in their souls."[23] Here, the paradoxical effects of French universalism are not simply political and social but *psychic* in the sense that they make those excluded physically ill. It is worth noting that these early texts of Fanon were also written during the Fourth Republic, the regime whose constitution Aimé Césaire and Léopold Senghor had helped redact, which extended citizenship across the French Empire.[24] Fanon's assertion that racism was inseparable from French universalism—a statement that he would repeat and develop in his later writings—thus appears particularly forceful in this period. As Fanon implied, the process of abstraction

Frantz Fanon and the Decolonization of Institutional Psychotherapy 55

demanded by assimilation had the extremely concrete and material effect of making an entire segment of the population sick.

"The North African Syndrome" first appeared in 1952, in a special issue, "North African Proletariat in France," in the journal *Esprit*, where he had published a few months earlier another essay, "The Lived Experience of the Black Man"—which eventually became the fifth chapter of *Black Skin, White Masks*. Founded in 1932 by the philosopher Emmanuel Mounier, *Esprit* was one of the most prestigious postwar publications, one of the main platforms for a left-leaning social Catholic intellectual current that sought to forge a third way between liberalism and communism. The two *Esprit* articles gave Fanon—who was only twenty-seven years old at the time—an immense exposure and brought his ideas out of the world of psychiatry onto the mainstream French intellectual scene.[25] *Esprit* was in many ways a perfect conduit for Fanon since the journal had long been critical of French colonial policy and since it had also taken an interest in psychiatry, as evidenced by the December 1952 issue, "The Misery of Psychiatry," to which Bonnafé, Tosquelles, Daumézon, Le Guillant, and others at Saint-Alban had contributed. It was through *Esprit* that Fanon found a publisher for *Black Skin, White Masks*, which Jean-Marie Domenach, the journal's editor-in-chief, passed on to Francis Jeanson at Éditions du Seuil. As Fanon's biographer David Macey suggests, *Black Skin, White Masks* would probably have been a difficult book to publish because of its juxtaposition of clinical data, literary allusions, philosophical analyses, and personal reflections.[26] Jeanson overcame his initial hesitation and agreed to work with Fanon on his manuscript. After convincing him to change his title from "Essay for the Disalienation of the Black Man" to *Black Skin, White Masks*, Jeanson wrote a preface celebrating Fanon's humanism, and the book appeared in French bookstores in the spring of 1952.

Fanon wrote *Black Skin, White Masks* while he was finishing medical school. As he indicated in one of his early chapters, he had originally intended to submit the manuscript as his medical thesis, but Dechaume was quick to reject it on the predictable grounds that it defied all existing academic and scientific norms.[27] It is in this context that Fanon turned to the more conventional topic of Friedreich's disease, somewhat reluctantly and hastily, so that he could graduate. As his initial title suggests, the question of "disalienation"—with its double meaning in French as both a social and a psychic process—was at the heart of *Black Skin, White Masks*. As Fanon wrote in his introduction, even though his analysis was primarily psychological, "it remains, nevertheless, evident that . . . the true disalienation of the black man implies a brutal awareness of the social and economic realities."[28] If racism did indeed produce an inferiority complex, Fanon continued, it began as an economic process that was later internalized, "epidermalized"—inscribed in the body and in the skin.

In *Black Skin, White Masks*, as in his medical thesis and in his article "The North African Syndrome," Fanon turned to a wide array of texts and disciplines to study the phenomenon of racial alienation. He referred to his book as a "clinical study," and in that sense, we can read it in line with these two other works, as a complementary text—one of three attempts to explore the question of causality in mental illness and to elaborate a theory of subjectivity that drew on psychiatry, psychoanalysis, phenomenology, and politics. Fanon's subject was defined by a structure of conscious and unconscious relations with others rather than by biological essentialism or brain chemistry. This structural analysis allowed Fanon to stress the importance of the social, the permeation of structural racism, and also the foundational role of alterity in the construction of the self.[29] Fanon began his book by highlighting his debt to Freud but also by signaling the methodological limits of his approach: "Reacting against the constitutionalizing trend at the end of the nineteenth century, Freud demanded that the individual factor be taken into account in psychoanalysis. He replaced the phylogenetic theory by an ontogenetic approach. We shall see that the alienation of the black man is not an individual question. Alongside phylogeny and ontogeny, there is also sociogeny. . . . Let us say that here it is a question of sociodiagnostics."[30] This statement confirmed much of what Fanon had argued in his thesis and in *Esprit* concerning the inseparability of the biological, the psychological, and the social. As he continued in his introduction, "the black man must wage the struggle on the two levels," the political and the psychic, and "any unilateral liberation is flawed."[31]

But aside from Freud, Fanon's critique in *Black Skin, White Masks* had multiple targets. His anger was first and foremost directed toward racism, toward the kind of essentializing and dehumanizing racism that Fanon had so often experienced in France—his own *Erlebnis*. Fanon described racialization as a process of interpellation, as an encounter with an Other, with the gaze of an Other, that was performed and repeated, a process that "locks man in his body" and makes the black man responsible "not only for [his] body but for [his] race and [his] ancestors."[32] Turning to Jean-Paul Sartre's phenomenology and to *Anti-Semite and Jew*, Fanon explained that just as anti-Semitism produced the "Jew" as a category, "it is the racist who creates the inferiorized."[33] From Sartre, Fanon took up the idea that there were no fixed essences and that we become who we are through our interactions with others. But unlike Sartre, who failed to acknowledge that "the Jewishness of the Jew . . .

Frantz Fanon and the Decolonization of Institutional Psychotherapy   57

can go unnoticed. He is not integrally what he is," Fanon claimed that the black man was "not given a second chance. [He] is overdetermined from the outside. He is a slave not to the 'idea' others have of [him] but to [his] appearance."[34] How then, Fanon asked, could we imagine a disalienated subjectivity given these dynamics of racial formation?

In order to answer this question, Fanon proceeded negatively by criticizing three other models of subjectivity that, according to him, could not make sense of the lived experience of race and could not provide a viable antidote to racism: abstract universalism, *négritude*, and the psychology of race proposed by one of his contemporaries, the psychoanalyst Octave Mannoni. Fanon began by dismissing abstract universalism, the underlying principle of the Fourth Republic and of French republicanism more generally. Refusing to *see* race and to recognize difference—what we would call today color blindness—did not make racism disappear. Neither the "old universalisms" nor the "old humanisms" of the Enlightenment, he contended, could eliminate racism. Neither could the "appeals for reason or respect for human dignity change reality."[35] Furthermore, the negation of racial difference was psychically toxic for the racialized subject, who experienced this process as a form of what Sartre called bad faith or inauthenticity. According to Fanon, this "bad faith" was best exemplified by the work of his fellow Martinican, the writer Mayotte Capécia.[36]

If Fanon insisted on the fact that abstract universalism could not effectively combat racism, he was equally suspicious of all forms of reverse essentialisms: "Blacks [who] want to prove at all costs to the Whites the wealth of the black man's intellect and equal intelligence."[37] Being black, Fanon stated, was not anchored in a civilizational essence. As he put it: "my black skin is not a repository for specific values."[38] Fanon's prime example of this kind of naïve and ahistorical self-affirmation that he considered deeply problematic was *négritude*. He described this intellectual movement as a romanticism, a primitivism, and a nostalgia for an untainted past that, he contended, had been forever decimated by colonialism. This was the first sketch of Fanon's critique of *négritude*, which he would develop in his later writings. As many commentators have pointed out, Fanon's relationship to *négritude* was complex. Some have drawn our attention to Fanon's oedipal struggle against Aimé Césaire, his high school teacher at the Lycée Schoelcher in Fort-de-France, whom he greatly admired but with whom he also vehemently disagreed, especially regarding the goals and means of decolonization and departmentalization. Others have emphasized Fanon's antipathy toward Léopold Senghor's spirituality and the uncritical celebration of traditional African values in a journal such as *Présence africaine*.[39] In *Black Skin, White Masks*,

Fanon was especially harsh toward Sartre and his own rendition of the project of *négritude* in "Black Orpheus," his 1948 preface to Senghor's anthology of poetry. For Sartre, *négritude* was not an end but a means, an intermediary step in the dialectic, "the moment of negativity" that would eventually open up to a society without race or racism.[40]

Fanon's conclusion to *Black Skin, White Masks*, which foregrounds the question of history and temporality, can thus be read as a response to these two visions of race: the fetishization of the past that Fanon attributed to *négritude* and Sartre's reading of black consciousness as "potentiality" striving toward the universal.[41] Instead, Fanon advocated a model of subjectivity shaped by the past but radically open toward the future: "disalienation will be for those Whites and Blacks who have refused to let themselves be locked in the substantialized 'tower of the past.' . . . I am a man, and I have to rework the world's past from the very beginning. I am not just responsible for the slave revolt in Saint Domingue. . . . In no way do I have to dedicate myself to reviving a black civilization unjustly ignored. I will not make myself the man of any past. I do not want to sing the past to the detriment of my present and my future."[42] To be sure, Fanon added, it would be of "enormous interest to discover a black literature or architecture from the third century before Christ. We would be overjoyed to learn of the existence of a correspondence between some black philosopher and Plato." But this discovery would in no way "change the lives of the eight-year-old kids working in the cane fields of Martinique or Guadeloupe."[43] Racism, in other words, was a structural phenomenon, deeply tied to capitalism and colonialism. The attempt to imagine an unspoiled past that would lead to an uncorrupted future was simple disavowal, alienation in Marx's sense of the term.

Given the inability of liberal pluralism and of *négritude* to make sense of the lived experience of race, psychoanalysis emerged as a third possibility. Fanon was especially interested in Octave Mannoni's book *Psychologie de la colonisation*, published a few years before *Black Skin, White Masks*, in 1950. He praised the work as one of the first attempts to use psychoanalysis to think through race. Ultimately, however, Fanon rejected Mannoni's thesis as "dangerous."[44] Mannoni wrote *Psychologie de la colonisation* in the aftermath of the 1947–48 anticolonial uprising in Madagascar, one of the bloodiest episodes of French colonial history, in which French troops killed over 100,000 Malagasy.[45] Mannoni, who eventually undertook an analysis with Lacan in 1947 before he became a psychoanalyst himself, had lived in Madagascar for over twenty years, working first as a philosophy teacher and later as the director-general of the information service. His hope in *The Psychology of Colonization* was to make sense of the rebellion with the tools offered by psychoanalysis, ethnology, and anthropology. As one of the first efforts to understand how colonialism shaped psyches on a collective level, this book could only attract Fanon's interest.

Mannoni's argument rested on the hypothesis that two types of personality coexisted in Madagascar: a Malagasy personality, characterized by its subservience to ancestors and authority figures; and a colonizer personality shaped by a series of childhood complexes including an inferiority complex that the colonizer would seek to overcome through the colonizing mission. In the first stages of colonization, Mannoni suggested, these two personalities complemented each other: the colonizer provided social security and psychic stability to the colonized. However, in the decade that preceded the revolt, this balance—the "psychology of colonization"—was upset by various events including the Second World War and the anticolonial movement. Faced with the weakness of their parents/colonizers, the Malagasy felt abandoned, acted irrationally, and began to revolt. The rebellion, Mannoni concluded, was caused by the crisis of these two personality models at a particular historical conjuncture.

Fanon embraced Mannoni's book for understanding that "the problem of colonization . . . comprises not only the intersection of historical and objective conditions but also man's attitude toward these conditions."[46] The psyche, as he repeatedly argued, must be a central object of study in any attempt to understand colonialism. However, according to Fanon, the main problem with Mannoni's thesis was his assumption that "the inferiority complex exists prior to colonization."[47] For Fanon, this kind of argument was reminiscent of those in mainstream psychiatry that presumed the existence of a constitutional deficiency instead of examining the patient's social, political, and psychological history. Mannoni, in other words, despite his avowed commitment to antiracism, ended up promoting ideas dangerously close to the racist theses propagated by colonial psychiatry.

The critique of Mannoni allowed Fanon to clarify his own understanding of subjectivity as structural—as opposed to natural or essential—and as fundamentally shaped by the social and political context. What ultimately determined the "psychology of colonization" according to Fanon was not a childhood complex or one's relationship to one's parents and ancestors but the fundamental violence of colonialism and of racism—something that Mannoni seemed to have "forgotten."[48] As Fanon declared: "Once and for all we affirm that a society is racist or it is not."[49] Racism was not limited to a few "bad apples" in the system: it was a structural phenomenon. Thus, Fanon explained, South

60   CHAPTER TWO

Africa was racist not because of some disgruntled petty official or small traders: "it's because the structure of South Africa is a racist structure."[50] Similarly, the situation in Madagascar could not be understood outside of French colonialism and French racism. France was not, as Mannoni claimed, "unquestionably one of the least racialist-minded countries in the world"; it had, like all of Europe, "a racist structure" that produced a structural "psychology of race."[51]

Fanon's Encounter with Institutional Psychotherapy: Saint-Alban

As I have suggested, Fanon's early texts all wrestled with the problem of causation in psychic life. Against the biological determinism that he deplored in psychiatry, the essentialism that he perceived in *négritude*, and the implicit imperialism underlying the psychological model proposed by Mannoni, Fanon developed a theory of a subjectivity that was linked to the social and the political through a structural relationship. While these works were primarily anchored in Fanon's philosophical and scientific readings, it was his medical practice at Saint-Alban and later in North Africa that confirmed his theory of psychic causation. Fanon first heard about Saint-Alban through Paul Balvet, who, as we saw in chapter 1, had taken over the directorship of the hospital in 1937, recruited Tosquelles from the refugee camp in Septfonds, and was central to the Saint-Alban experiment. Fanon met Balvet through one of his classmates, who was a family friend of his and who lived in Balvet's home in Lyon. According to David Macey, Fanon was a frequent dinner guest at the Balvet household, and he enjoyed discussing psychiatry and Surrealism with Balvet.[52] After finishing medical school, Fanon accepted a short residency in the psychiatric hospital of Saint-Ylie of Dole in the Jura where, as the only resident for a hundred and fifty patients, he was exposed to the dire conditions of French psychiatric hospitals.[53] After a brief—and equally demoralizing—return to Martinique as a temporary locum at the Colson hospital, Fanon arrived at Saint-Alban in April 1952, in the midst of the psychiatric revolution that came to be known as institutional psychotherapy—but that Fanon more frequently referred to as *socialthérapie*.[54]

Fanon never wrote directly about his experience at Saint-Alban, but we know from Tosquelles, who devoted two essays to Fanon's psychiatric legacy, that he was an enthusiastic participant in the various social activities of the hospital. During his fifteen months there, Fanon relied on the structure of the Club and the meetings to imagine different vectors of transference to "heal" the collective. He helped set up plays, musical productions, and ergotherapy stations, and he wrote several pieces for the hospital's newsletter *Trait d'union.*[55] In an editorial titled "Yesterday, Today, and Tomorrow" dated March 6, 1953, Fanon insisted on the importance of historicity in the constitution of the self (see fig. 1.10). In another piece, "The Therapeutic Role of Engagement," he urged nurses to stop treating psychosis as "chronic" and to focus instead on the singularity of each patient.[56]

During this time, Fanon also co-wrote two papers with Tosquelles, which they presented at the national congress on psychiatry and neurology, papers in which they praised the virtues of electroshocks, insulin shocks, and narcotherapy. According to Fanon and Tosquelles, mainstream psychiatry used these procedures indiscriminately, as an end rather than a means. Instead, the authors advocated a limited use of these techniques as tools to "shake up" the patient's personality, which institutional psychotherapy could help reconstruct. To support this claim, Fanon and Tosquelles cited Lacan, for whom the personality was never a fixed essence but always constructed and thus potentially "reconstructable."[57] As Tosquelles recalled in a later interview, Fanon was fully immersed in the Saint-Alban adventure, which he embraced as an alternative to the dry version of organicist psychiatry that he had encountered in Lyon. Saint-Alban was the site of a "hypothesis," to use Tosquelles's term, "a space 'opened' from within and from outside," a hypothesis that stipulated that if you could assemble a group of people in an open space, some crazy and some not, and give them the means to articulate and rearticulate who they were and how they were shaped by history, they could, eventually, feel better.[58]

Institutional Psychotherapy in North Africa

In June 1953, Fanon passed the exam to become medical director of public psychiatric hospitals (*médecin-chef*) and immediately applied in the centralized system of the French Ministry of Health for a position in Guadeloupe.[59] This particular post, however, would not become vacant until later in the year, and so Fanon applied to the only other job outside of metropolitan France, at the hospital Blida-Joinville, the "capital of madness" of Algeria (fig. 2.1). Fanon's candidacy was accepted in October 1953 while he was working as a substitute doctor at a hospital in Pontorson, a small town in Normandy. Once again, Fanon was struck by the backwardness of French psychiatry. The patients at Pontorson spent their days immobilized, locked up, and treated like animals by a medical staff that appeared fundamentally afraid of them. In Normandy, Fanon was also confronted with the racism of his fellow doctors. From the moment he arrived at Pontorson, he tried to implement

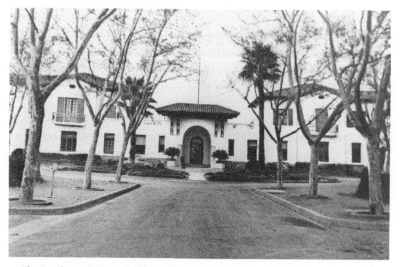

2.1 The Psychiatric Hospital of Blida-Joinville
© Fonds Frantz Fanon/IMEC

the theories and practices that he had learned at Saint-Alban. Breaking the walls of the hospital in order to integrate it into the community had been especially important for the founding fathers of Saint-Alban. Thus, in line with this vision of an "open door" institution and of a psychiatry "outside the walls," Fanon authorized twenty-nine of his patients to attend the Wednesday morning market, accompanied by a few nurses. The director of the hospital refused to sign the order, and the following morning, the hospital patients launched a general strike.[60] Fanon was eventually forced to back down, but his relations with his superiors deteriorated rapidly.[61]

Fanon arrived in Algeria in November 1953, after these successful and unsuccessful experiences, deeply marked by his desire to revolutionize psychiatric care. The hospital of Blida-Joinville was the largest psychiatric institution in North Africa. The idea of creating a state-of-the-art facility to treat the mentally ill in Algeria first emerged in 1912 at a congress of French alienists and neurologists. The project was later spearheaded by Antoine Porot, the chair of psychiatry at the medical school of Algiers, the principal architect of French Algeria's network for psychiatric care, and one of the figures whom Fanon attacked throughout his life as emblematic of colonial medicine's racism. As Richard Keller has shown, the Blida hospital, which had opened in 1938, encapsulated many of the paradoxes inherent in the project of French colonial medicine: it was modernizing while racializing, reforming while conservative. As Keller put it, Blida "served as a vessel for impassioned discussions over the relationship between colonialism and medicine, and over the nature of the French colonial project in Algeria itself."[62]

Porot was an equally complex figure, someone who considered himself a true reformist, the "Pinel of Algeria," who fought tirelessly to create a health system independent of the metropole while positing at the same time some of the most racist theories about "native" psychology.[63] As Fanon recalled, Porot was the first to sketch a psychiatric approach to the Muslim in his 1918 "Notes on Muslim Psychiatry." According to Porot, the North African *indigène* suffered from a genetic immaturity that had become fixed on the brain. Porot characterized North African behavior in the following terms: "none or hardly any emotivity; credulous and suggestible to the utmost; tenacious obstinacy; mental puerilism without the curiosity of the western child; a propensity for accidents and pithiatic [hysterical] reactions."[64]

By the time Fanon was recruited at Blida, the hospital was overcrowded with two thousand patients for eight hundred beds, underfunded, and in desperate need of restructuring. As many testimonies—including Fanon's—confirm, living conditions at Blida were truly dehumanizing. Patients wandered in rags when they were not tied to their beds or to trees in the garden. Like Saint-Alban before the war, the hospital looked and felt essentially like a prison.[65] But Blida suffered not only from the set of infrastructural problems common to most French psychiatric institutions in the afterwar period: it also functioned as a microcosm of Algerian colonial society with all of its racial segregation and discrimination. Medicine as a field of study was still mainly restricted to Algeria's white population, and when Fanon arrived, none of the psychiatrists working at Blida were of Arab descent. The patients were divided into gender-specific pavilions, some reserved for Europeans and the others for Muslims. Upon his arrival at Blida, Fanon joined four other supervising doctors (*chefs-de-service*) who were not in the least interested in psychiatric innovation or in anticolonial activism. One of Fanon's new colleagues, in fact, Dr. Ramée, had been a student of Porot's, and he remained a strong advocate of the theory of Arab primitivism promoted by the Algiers School. Another of these doctors was Raymond Lacaton, the addressee of Fanon's "Letter to a Frenchman," which was later republished in *Toward the African Revolution*. For Fanon, Lacaton was symptomatic of the blindness that characterized the French settler population—the *pieds noirs*—right before the war. Lacaton, "laughing," told Fanon he was leaving because "the atmosphere is getting rotten." Yes, as Fanon put it, "for eight years you have been in this country. And no part of this enormous wound has held you back in any way. And no part of this enormous wound has pushed you in any way."

Lacaton, like Fanon's other colleagues, had "not understood," had not "wanted to understand what has happened around you every day."[66]

From the moment he arrived at Blida, Fanon was vocal about his objections to colonialism and to the way psychiatry was practiced—which made working with his colleagues arduous. As he recounted in a letter to his friend Maurice Despinoy, a psychiatrist whom he had met at Saint-Alban and who had moved to Martinique, it was very difficult to practice institutional psychotherapy at Blida when people had a completely different "understanding of psychiatry and the mental life of the patients." As an example, Fanon mentioned that his desire to institute bi-monthly meetings was received with generalized apathy on the part of the patients and the staff: "No overall project, no collaboration, no cooperation; and the worst is that at the start of meetings, everyone is already tired as if all dialogue was simply in vain."[67] As a result, Fanon began to surround himself with a group of young interns that included Alice Cherki, Jacques Azoulay, Charles Géronimi, and François Sanchez, all intrepid, politically engaged, and enthusiastic about the possibility of using psychiatry to advance a decolonial revolution.[68] With the help of these interns, Fanon applied some of the techniques that he had learned at Saint-Alban in a "fifth division," which he supervised. This division was composed of four pavilions, one of European women and three of Muslim men.

As he had learned from Tosquelles and from Simon, institutional psychotherapy needed to "cure the hospital" (*soigner le personnel soignant*) before it could begin to cure its patients. The staff thus played an essential role in this mission, and Fanon insisted on the importance of training his nurses and interns, just as Tosquelles had at Saint-Alban (fig. 2.2).[69] To that effect, he organized classes and seminars for his employees and encouraged them to record their daily observations in diaries. He urged them to eat with the patients—something that had been previously forbidden (fig. 2.3).[70] He insisted on removing all uniforms to fight against depersonalization. He set up a café, Le Café Bon Accueil, modeled on the Club Paul Balvet at Saint-Alban. As Fanon put it, the café was a "space to re-learn the gestures of the outside" and to "institute the social."[71] He organized daily meetings, built a library, set up ergotherapy stations—weaving, pottery, knitting, gardening—and promoted sports, especially soccer, which, he argued, could play an important role in the resocialization of patients. He planned field trips to the beach, arranged parties and holiday celebrations, encouraged drama, singing, and other artistic productions, screened a series of movies, and invited professional singers to perform at the hospital.[72]

These various activities, developed to reconstitute "the social archi-

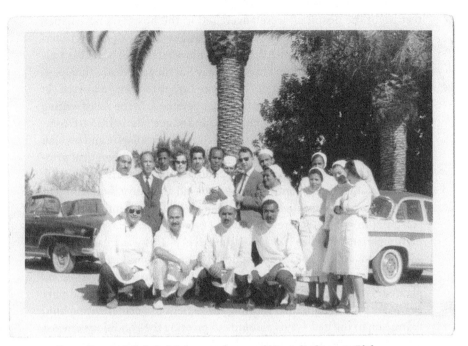

2.2 Frantz Fanon, sixth from left in second row, and his medical team in Blida
© Fonds Frantz Fanon/IMEC

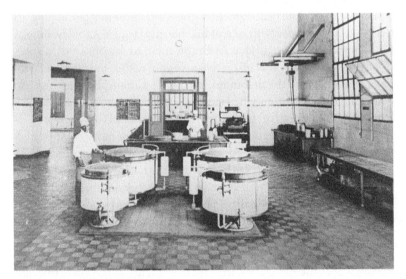

2.3 The kitchen of the Blida hospital
© Fonds Frantz Fanon/IMEC

tecture of the hospital," were advertised in the hospital's newspaper, *Notre journal*, which was printed by the patients in one of the ergotherapy stations.[73] As at Saint-Alban, these newsletters had a double purpose: they advertised the events of the day but they also had a therapeutic goal. As one editorial put it: "To write means to want to be read. In the same stroke it means to want to be understood. In the act of writing there is an effort being made; muddled and vague [thoughts] are combatted, surpassed."[74] Finally, the newsletters allowed Fanon and his staff to communicate with the patients and to explain the theoretical principles that underlay institutional psychotherapy: "If we are not careful, the hospital establishment which is above all a curative establishment [*établissement thérapeutique*] is gradually transformed into a barracks [*caserne*] in which children-boarders [*enfants-pensionnaires*] tremble before parent-orderlies [*infirmiers-parents*]."[75] This was in accordance with Fanon's reflections in more scholarly publications during this time, including an article on agitation for the journal *Maroc médical*. As he explained, isolating agitated patients in solitary confinement could only aggravate their symptoms: "shutting the patient in a cell, isolating him, fixing him to the bed—this amounts to printing the conditions of existence for hallucinatory activity."[76] Instead, the hospital needed to function as a healing collective, as the knot of social relations, the site of production of "disalienating" forces (*forces productives désaliénantes*).[77]

Fanon meticulously documented these practices in a fascinating article that he co-wrote with one of his interns, Jacques Azoulay, in 1954 for *L'Information psychiatrique*. As Fanon and Azoulay observed, institutional psychotherapy was instantly successful within the ward of European women. From the first months, "the very atmosphere of the ward had changed. . . . Not only had asylum life become less distressing for many, but the rhythm of discharges had already markedly increased."[78] In the Muslim men's section, however, things were more complicated. Fanon and Azoulay described their first months as a "total failure."[79] The meetings designed to plan the parties, the movies, the newsletter— meetings conceived to "transform that abstract and impersonal multitude into a coherent group driven by collective concerns"—did not interest the patients in the least.[80] The sessions were eventually shortened, but the patients remained indifferent and the staff resented the meetings as an additional burden. Fanon and Azoulay were also disheartened to realize that the newsletter, the "social cement" of the collective, did not appeal to these male patients who cared neither to read nor to contribute to it. In the first months, only one text had been written by an Arab patient. In the ergotherapy sessions, the patients remained still, "unoccupied, completely indifferent to the accomplishment of shared

Frantz Fanon and the Decolonization of Institutional Psychotherapy   67

work [*travail commun*]."[81] Neither the theater nor the movies managed to capture their attention. As Fanon and Azoulay concluded, after three months and despite their sustained efforts, they were unable to get the Muslim patients involved in the collective life that was flourishing in the European pavilion. Instead, the atmosphere in the Arab quarters was "oppressive, stifling [*irrespirable*]."[82]

In the second half of their article, Fanon and Azoulay tried to come to terms with the reasons behind this failure: "We naively considered our division as a whole and believed we had adapted to this Muslim society the frames of a particular Western society. . . . We wanted to create institutions and yet we forgot that all such approaches must be preceded by a persistent, real, and concrete interrogation into the organic bases of the indigenous society. How can we have been so misguided as to think that a Western-inspired social therapy [*socialthérapie*] could be simply applied to a ward of Muslim patients? How was a structural analysis possible if we bracketed the geographic, historical, cultural, and social frameworks?"[83] As Fanon and Azoulay made clear, their attempt to impose a Western grid in Algeria was a form of violence that was ultimately complicit with imperialism. Instead of "adopting a policy of assimilation," psychiatry needed to embrace a "revolutionary attitude"—it needed to shift from a "position in which the supremacy of Western culture was evident, to one of cultural relativism."[84] As Fanon and Azoulay specified, the "cultural relativism" they were advocating was not the cultural relativism of ethnopsychiatry as practiced by Porot and the Algiers School. Rather, what they had in mind was to consider Algeria as a "total social fact" in Marcel Mauss's sense, to pass "from the biological level to the institutional one, from natural existence to cultural existence."[85] The point was not to return to a traditional Algerian society untouched in the past but rather to observe, to take into account its irreversible transformation under colonialism, and to invent a new set of institutions.

In their attempt to discern this "total social fact" and to understand which institutions would support a true "national culture," Fanon and Azoulay began to travel throughout Algeria. Little by little, they came to understand why this initial form of institutional psychotherapy had failed in Blida. The first obstacle that they mentioned was the language barrier and the fact that none of the doctors—including Fanon—spoke Arabic. Moreover, most of the Muslim patients were illiterate and so reading and writing in the newsletter was simply not an option. For most of the Muslim patients, Fanon and Azoulay observed, social gatherings were primarily religious or familial so it was difficult to get them excited about the abstract idea of a party. A majority of these patients had never been exposed to the theater, which existed only in large ur-

68   CHAPTER TWO

ban centers. Instead, Fanon and Azoulay noticed that the more per-
vasive form of entertainment in Algeria was professional storytellers
who traveled from village to village and recited epic poems grounded
in the local folklore. Similarly, Fanon and Azoulay understood that the
kinds of activities proposed in the ergotherapy stations, weaving for example, were disparaged as intrinsically feminine. Finally, they realized
that if the patients seemed uninterested in the movies that they were
screening, it was because their plots were too "Western." If they avoided
playing the games that were being proposed (like hide-and-seek), it was
because these were not familiar.

With this new knowledge, Fanon and his interns began to adapt institutional psychotherapy to the Algerian context. They changed their
movie selection and privileged action-filled films; they picked games
that were recognizable to Algerians; they celebrated the traditional
Muslim holidays; they invited Muslim singers to perform in the hospital; and they hired a professional storyteller to come speak to the patients. What Muslim men most seemed to enjoy doing after work was
gathering amongst themselves in a café where they could play cards or
dominos. Thus, Fanon and his team inaugurated the Café maure, which,
they claim, rapidly became a popular socializing space. Each day, the
number of patients involved in these activities grew, and soon enough
institutional psychotherapy had changed the social fabric of the hospital: it had literally *instituted* the social. As Fanon concluded, this was
"only a beginning, but already we believe we have eliminated the methodological errors."[86] Unlike the "assimilated psychiatry" that Fanon had
arrived with, this was a truly disalienated and disalienating psychiatry.

Day Hospitalization in Tunisia

Fanon was expelled from Algeria in January 1957 soon after sending his
letter of resignation to Lacoste. France was officially at war by then and
Fanon still worked in a public hospital, as a public servant, so French authorities were quick to react. After transiting through Paris, Switzerland,
and Italy, he accepted a position in Tunisia—which had achieved independence in 1956—at the hospital of La Manouba, outside of Tunis.
There, he was confronted with the same kinds of resistances to his psychiatric practices, in addition to the racism of his Tunisian colleagues.
By now, however, he was used to it, and he was much more experienced.
During these first months in Tunisia, Fanon deepened his links with the
FLN. Every week, he was part of a convoy of doctors sent to treat Algerian combatants and refugees who were hidden in a farm near the border. Some of these patients later became case studies in the last chapter

of *The Wretched of the Earth*.[87] As Fanon observed, once again stressing the structural link between the psychic and the political, the war had become a "breeding ground for mental disorders."[88]

Given his frustrations at La Manouba, Fanon happily accepted the directorship of an outpatient facility (*centre psychiatrique de jour*) at the Charles-Nicolle General Hospital in Tunis, which had a more cosmopolitan and more receptive staff. This was the last post for Fanon, the last site of psychiatric experimentation before he died of leukemia in the United States, in December 1961. It was also during these last years that Fanon wrote most of his political texts, which were published by François Maspero, an editor sympathetic to anticolonialism and third-worldism but also to psychiatric reform.[89] These included a series of articles for the FLN newspaper *El Moudjahid*, conference papers, and political speeches that were gathered in *Toward the African Revolution*, published posthumously in 1964; *The Year Five of the Algerian Revolution* in 1959; and finally, his most famous book, *The Wretched of the Earth*, in 1961. After a serious accident at the Moroccan border that left his upper body in a cast, Fanon chose to dictate *The Year Five* and *The Wretched of the Earth* to Marie-Jeanne Manuellan, a social worker who was one of his assistants at the Charles-Nicolle day center. Fanon and Manuellan would meet from seven to nine in the morning before Fanon began his consultations of the day. Fanon would speak and Manuellan would type. As Manuellan recalls, Fanon liked to repeat that madness was a "pathology of freedom" and that the goal of psychiatry was to produce free men.[90] More generally, we could say that Fanon's political works were literally intertwined with his psychiatric practice, from a theoretical standpoint but also at the very concrete level of production.

At the day center, Fanon continued to experiment with institutional psychotherapy, but this time outside the walls of the hospital. Like other psychiatrists in France—including Philippe Paumelle and the movement around the *psychiatrie de secteur*—Fanon praised the virtues of an "open door" model of care. As he saw it, day hospitalization offered two main advantages: it allowed the patient to remain within his familial and professional milieu; and it did not mask the various psychiatric symptoms produced by familial, social, or professional conflicts that hospitalization often concealed.[91] Day hospitalization as Fanon conceived it was perfectly in line with the principles of institutional psychotherapy: it was psychiatry without doors, without gates, without handcuffs, and without uniforms. As he had done in Blida, Fanon interspersed the various social activities with forty-minute one-on-one psychoanalysis sessions and with group therapies—*sociodrames*—inspired by the work of Jacob Moreno.[92] As a "pathology of freedom," madness placed the patient in a "world in which his or her freedom, will and desires are constantly broken by obsessions, inhibitions, countermands, anxieties." As Fanon continued, "classical hospitalization considerably limits the patient's field of activity, prohibits all compensations, all movement, restrains him within the closed field of the hospital and condemns him to exercise his freedom in the unreal world of fantasy."[93] Instead, *socialthérapie* (or institutional psychotherapy) forced the patients "to verbalize, to explain . . . to take a position"; it "wrests patients from their fantasies and forces them to confront reality on a new register."[94]

Decolonizing Institutional Psychotherapy

How, then, were Fanon's last experiences with institutional psychotherapy, first in Blida and later in Tunisia, related to his well-known political writings? As Fanon famously—and controversially—suggested in the first chapter of *The Wretched of the Earth*, violence was necessary in the process of decolonization because of the structural violence that pervaded the colonial context, the "atmospheric violence, the violence rippling under the skin [*à fleur de peau*]."[95] As he repeated throughout his work, colonial violence was always political, social, and psychic at once, and the kind of decolonial violence that he was encouraging needed to operate on all three levels. As he put it, violence unified the people in the struggle against a colonial power: it was "enlightening" politically, and "at an individual level, violence is a cleansing force."[96] In some ways, the violence that Fanon called for in *The Wretched of the Earth* functioned similarly to the electroshock that Fanon had praised at Saint-Alban. Violence was a means to "shake up" the psyche and the social before the work of reconstruction could begin. In both cases, violence was regenerative: the stepping stone for a new order.

Unlike *The Year Five of the Algerian Revolution*, which in many ways was written for a French public, a public that Fanon wanted to make aware of the horrors of colonialism, *The Wretched of the Earth* was primarily directed toward the nascent Third World, the African, Latin American, and Asian populations who were fighting for independence during the Cold War. As Sartre succinctly put it in his famous preface aimed at a European readership, *The Wretched of the Earth* "often talks *about* you, but never *to* you."[97] Throughout his book, Fanon insisted on the structural imbrication of European liberalism and colonialism. Western universalism and humanism had been constituted through colonial and racial violence, through the "pathological dismembering of [man's] functions and the erosion of his unity," through systematic "racial hatred, slavery, exploitation, above all . . . bloodless genocide."[98] Europe, as such, could not serve as a template for social, political, and cultural reconstruction in the wake of decolonization. "Come, comrades," Fanon wrote in the last pages of his book:

> The European game is finally over, we must look for something else. We can do anything today provided we do not ape Europe, provided we are not obsessed with catching up with Europe. . . . It is all too true, however, that we need a model, schemas, and examples. For many of us the European model is the most elating. But we have seen in the preceding pages how misleading such an imitation can be. European achievements, European technology and European lifestyles must stop tempting us and leading us astray.[99]

"Let us decide not to imitate Europe," Fanon concluded, "let us not pay tribute to Europe by creating states, institutions, and societies that draw their inspiration from it."[100]

The task of rethinking and remaking institutions was thus central not only to Fanon's psychiatric work but also to his political project. Just as Fanon sought to create new institutions within the confines of the hospital, institutions that could turn a segregated and deeply colonial environment into a healing community, he tried to imagine new institutions to uphold the rising Third World. In this sense, one way to read *The Wretched of the Earth* is as a quest for the "model, schemas, and examples" that could also help to disalienate and reconstruct the postcolonial social. Fanon never offered a definitive or prescriptive answer to this search, just as institutional psychotherapy never specified the content of its method. It seems, however, that his concept of the nation, of national liberation and national culture, comes close.

While Fanon never put forth a precise definition of national culture, much of *The Wretched of the Earth* was devoted to disputing what it should *not* be. As the passage above makes clear, national self-determination could not result from the simple application or projection of the historical Western model of the nation-state at the political or at the cultural level. Politically, neither liberalism nor Marxism could pave the way, and Fanon repeatedly urged the Third World to abandon the fantasy that it needed to "choose between the capitalist system and the socialist system."[101] Similarly, Fanon criticized "assimilated intellectuals" trained in the metropole who embraced the Western canon and wished to simply apply it to the postcolonial realm.[102] Fanon, however, was equally harsh against the many intellectuals and politicians who preached a return to "tradition" and who sought to rehabilitate and revalorize precolonial civilizations. As he maintained, reverse essentialism—which, according to him, crucially hindered *négritude*, Arabism, and tribalism—was merely "irresponsible."[103] The naïve glorification of a past untainted by colonialism and "increasingly cut off from reality" was as politically dangerous as the cooptation of the European canon.

It is in opposition to these forms of political and cultural self-determination that Fanon put forth his notion of "national culture," which he described as synonymous with combat and with national liberation. Rather than encompassing a particular content, national culture provided a theoretical framework: it was to be grounded in the past and in local tradition while being radically oriented toward the future; it was culturally specific and yet universal; it could serve as an instituting vector for both the subject and popular will. As examples of this national culture, Fanon listed storytellers—also important in his revised version of institutional psychotherapy at Blida. As he put it in *The Wretched of the Earth*, storytellers could mobilize the people by giving them epics geared toward the present and the future, as opposed to tales frozen in time: "The present is no longer turned inward but channeled in every direction."[104] Other examples of national culture included artisanship, wood carving, ceramics, and pottery—activities that were, again, all central at Blida. As Fanon conceived them, these activities were no longer trapped by "formalist paradigms" but rather had succeeded in "bringing faces and bodies to life" and in "inspiring concerted action."[105] As Fanon concluded: "In the colonial context, culture, when deprived of the twin supports of the nation and the state, perishes and dies. . . . The nation is not only a precondition for culture, its ebullition, its perpetual renewal and maturation. It is a necessity."[106]

Within Fanon's political work, the nation played a role similar to that of institutions in the psychiatric practice that emerged in Blida. Institutional psychotherapy, as Fanon revised it after his experience in Algeria, was also anchored in the language, customs, and everyday life of the people while remaining open to the future. It could provide the necessary tools to diagnose but also to combat the political, social, and psychic violence of racism and colonialism. If Fanon insisted on the centrality of institutions to reconstitute the social within the psychiatric hospital, he also advocated the nation as integral to what the political theorist Adom Getachew has recently named "worldmaking after empire."[107] Neither institutional psychotherapy nor national self-determination was ever meant to operate as a rigid template or grid that could be applied indiscriminately and independently of context. Rather, they were to function more as an ethics, as a practice of everyday

Frantz Fanon and the Decolonization of Institutional Psychotherapy   73

life that could prevent the appearance of "concentrationisms" and ultimately lead to a freedom that would be collective and personal at once.

As I have suggested, Fanon embraced institutional psychotherapy as a theory and as a practice for several reasons. First, it offered an appealing alternative both to the biological essentialism of the psychiatry that he was confronted with in medical school in Lyon and to the racism of the colonial psychiatry dominant in Algeria. Second, institutional psychotherapy gave Fanon a model of subjectivity in which the psychic, the social, and the political could be examined together. Since racism and colonialism always operated on all these levels, psychiatry could provide the necessary tools to identify and to fight against this form of political, social, and psychic violence. Third, and finally, institutional psychotherapy insisted on the role of institutions in the process of alienation and disalienation of the political, the social, and the subjective.

But Fanon took institutional psychotherapy as it was conceived in Saint-Alban one step further. If the explicit goal of institutional psychotherapy was to scrutinize all social and psychic formations, to unearth remaining traces of authoritarianism, to prevent reification and stagnation—to systematically "defamiliarize, de-oedipalize, decode, and deterritorialize," to use the vocabulary that Deleuze and Guattari would claim a few years later, then Fanon's work in North Africa was perhaps the most perfected example of institutional psychotherapy.[108] Instead of simply applying a model that he had learned in the metropole and that was clearly not working in the colonial context, Fanon "deterritorialized" and transformed the practices and the theories themselves. In this sense, his psychiatric work was radical not necessarily for its content but for forcing us to "decolonize" intellectual history and to rethink the supposedly European parameters of the history of medicine, psychiatry, and what is generally referred to as "French theory."

CHAPTER 3

Félix Guattari, La Borde, and the Search for Anti-oedipal Politics

Jean Oury arrived at Saint-Alban on September 3, 1947. For the twenty-three-year-old medical student, 1947 had been an important year. Oury had been gravitating toward psychiatry, especially after his encounter with Julian de Ajuriaguerra, René Angelergues, and Georges Daumézon, three of the most innovative professors in the world of French psychiatry, who had followed the initial steps of institutional psychotherapy closely. During the first semester of 1947, Oury attended a series of talks at the École Normale Supérieure, and it was in this context that he encountered François Tosquelles, and a few months later, Jacques Lacan. In both cases, he was instantly seduced. He contacted Lacan to begin an analysis with him and wrote to Tosquelles to apply for a residency at the Saint-Alban Hospital.[1] Oury thus actively participated in the first years of the Saint-Alban experiment, in the meetings, the Club, the journal, the ergotherapy stations, and all the other attempts to "disalienate" the asylum and the community more broadly.

For Oury, the creative effervescence palpable at Saint-Alban offered a perfect complement to his previous political engagement. In 1936, when he was only a teenager, he had enthusiastically taken part in the Front Populaire strikes alongside his brother, Fernand Oury. He attended meetings and brought sandwiches to the workers at Hispano-Suiza, the automobile factory where their father worked. Soon, however, the Oury brothers became disillusioned with the rigidity of the French Communist Party (PCF) and, like Tosquelles, with Stalinism more generally, and they turned to smaller anarchist-Trotskyite currents. More specifically, Jean and Fernand Oury became active in the network of youth hostels (*auberges de jeunesse*) that blossomed in the 1930s and that allowed young people to travel throughout France by offering inexpensive lodging. Unlike the scout movement associated with Catholicism

Félix Guattari, La Borde, and the Search for Anti-oedipal Politics   75

and conservatism, the *auberges de jeunesse* became a space of innovation for leftist ideals. Similarly, around the same time, Oury became involved with the *caravanes*, a web of summer camps geared toward the children of workers. In both cases, Oury was drawn to the spirit of common enterprise—what Félix Guattari would later call the *complexe de 1936*—a vision of self-managed collective life that he would find again in the social organization of Saint-Alban.[2] Working at the intersection of medicine and politics, the doctors and the staff of Saint-Alban appeared invested in a similar project of thinking and rethinking institutions, of imagining a different, more horizontal and less hierarchical, collectivity.

In 1949, after two years as a resident at Saint-Alban, Jean Oury accepted a position at the psychiatric clinic of Saumery, a private establishment in the Loire region. Working conditions were harsh, as in most hospitals after the war, with only twelve beds for a population of 250,000.[3] Yet Oury tried to implement some of the practices of institutional psychotherapy that he had learned with Tosquelles and his colleagues. It was at Saumery that Félix Guattari first met Oury (fig. 3.1). Guattari, who was bored with his studies to become a pharmacist, was sent to Saumery by Fernand Oury, who had been his high school teacher.[4] Like his brother, Fernand Oury was active in the youth hostel and summer camp movements. He was also a disciple of the famous pedagogical reformer Célestin Freinet, an admirer of his Mouvement de l'École moderne, and an avid reader of John Dewey. In the late 1950s, Fernand Oury would summarize his pedagogical ideas under the label "institutional pedagogy." As its name indicates, institutional pedagogy was close to institutional psychotherapy, and there were many overlaps between the two currents. Aïda Vasquez, for example, who in 1967 co-wrote with Fernand Oury *Toward an Institutional Pedagogy* (published by François Maspero), worked as a psychoanalyst at La Borde. Like institutional psychotherapy, institutional pedagogy was anchored in the praxis of the classroom experience, and it tried to consider the effect of institutions on the unconscious, the symbolic laws of the classroom, the desires of the students and teachers, and the transferential relationships among them.[5]

At Saumery, Jean Oury began to constitute a network of nurses, doctors, and friends—including Guattari—who shared his political and theoretical aspirations. The group traveled to the clinic from Paris every weekend to work with the psychotic patients, lead workshops, and help with the medical care. After four years of fighting the clinic's administration, which had little interest in or patience for the medical and social innovations of institutional psychotherapy, Oury and his friends decided to leave Saumery. Taking along several of their patients, they

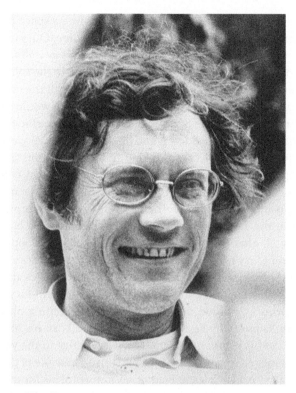

3.1 Félix Guattari
© Bruno, Emmanuelle, Stephen Guattari/IMEC

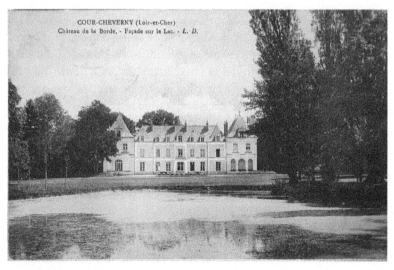

3.2 Postcard of the Château de La Borde
© Public Domain

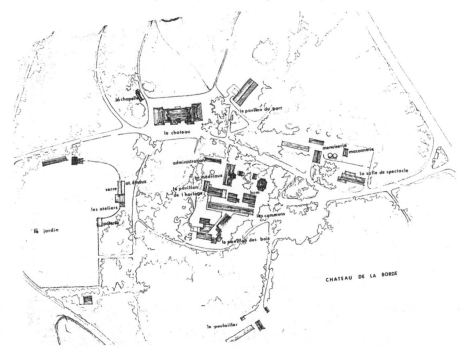

3.3 Map of La Borde
© Revue Recherches N°21, mars 1976, Histoires de La Borde. 10 ans de psychothérapie institutionnelle à la clinique de Cour-Cheverny, 1953–1963

searched for a new location in which they could continue experimenting with radical psychiatry. In 1953, they arrived at La Borde, a rundown castle surrounded by a large wooded property, which was listed for sale (figs. 3.2 and 3.3). After gathering loans wherever he could, Oury bought the property and moved in with his patients, a close circle of friends, and colleagues. In 1955, Guattari relocated to La Borde permanently, with his partner Micheline Kao. In the years that followed, La Borde became a legendary pilgrimage site within the French intellectual world. Medical students, philosophers, anthropologists, political activists, psychoanalysts, artists, and filmmakers—the "barbarians" or the "invaders" as Oury called them—traveled back and forth from Paris, some staying for months or years, living with the psychotic patients, while thinking about the relationship between the political and the libidinal.

This chapter focuses on the cosmology of La Borde from the 1950s to the 1970s and more precisely on the intersections of psychoanalysis, philosophy, and politics in the works of Jean Oury and Félix Guattari. By pausing on the operations of daily life at La Borde, I wish to show that psychiatry played a fundamental role in Guattari's work and activism, especially in *Anti-Oedipus: Capitalism and Schizophrenia*, which Guattari co-wrote with Gilles Deleuze in 1972. The "anti-oedipal" politics that Guattari defended—his schizoanalysis—were very much inspired by the theory and the praxis of institutional psychotherapy. The point was not to destroy all institutions (as much of antipsychiatry argued and as many readers of *Anti-Oedipus* still mistakenly maintain), but to reimagine them as horizontal and temporary, to "deterritorialize" them. Like Tosquelles, Bonnafé, and the other "founding fathers" of institutional psychotherapy, Oury and Guattari were convinced that psychic and social alienation were intimately tied. Subjectivities, they argued, were never simply centered on the individual—they were always shaped by the social and the political. Furthermore, they contended, all institutions, all collectivities, and all subjectivities had the potential to become authoritarian or totalitarian—"small kingdoms," in the words of Oury. Thus, a disalienated political and medical practice needed to focus on tracking down these latent "concentrationist" tendencies by mobilizing individual and collective desires, fantasies, and transferences.

As we saw in chapter 1, Tosquelles had come to this conclusion not only through his medical and intellectual trajectory, but also through his life experience, especially after his encounter with fascism, first in Spain and later in France during the Second World War. Twenty years after the end of the war, Guattari's context was very different. As Michel Foucault put it in his preface to *Anti-Oedipus*, the immediate threat was no longer the "historical fascism" of Hitler and Mussolini but rather "the fascism in us all, in our heads and our everyday behavior, the fascism that causes us to love power, to desire the very thing that dominates and exploits us."[6] In other words, Guattari's question was no longer "how was fascism able to succeed?" but "why is fascism *still* so appealing?" As the political context of the Cold War had made clear, fascism had not been eradicated, even with the advent of Marxist-socialist revolutions in many parts of the world. Institutional psychotherapy thus offered Guattari a lens to consider why alienation persisted and why so many people still *desired* "fascism," the term that in his work functioned as a proxy for authoritarianism, domination, and oppression. Working at La Borde taught Guattari that libidinal economy and political economy were inseparable. Therefore, the goal of the "anti-oedipal politics" that Guattari longed for—an "ethics" rather than a theory, as Foucault would later say—was to decolonize or "disalienate" the unconscious, the familial, the social, and the political, all at once.[7]

Daily Life at La Borde

As with Saint-Alban and with Fanon's hospitals in North Africa, daily life at La Borde was organized around the assumption that theory and praxis were intrinsically connected. In the words of Oury, La Borde was not a philosophy but rather a "site of crystallization, a praxical site [*lieu praxique*]."[8] On the eve of the official opening of the clinic, on April 1, 1953, Oury and his colleagues promulgated a "Constitution of the Year I"—in a witty reference to the 1793 constitution, the most radical constitution of the revolutionary period. As its authors declared, their first goal was to turn La Borde into a "therapeutic group." Everything pertaining to the organization of the clinic (administration, management, entertainment . . .) needed to be governed by this fundamental principle.[9] As the constitution specified, administrative decisions at La Borde depended on a management group that met monthly and that included the general director and owner of the clinic (i.e., Jean Oury), who had veto power during the general meetings. This form of "democratic centralism" was necessary for the effective functioning of the clinic, but any potential authoritarianism or closure was to be avoided by a second principle: the "precariousness of statutes." This meant not only that elected officials could be recalled, but also that the daily tasks (cleaning, cooking, working at the café, entertainment . . .) were open to redefinition: "Taking responsibility for a task is not only making sure it is executed, it is also connecting it to others, denaturalizing it, reinventing it."[10] In order to avoid excessive specialization and compartmentalization of roles, all staff rotated regularly, so that nurses could wash dishes, garden, or cook, just as patients could take part in the administrative decisions. All employees, including the doctors, received the same salary. As the Constitution explained, the point of this "communitarian organization" was to destabilize fixed identities, the kinds of identities invested in stable definitions of "name, age, profession, salary, sex," and to produce "other 'dis-egoized' sites of investment [*lieux d'investissements 'démoïsés'*]."[11]

Oury—and especially Guattari who was in charge of overseeing this system of rotation for almost ten years—called it "the grid" (*la grille*). The grid was, simply put, a double-entry chart with a timetable, the names of each staff member, and the work that was assigned to him or her each day (fig. 3.4). As Guattari put it, the grid was conceived as an instrument of "disorganization," as a way to introduce chaos into social relations and as the only remedy against "the bureaucratic routine and the passivity generated by the systems of traditional hierarchy."[12] Fur-

Name	(start)	8h–13h	13h–21h
Emma		Plateaux	Surv. Repas · SCAJ · Atelier Kalo-Gouter · R de 6 h · Tilleul
Oscar		Bur. Administratif · Secr. du Club	SCAJ · Bureau Administratif · R de 6 h
Clémence Journel	5 heures	2ᵉ étage · Soins Ménage	
Nadine			
Saïto		Comité Menus · S. de Table · Plateaux	Service de Table · R de 6 h · Serv. de Table
Esther		Insuline	Surv. Repas · Gouter Insuline · R de 6 h · Surv. Repas
Mlle Paupinelle		Infirmerie	Atelier Couture · Surv. Repas
Arianne		Electroencéphalogrammes	
Hélène	6 h 30 Insuline		SCAJ · Bureau Administràtif · R de 6 h ?
Croizart			SCAJ
Paméla		Bur. Administratif-Permanence	Bureau Administratif-permanerice
Lelond		At. Dessins · Secr. du Club	SCAJ · Promenade At. Dessin · R de 6 h · Nuit
Blandine		1ᵉ étage · Soins Ménage	Grille · R de 6 h
Jocelyne		1ᵉ étage · Soins Ménage	Cuisine
Pauline		Ménage Rez de Chaussée Chateau	Lingerie
Georgette	Congé		
Mathilde		Infirmerie	Infirmerie · R de 6 h · Infirmerie
Giuseppe		Atelier Mime	SCAJ · Courses en ville · R de 6 h
Bertha	Congé		
Carole		2ᵉ étage · Soins Ménage	Comité bar Gouter · Comité Entreprise · Plateaux
Séverine		Ménage rez de chaussée	Promenade Atelier Grand salon
Pascal Dega		Pharmacie	Pharmacie
Barbara		Secrétariat	Secrétariat · R de 6 h
Nicolas Journel		Poulailler	Poulailler
Valjan		Chauffe	Poulailler · R de 6 h
Amandine	Congé		
Jérôme Fotana	1/2 Congé		SCAJ · Comité bar Volley-ball · R de 6 h
Blanche		Lingerie	Lingerie
Guillaume	7 h Cuisine	Comité Menu · Cuisine	Cuisine
Anna		Cuisine · Menu	Cuisine · Cuisine
Eliane Fraisier		Atelier pluche	Atelier Vannerie · R de 6 h
Claudien		Voirie-Poubelles	SCAJ · Atelier Imprimerie · R de 6 h
Honorine		bur. dr Odin · Ménage · Sanitaires	Ménage de la salle à manger (vitres parquet)
Dr Zarka			
Dr Biellent			
Antoinette		Caisse dépots S. de T.	S. de T. · SCAJ · Atelier poterie · R de 6 h · Service de Table
Ramon		Entretien	Entretien · R de 6 h

3.4 The "Grid" (la "Grille") at La Borde
© Revue Recherches N°21, mars 1976, *Histoires de La Borde. 10 ans de psychothérapie institutionnelle à la clinique de Cour-Cheverny, 1953–1963*

thermore, like every other activity at La Borde, the grid presented a forum through which staff members could discuss their feelings, desires, and fears, by talking and "incessantly questioning" all activities and all personnel relationships. The idea was, once again, that the grid would contribute to the process—so crucial to Tosquelles and his colleagues at Saint-Alban—of "curing" or "disalienating" the hospital and the medical team.[13]

As at Saint-Alban, the organization of collective life at La Borde relied on various subcommittees: one in charge of drawing up menus, another that handled economic matters, a laundry and cleaning team, a medical committee, and perhaps the most important one, the "Club." Modeled on the Saint-Alban "Club Paul Balvet," the Club at La Borde was a self-managed association, a union designed for the patients to organize their life-in-common. It was a physical space where patients could meet and gather, a "point of reference not subjected [assujetti] to the hospital hierarchy."[14] It also had, however, a theoretical purpose as a "machine to foment desire." In the words of Anne-Marie Norgeu, who worked at La Borde for several years, the Club was the "masterpiece of the institutional machinery."[15] It provided a microcosm to observe and to work with the psychotics' relations of transference, what Oury called their "dissociated transference," a transference attached to many points of reference and not just to another person.[16] Just as with the grid, Guattari played a central role in setting up the Club. As he recalled, because of his youth activism with the *auberges de jeunesse*, he "knew how to lead a meeting, structure a debate, encourage the silent people to speak up, propose practical decisions, and put in place the previously decided tasks."[17] These were all skills that Oury cherished, especially in the first years of La Borde.

The days at La Borde were punctuated by various meetings: meetings of the Club, meetings within the subcommittees, training meetings for the staff, and daily meetings that the entire clinic—including the patients—was invited to attend. Since daily life was meant to be self-managed, any member of the community could propose a project, an activity, an event that would be discussed with the entire group. The meetings thus had a specific and practical organizational purpose but also a larger theoretical goal. As one participant described this, at La Borde, "meetings proliferated": "Knots, intersections, crossroads, they stir the entire population of the clinic. Sites of speech, they accelerate the exchange of ideas, of information. They allow new questions to emerge. By their very dynamism, they contribute to questioning of each role and modifying habits."[18] The function of the meetings was not simply to "mold" existing subjectivities but to produce new ones.[19] Self-management did not mean "everything goes"—a kind of *laisser-faire* in the words of Oury—but it opened up the possibility of generating different laws and a new symbolic.

As at Saint-Alban, the Club of La Borde was in charge of organizing all sorts of activities for the patients, activities that would be written down on a large blackboard and advertised through the clinic's various journals and newsletters: *La Borde Éclair*, *Cluboscope*, *Nouvelles labordiennes*. In one issue from July 2, 1967, for example, *La Borde Éclair* listed several possible sporting events (ping-pong, tennis, swimming, volleyball, punching-ball), as well as a film series that included movies by Luis Buñuel, Alfred Hitchcock, Agnès Varda, Andrzej Wajda, Michelangelo Antonioni, and Jean-Luc Godard.[20] Other ergotherapy workshops or *ateliers* involved art making, bookbinding, gardening, sculpture, printing, and theater. Each day, around forty activities were proposed to the hundred or so patients, supervised by seventy staff personnel (*moniteurs*) and interns.[21] In Nicolas Philibert's 1996 documentary on La Borde, *La moindre des choses*, we can observe a group of patients rehearsing for a production of the play *Opérette* written by Witold Gombrowicz, the Polish experimental playwright whose work is often praised for its deep psychological analysis.[22] The choice of movies and plays suggests once again that for the practitioners of institutional psychotherapy, form and content were intimately linked: what was being said, read, or seen was as important as the act of saying, reading, or seeing. In line with this principle, the patients had access to the clinic's rich library, which included, aside from literature and poetry, many works of psychoanalysis, histories of psychiatry, philosophy, and anthropology, from classics to the most recent publications.

Jean Oury's Clinic of Psychosis

As we saw in previous chapters, Jacques Lacan's work—especially his thesis on psychosis—was foundational to the development of institutional psychotherapy.[23] The second generation of institutional psychotherapy was equally indebted to Lacan, perhaps even more than the first, since Lacan's ideas had become better known after the 1950s and since La Borde's proximity to Paris facilitated access to his seminars.[24] Many of the La Borde psychiatrists and psychoanalysts were in analysis with Lacan.[25] This was the case of Oury and Guattari, who both took the train to Paris every Wednesday to see him in his private practice and, later that day, to attend his seminar. Like the doctors of Saint-Alban, the psychiatrists of La Borde did not hesitate to prescribe medications and neuroleptics, which, they maintained, could significantly alleviate psychotic symptoms. And like Fanon, Oury praised the controlled use of electroshocks as tools to trigger psychic reconstruction. In his words, electroshocks could be useful as long as psychiatry did not become a "veterinary medicine" but remained a "human science."[26] For Oury, all medical treatment needed to involve the kind of social or group activities practiced at La Borde, as well as one-on-one analytic sessions. As he put it, psychiatry and psychoanalysis needed to be "constantly integrated into one another."[27] Psychoanalysis was, for him, the "alphabet" of psychiatry.[28]

One of the main tenets of institutional psychotherapy was that alienation constituted one of the fundamental dimensions of human existence, whether one was considered "normal" or "crazy." Yet, in his theoretical writings, Oury was careful to think through the specificity of psychosis, the ways in which the mental and social alienation characteristic of psychosis was radically different from that of neurosis. In this struggle to understand the etiology, the manifestation, and the treatment of psychosis, Lacan's work was, for Oury, absolutely key. As Oury lamented throughout his life, institutional psychotherapy was often mistaken for antipsychiatry, in its British, Italian, or American versions, and as represented by the work of Franco Basaglia, David Cooper, R. D. Laing, or Thomas Szasz. Oury and Guattari both stressed the crucial differences between antipsychiatry and institutional psychotherapy as they maintained that mental alienation—or madness—could never be reduced to a reaction against social, political, or familial oppression. Oury's insistence on the singularity of psychosis also led him to criticize authors such as Robert Castel, Michel Foucault, and at times even Guattari, all of whom he accused of sharing antipsychiatry's fascination with madness as a form of social and political resistance. Psychosis, Oury argued, was never simply a cultural construction, just as it was never the pure product of biology or brain chemistry. Rather, psychosis needed to be understood as a *psychic* issue, one that involved neurological, familial, and social factors. According to Oury, nobody had understood this better than Jacques Lacan.

Oury drew on many of Lacan's concepts, but most important, he relied on his notions of the Real, the Imaginary, and the Symbolic, which had helped Lacan understand psychosis as a *structure* different from two other structures: neurosis and perversion. Lacan began to study this triangulation of Real, Imaginary, and Symbolic early on in his work, perhaps even as early as 1936 when he first presented his theory of the "mirror stage" at an International Psychoanalytic Association (IPA) congress. The mirror stage described the reaction of a baby from six to eighteen months, who, despite his lack of physical coordination, recognized himself in a mirror. The child, who was carried by his parent, experienced his body as fragmented. Yet the image he perceived was whole, integrated, and contained. This contrast produced a feeling of jubilation but also of conflict and aggression, which the child attempted to overcome by identifying with the image. For Lacan, the mirror stage described the structure of neurosis: the unconscious, self-defined by the free play of the drives, identified with an ideal I, the ego, or the social self. Identity formation thus proceeded from this constitutive ambiguity, which led to a sense of alienation: even in neurosis, identifications were based on self-recognitions that were always already misrecognitions. The mirror stage, as Lacan would later argue, also marked the subject's entry into language. There was an imaginary dimension to this double process of language acquisition and identity formation, resulting from the sense of mastery, autonomy, and wholeness.[29]

Lacan reworked his concepts of the Imaginary, the Symbolic, and the Real in his 1953 IPA paper "The Function and Field of Speech and Language in Psychoanalysis," also known as the Rome Discourse. In this paper, Lacan turned to Claude Lévi-Strauss's *Elementary Structures of Kinship*. According to Lacan, Lévi-Strauss had posited a structural equivalence between the subjective, the familial, the social, and the linguistic, all of which were mediated by the prohibition of incest, the "Law" with a capital *L* as Lacan designated it.[30] Lacan's notion of castration operated similarly to the incest prohibition: no object could ever fully satisfy desire, not even the mother or the child, but other "small objects" (*objets petit a* as opposed to the big A *Autre*/Other) could come into being. Although these *objets a* generated desire, they remained unobtainable. The structural lack of the object—the impossibility of having the full thing, *das Ding*—was once again analogous to the structural inability to ever have a full, transparent, immediate language. Just as Lévi-Strauss suggested that man could never return to a state of nature—which was by definition always already foreclosed—Lacan indicated that humans (unlike animals) could never lead a purely instinctual existence.

Throughout the 1960s and 1970s, Lacan began to represent the Imaginary, the Symbolic, and the Real as a "Borromean knot" to illustrate the mutual implication of these terms, all defined in relation to castration and to language. The Imaginary, illustrated by the mirror stage, described the identification of the ego and the specular image, the reflection of one's own body. The Imaginary was the realm of synthesis, plenitude, and duality, but also of alienation and illusion. The Symbolic was always already implicated in the Imaginary, as the image of the parent holding the child implied. If the Imaginary was the realm of the signified, the Symbolic was the realm of the signifier, of the "Other," and of radical alterity. The law that regulated desire in the Oedipus complex and that mandated the prohibition of incest was also located in the Symbolic. In this context, Lacan developed the notion of the *nom-du-père* (name-of-the-father), based on the homophony *nom* as "name" and *non* as "no." Here, Lacan sought to expand Freud's understanding of the role of the biological father in the Oedipus complex as the one who breaks the dual identificatory relation between mother and child, in order to designate broader structures of authority: other people but also institutions such as the school, the army, and the law. Finally, the Real designated what escaped from both the Imaginary and the Symbolic, the undifferentiated, the traumatic, the impossible, that which could not be expressed in language but always returned—in the form of a symptom, a slip of the tongue and parapraxis more generally, a dream, or in acting out for example.

Oury relied extensively on Lacan's typology, but he adapted it and perfected it in light of his extensive clinical experience with psychotics.

Like Lacan, Oury considered psychosis a structure that resulted from the foreclosure of the signifier, a "hole" or "lesion" in the Symbolic order and the absence of the name-of-the-father. Just as the psychotic was unable to function in the social, he was unable to "signify" linguistically, to be understood. As Oury put it, "the foreclosure of the name-of-the-father is what invalidates any possibility of gathering"—the gathering of the drives that occurs in neurosis at the level of the mirror stage—"in other words, it is what makes desire impracticable." Furthermore, Oury continued, "the name-of-the-father is what allows syntax. In the schizophrenic existence, we can say that the syntax is broken."[31] In neurosis, a signifier was attached to a particular signified. Most neurotics realized that this attachment was arbitrary and ultimately unsatisfactory, but the link remained. In psychosis, however, signifiers appeared to be free-floating, not attached. As Oury explained it, once again referring to Lacan, instead of *parole*, psychotics had *lalangue*, "a deposit of signifiers in a state of purity, that is to say, nonarticulated."[32] In this sense, Oury claimed that the schizophrenic "poses, quietly, the impossible question of the referent" by highlighting this intrinsic discrepancy between signifier and signified—a discrepancy that Ferdinand de Saussure had already pointed to when he came up with these concepts in the early twentieth century.[33]

In the words of Tosquelles, schizophrenia represented a "collapse of transcendence"—a collapse, in other words, of the Law.[34] According to Oury, neurotics came to a confrontation with the Symbolic through the process of castration, which led to the encounter with the Other, the name-of-the-father who said "No" and imposed the Law. Castration, as Oury put it, was the "access road to the Symbolic."[35] Unlike neurotics, however, psychotics lived in the domain of the Real, with a shattered Symbolic.[36] As Oury expressed it in another formulation, in schizophrenia, one of the rings in the Borromean knot was broken: "at this moment, the entire chain breaks and there is no longer an *objet a*. . . . There are only bits of bodies, bits of existence, memories, that replace the *objet a* so that it all holds more or less together."[37] On the one hand, psychosis for Oury emerged as a problem of desire, as an impossible or "unrealizable" (*impraticable*) desire.[38] On the other hand, the psychotic body was experienced as "dissociated" or "scattered." The mirror, which in Lacan's schema "gathered" or "tamed" the uncontrolled drives, no longer served this purpose in psychosis—instead, it constituted a "point of horror."[39] The mirror stage thus represented the "first alienation" in psychosis according to Oury, but a different alienation from that of neurosis: "alienation in the mirror" (and in the body) and "in language."[40]

Aside from Lacan, Oury drew his theoretical understanding of dissociation from two other psychiatrists who remained crucial references throughout his life: Eugen Bleuler, the Swiss contemporary of Freud, and Gisela Pankow, a German-born French psychoanalyst and psychiatrist. From Pankow, Oury retained the notion that schizophrenia manifested itself as a difficulty or trouble at the level of the body, at the level of "incarnation."[41] Indeed, for Pankow—who had also followed Lacan's seminars at Sainte-Anne closely—the Law constituted the ontological foundation of the human being, the condition of his structuration, his encounter with the Other and with the social.[42] From Bleuler, Oury borrowed the idea of a "dissociated transference" in psychosis, a process close to what Tosquelles called "multi-referential transference." While in neurosis transference functioned on an intersubjective level (in which the analyst was the Other), transference in psychosis was necessarily collective. As Oury reminded us, the absence of transference with the analyst was one of the main reasons that led Freud to assert that psychoanalysis could not be an effective treatment for psychotic patients.[43] Freud, Oury suggested, had simply not understood that transference could in fact be collective.

The great invention of institutional psychotherapy was the possibility of implementing and working with this dissociated transference. The "trick" of institutional psychotherapy, as Oury wrote, was to have taken into account, through the controlled implementation of multiple relations, "that which is characteristic of the schizophrenic existence": "the dispersal, the dissociation of transference, the attachment of things and words, so that the organization of a group, the establishment of a system of partial responsibilities (bar, theater, library, entertainment) manage to become 'representative' at an unconscious level."[44] In another formulation, Oury explained that through institutional psychotherapy, "the mirror of the world" came to substitute for the "primary narcissistic mirror."[45] Thus the Club, but also the collectivity more generally, could orient and resituate these multiples transferences and foster new forms of desire that could ultimately give patients the impetus to live.

Anti-Oedipus as Institutional Psychotherapy

While Oury's theorization of psychosis borrowed heavily from Lacan's, Guattari differed from Oury and Lacan on several key issues, perhaps most significantly on their starting point: their understanding of subjectivity, which was tied to their definitions of desire. Whereas desire for Oury and Lacan was always lacking (because subjectivity was premised on castration), Guattari considered desire as fullness and plenitude, as fundamentally productive (as opposed to negative). This vision of desire guided Guattari's most significant philosophical contribution, the two-volume work that he co-wrote with Gilles Deleuze, *Capitalism and Schizophrenia*. The first volume, *Anti-Oedipus*, published in 1972, can thus be read in two ways. On the one hand, it came as the culmination of Guattari's two decades of work at La Borde. It can thus be interpreted as a philosophical translation of institutional psychotherapy, or more precisely, of "institutional analysis," the term that Guattari used to describe the application of institutional psychotherapy to politics and social thought more broadly. On the other hand, *Anti-Oedipus* was also a strong engagement with—and ultimately a strong rejection of—Lacanian psychoanalysis, and thus, a complex debate with both Lacan and Oury.

Guattari's ambivalence toward Lacan is one of the reasons why *Anti-Oedipus* remains such a difficult book: the critique of Lacanianism—especially of what Guattari referred to as "Lacanian orthodoxy"—was articulated through some of Lacan's most important concepts, including structure, signifier, phallus, castration, desire, and others. Thus, while Deleuze and Guattari repeatedly praised Freud for his definition of desire as libido, they criticized him for constricting this libido through the prism of the family, for "alienating" this desire through the Oedipus complex, and for privileging neurosis at the expense of psychosis.[46] Similarly, Deleuze and Guattari recognized Lacan's crucial intervention in his "return" to Freud against the dominance of behaviorism and ego psychology. Lacan had indeed reclaimed the unconscious as the basis of subjectivity and as the primary medium for the psychoanalytic practice, and he had linked both psychoanalysis and the unconscious to language in his 1953 "Rome Discourse."[47] At the same time, much of *Anti-Oedipus* revolved around the refutation of Lacan's structuralism, which solidified the inscription of "Lack"—lack of desire, lack of object, lack of full and transparent language—at the heart of subjectivity.[48]

Even though Guattari remained at La Borde until his death in 1992, he began to distance himself from Oury and from what he referred to as the "Lacano-Labordian complex" around May '68 for both theoretical and political reasons. Around this time, Oury also made various disparaging comments about Guattari's naïve interpretation of desire and his obsession with the power of the erotic. In the words of Oury, for Guattari and his friends, "desire just seemed to be there, you just needed to kneel down to pick it up." Clinically, especially with psychosis, this was simply absurd.[49] Furthermore, Oury blamed *Anti-Oedipus* for spreading the idea of a "schizo-fashion"—the belief that there could be a certain glory and happiness to the schizophrenic condition.[50] Even though Guattari remained skeptical of antipsychiatry throughout his life, Oury

88   CHAPTER THREE

suggested that several of the arguments in *Anti-Oedipus* appeared dangerously close to those of antipsychiatry, arguments that were especially appealing to the more libertarian currents that flourished after May '68.

But Guattari and Oury's disagreements were not only theoretical; they were also political. Throughout his life, Guattari drifted from one group to another, some close to Trotskyism, others to Maoism, others to thirdworldism. All were anti-Stalinist and anti-authoritarian: Voie communiste from 1955 to 1965, Opposition de gauche in 1966, Mouvement du 22 mars during May '68.[51] Neither Oury, nor Lacan, nor Tosquelles for that matter, shared Guattari's enthusiasm for the "molecular revolutions" that had been sparked by May '68. In the words of Tosquelles, "nothing had happened in May '68."[52] Or as Lacan warned his students at the University of Vincennes—many of whom were Maoist devotees who had been decisive players in the wave of strikes and protests—revolutionary aspirations always resulted in the imposition of the "discourse of the master."[53]

Yet May '68 was central to the conception and the production of *Anti-Oedipus*. Deleuze and Guattari met in 1969, a few months after the events.[54] Deleuze, a philosophy professor who had written monographs on Hume, Nietzsche, Kant, Bergson, Proust, Sacher-Masoch, and Spinoza, had just accepted a position at the newly opened campus of the University of Paris VIII, also known as "Vincennes." Vincennes was created in direct response to the student uprising of 1968. Among other issues, the students had demanded a greater degree of curricular flexibility, and they had pressed for more involvement in the administration of the university. Vincennes was thus conceived as an experimental center to test out these pedagogical innovations. Students could be accepted without the French high school degree (the *baccalauréat*), and they were encouraged to take classes in various disciplines. Teaching at Vincennes tended to be organized in smaller seminars, in contrast with most other French universities, which still privileged large lectures. Workers and older students were allowed to enroll in classes.

These reforms, however, were not simply logistical: on a theoretical level, Vincennes offered the possibility of reconceiving the student-teacher relationship along more horizontal lines.[55] Aside from Deleuze, Vincennes included among the members of its faculty François Châtelet, Michel Foucault, Jean-François Lyotard, Alain Badiou, Georges Lapassade, René Schérer, Robert Castel, and many others who, if they were not directly involved in leftist politics, were at least invested in the project of rethinking structures of power and domination in their scholarship. We can thus point to several parallels between Vincennes and La Borde. Both projects were animated by the conviction that theory and

Félix Guattari, La Borde, and the Search for Anti-oedipal Politics   89

praxis were intimately tied, and both sought to foster a more democratic, self-managed, nonauthoritarian community, whether it be within
the walls of the asylum or the university. In this sense, *Anti-Oedipus* was,
as the sociologist Robert Castel has put it, very much the child of "La
Borde and Vincennes."[56]

As Deleuze and Guattari repeated in various interviews, their collaboration on *Anti-Oedipus* was born out of a set of specific circum-
stances around the "questions left unanswered" by the "aborted revolution in May '68." Their starting point, they claimed, was to consider
"how during these crucial periods, something along the order of desire was manifested throughout the society as a whole, and then was
repressed, liquidated, as much by the government and police as by the
parties and so-called workers unions and, to a certain extent, the leftist
organizations as well."[57] May '68 was indeed, in their eyes, an "aborted
revolution" to the extent that the workers had chosen to negotiate with
the government. Rather than taking the revolution to its most radical
consequences as many of the student groups demanded—even if these
demands were not articulated particularly clearly—worker unions and
representatives had chosen to settle for better salaries and better working conditions, culminating in the Grenelle Agreements of May 27, 1968.
Whatever shape it would take, a "total revolution" was, according to
most of the extreme left, clearly "in the interest" of the working classes
in social and economic terms. Yet workers systematically voted against
their interests and sabotaged their potential emancipation.

To be sure, Deleuze and Guattari were not the only intellectuals who,
during the 1960s and 1970s, worried about this question of what Etienne
La Boétie many centuries before had referred to as "voluntary servitude." To a large extent, Louis Althusser's essay on "ideological state
apparatuses" (ISAs), Michel Foucault's concept of *assujettissement* (sub-
jection but also subject-formation), and Pierre Bourdieu's notion of *ha-
bitus* wrestled with similar questions concerning the modalities of alienation in the very production of subjectivity. Why did people continue
to desire their oppression, or, in Spinoza's formulation cited several
times throughout *Anti-Oedipus*: "why do men fight *for* their servitude
as stubbornly as though it were their salvation?"[58] For these various
thinkers, this process could not simply be understood socially or politically as coming from the "outside" or from "above," from a ruling class
who controlled everything. Rather, alienation needed to be addressed
at the level of the unconscious. Ideology and subjectivation were *constitutive* of the subject—hence, the enormous difficulty of figuring out
how to say "no" to ideology or how to step outside of these structures of
power.

For Deleuze and Guattari, the name of this insidious process that stifled, trapped, and repressed man's innate desire was "oedipalization." At the subjective level, "oedipalization" privatized desire and channeled it toward the safe objects of the heterosexual reproductive family. On the social and political levels, it conditioned people to crave authoritarianism, conformity, and what they called "Fascisms." Both of these arguments were premised on the authors' definition of desire as the essence of man and on the idea that human subjectivity was coextensive with nature. Deleuze and Guattari borrowed this anthropology from Spinoza, an author that Deleuze had studied extensively in two previous books, *Spinoza et le problème de l'expression* in 1968 and *Spinoza: Philosophie pratique* in 1970.[59]

Spinoza's framework guided the opening pages of *Anti-Oedipus* in which Deleuze and Guattari establish an identity between production and consumption on the one hand and between man and nature on the other. Men are described as "desiring machines," constantly producing and consuming flows that connect them to one another.[60] Desire, for these authors, was thus eminently social: "We maintain that the social field is immediately invested by desire, that it is the historically determined product of desire, and that libido has no need of any mediation or sublimation, any psychic operation, any transformation, in order to invade and invest the productive forces and the relations of production. There is only desire and the social and nothing else."[61] From this passage alone, it is easy to notice the sharp contrast between this notion of desire and Lacan's elaboration of desire as structural lack. As Deleuze and Guattari further explained: "Desire does not lack anything: it does not lack its object. It is, rather, the *subject* that is missing in desire, or desire that lacks a fixed subject; there is no fixed subject unless there is repression."[62] In the second part of the book, Deleuze and Guattari turned their attention to the two discourses that they held responsible for convincing men to repress, mediate, or sublimate their innate desire: familialism and psychoanalysis, both of which, according to these authors, have buttressed each other, historically and theoretically.

As Deleuze and Guattari clarified, psychoanalysis was not responsible for the Oedipus complex. Society was. In their words: "the subjects of psychoanalysis arrive already oedipalized, they demand it, they want more."[63] But the authors accused psychoanalysis of being complicit with this form of familialism, of formulating its most elaborate justification, of lending it "the new resources and methods of its genius."[64] More precisely, Deleuze and Guattari blamed psychoanalysis for propagating three "errors" concerning desire: "lack, law, and signifier."[65] Constructing desire as lack "crushes all desiring-production"; welding it to law represses its strength (*puissance*); tying it to the signifier limits its "productive breaks-flows that never allow themselves to be signified within the unary stroke of castration."[66]

While these mechanisms of repression were already central in Freud's work, Deleuze and Guattari argued that they came to be consecrated with Lacan's turn to structuralism. Indeed, with Lacan, lack, law, and the signifier—all of which acquired capital initials—were no longer phenomenological but rather *structural* features constitutive of the subject that were neither historically nor geographically determined. This was especially true in the case of the Oedipus complex, which Lacan constructed as a structural invariant.[67] Directly referencing Lacan's notion of the name-of-the-father, Deleuze and Guattari thus wrote: "we are invited to go beyond a simplistic conception of Oedipus based on parental images, in order to define symbolic functions within a structure" in which "the traditional daddy-mommy are replaced by a mother-function, a father-function." This move, however, only consolidated "the universality of Oedipus beyond the variability of images; the fusing of desire even more strongly to law and prohibitions; and the pushing of the process of oedipalization of the unconscious to its limits."[68] According to Deleuze and Guattari, structuralizing these concepts produced a kind of psychoanalysis that was intrinsically transcendental, abstract, and metaphysical. In psychoanalysis, they explained, "the question of the father is like that of God: born of an abstraction, it assumes the link to be already broken between man and nature, man and the world, so that man must be produced as man by something exterior to nature and to man."[69] In other words, "psychoanalysis has its metaphysics—its name is Oedipus."[70]

For Deleuze and Guattari, the "analytic imperialism of the Oedipus Complex" had a series of consequences for the treatment (or nontreatment) of psychosis.[71] By defining psychosis as a resistance to the Oedipus complex (in the case of Freud), or as the foreclosure of the signifier and the absence of the name-of-the-father (in the case of Lacan), psychoanalysis "cloaks insanity in the mantle of a 'parental complex.'" In this way, Deleuze and Guattari argued, citing Michel Foucault's *History of Madness*, psychoanalysis has simply completed and perfected the task begun by nineteenth-century psychiatry "with Pinel and Tuke": the consolidation of bourgeois moralism.[72] As Deleuze and Guattari suggested, Freud's fundamental misunderstanding of psychosis was especially blatant in his interpretation of Daniel Paul Schreber's 1903 *Memoirs of My Nervous Illness*. Instead of exploring the richness of Schreber's deliriums (being sodomized by the rays of heaven, for example), Freud reduced Schreber's symptoms to a question of paternal deficiency, to a dysfunction of the Oedipus complex: "from the enormous political, social, and historical content of Schreber's delirium, not one word is retained."[73] Furthermore, Deleuze and Guattari pointed out, Freud failed to mention that Schreber's father invented and fabricated "astonishing little machines, sadistico-paranoiac machines . . . for restrictive use on children, for making them straighten up and behave." Why did these machines play no role whatsoever in Freud's analysis? What would have changed if Freud had treated Schreber's father not as "a head of family in an expressive familial transmission" but rather as "the agent of a machine, in a machinic information or communication?"[74]

For Deleuze and Guattari, Lacan was equally unable to grasp psychosis because of his "structural Oedipus" that "lead[s] us back to the question of the father" and that defined psychosis as a disfunction around the Symbolic. However, Deleuze and Guattari clarified, the important difference was not between the Symbolic and the Imaginary, but between the Real (the "real machinic element which constitutes desiring-production") and the "structural whole of the Imaginary and the Symbolic."[75] Nothing, in other words, was lacking in the Real, the privileged space of psychosis. Even antipsychiatry, which presented itself as a conscious critique of psychoanalysis, remained, according to Deleuze and Guattari, caught in the same trap: it was too complicit with this psychoanalytic familialism. Indeed, antipsychiatry too often sought to reduce psychosis to a reaction against "familial oppression." Furthermore, it modeled its therapeutic communities on a familial organization.[76] Thus, Deleuze and Guattari proposed to do away with the definitions that psychoanalysis had given us of neurosis and psychosis, both anchored in the Oedipus complex (neurotics being well oedipalized while psychotics refusing oedipalization). Instead, they urged us to focus our attention on the flux of desire and on the different modes of "territorializing" and "deterritorializing" this same desire.[77]

If the Oedipus complex had a series of consequences at the level of the individual, it also affected collective organization at its core. Deleuze and Guattari referred to Oedipus as "a means of integration into the group." It functioned by drawing upon the "nationalistic, religious, and racist sentiments" that flourished among "subjugated groups" (*groupes assujettis*).[78] Oedipus was, in this sense, different from ideology:

> There is an unconscious libidinal investment of the social field that coexists, but does not necessarily coincide with the preconscious investments, or with what the preconscious investments "ought to be." That is why, when subjects, individuals, or groups act manifestly counter to their class interests — when they rally to the interests and

ideals of a class that their own objective situation should lead them to combat—it is not enough to say: they were fooled, the masses have been fooled. It is not an ideological problem, a problem of failing to recognize, or of being subject to, an illusion. It is a problem of desire, *and desire is part of the infrastructure.*[79]

This idea that unconscious investments driven by desire could remain radically separate from the interests of the subject who desired could, for Deleuze and Guattari, explain the massive appeal of fascism: "It was not by means of a metaphor . . . that Hitler was able to sexually arouse the fascists," just as "a banking or stock-market transaction, a claim, a coupon, a credit, is able to arouse people who are not necessarily bankers."[80] These are flows, breaks in flows and fluctuations in flows, and in this sense, "an unconscious investment of a fascist or reactionary type can exist alongside a conscious revolutionary investment."[81] Desire thus *produced* reality, and fantasy was always a "group fantasy."[82] Libidinal and political economy, in other words, were one.

In these sections of *Anti-Oedipus*, Deleuze and Guattari drew heavily from the work of the psychoanalyst Wilhelm Reich, who had also spent much of his career trying to understand, as the title of his 1933 book indicated, "the mass psychology of fascism."[83] For Deleuze and Guattari, Reich was the first to understand that "psychic repression depended on social repression," the "first to raise the problem of the relationship between desire and the social field," and also "the first to reject the explanations of a summary Marxism too quick to say that the masses were fooled, mystified."[84] In their eyes, Reich demonstrated that "the masses were not innocent dupes; at a certain point, under certain conditions, they wanted fascism and it is this perversion of the masses that needs to be accounted for."[85] But Deleuze and Guattari departed from Reich when they argued that libidinal economy was not merely a prolongation of political economy but rather that the two were coextensive.[86] While Reich still clung to the ideal of a rational social production that he distinguished from the irrational element of desire, *Anti-Oedipus* identified the two: desire was the social field.

It is important to point out that the "Fascism" that Deleuze and Guattari alluded to so frequently in *Anti-Oedipus* was not simply the historical fascism in its German or Italian incarnations. As we saw in chapter 1, the first generation of institutional psychotherapy was also haunted by the specter of fascism, Spanish fascism in the case of Tosquelles, but also Vichy and Nazism—totalitarianism more broadly. By the time *Anti-Oedipus* appeared in 1972, however, the context had radically changed. As Deleuze and Guattari saw it, in the 1970s, the immediate threat was not only the return of authoritarian right-wing politics for which "Fascism" was a shorthand, but more important, what Foucault described as the "fascism in our heads," "the fascism that causes us to love power, to desire the very thing that dominates us and exploits us."[87] As Guattari would later put it, "We must abandon, once and for all, the quick and easy formula: 'Fascism will not make it again.' Fascism has already 'made it,' and it continues to 'make it.' . . . Fascism seems to come from the outside, but it finds its energy right at the heart of everyone's desire."[88] It was this "fascism in our heads," the fascism at the heart of desire, that Deleuze and Guattari held responsible for the failure of May '68, and more generally, for the impasse in which Western Marxism — especially French Marxism — found itself during the Cold War.[89]

Foucault understood this with impressive precision in his preface to the English translation of *Anti-Oedipus*, in which he praised Deleuze and Guattari for having written an "introduction to the non-fascist life," a "book of ethics, the first book of ethics to be written in France in quite a long time." How, Foucault asked, "does one keep from being fascist, even (especially) when one believes oneself to be a revolutionary militant? How do we rid our speech and our acts, our hearts and our pleasures, of fascism? How do we ferret out the fascism that is ingrained in our behavior?"[90] As we will see in the next chapter, Foucault was himself invested in a similar project in his own work as he sought to understand how power shaped and produced subjects and how this same power could be redirected toward less oppressive goals. For Foucault (unlike Guattari), the point was not liberation or emancipation — absolute freedom from power or from "fascisms" — but rather the manipulation or interception of these power flows. As he put it, "being anti-oedipal has become a life style, a way of thinking and living." Being anti-oedipal was, as institutional psychotherapy had shown, essentially a practice of everyday life. *Anti-Oedipus* was to serve as its philosophical complement. The revolution, which could only be immanent and materialist, could "proceed only by way of a critique of Oedipus."[91]

For Deleuze and Guattari, this "critique of Oedipus" began at the level of form, in the very writing and production of their text. As the authors explained in various interviews, *Anti-Oedipus* was based on their extensive correspondence and subsequent meetings. However, the performative nature of their writing and their commitment to "anti-oedipality" and "deterritorialization" are yet another reason for the difficulty of *Anti-Oedipus*. On the one hand, the book tried to enact the idea of "the unconscious as a machine, a factory; and a new conception of the delirium as indexed on the historical, political, and social world."[92] In this sense, the text's affective dimension was as important as its conceptual element.[93] On the other hand, *Anti-Oedipus* aspired to be a truly collective enterprise, not in the sense of adding two separate and distinct perspectives but in the sense of becoming one de-egoized voice, a true "assemblage" that would avoid all forms of closure. As Deleuze later explained: "what was important was the set of bifurcating, divergent, overlapping lines that formed this book as a multiplicity passing between the points, carrying them along without ever going from one to the other. . . . The lines respond to each other like the subterranean tendrils of a rhizome as opposed to the unity of the tree and its binary logic. It was truly a subjectless book with no beginning or end, and no middle."[94] Concepts would thus acquire an autonomous existence even when they were not necessarily understood by each author in the same way. In this sense, *Anti-Oedipus* was not a *dialogue* between two disparate entities. It was not, also, an example of communication: "never a homogenization, but a proliferation, an accumulation of bifurcations, a rhizome."[95] This ambition to create a book in which one no longer knew or needed to know who was speaking could again be compared to the "explosion" of roles that was so important to institutional psychotherapy. Ultimately, both sought to form a collectivity as an assemblage of differences.[96]

The systematic critique of "Oedipus" at the level of style was intimately connected to the book's philosophical and political ambition. Indeed, much of *Anti-Oedipus* was devoted to the assessment of the status quo, the political, the philosophical, the social, and the psychoanalytic status quo. However, Deleuze and Guattari also laid out, especially in the last section of the book, a goal, an alternative, which they called "schizoanalysis." Schizoanalysis, they immediately warned us, "has strictly no political program to propose."[97] In that sense, it was closer to the kind of ethics that Foucault described in his preface: suggestions, "lines of flights," indications for how to free desire and resist oedipalization. In the words of Deleuze and Guattari, schizoanalysis should remain "defamiliarizing, de-oedipalizing, decastrating, undoing theater, dream and fantasy; decoding, deterritorializing."[98] Or, in another formulation: "The task of schizoanalysis is that of tirelessly taking apart egos and their presuppositions; liberating the prepersonal singularities they enclose and repress; mobilizing the flows they would be capable of transmitting, receiving, or intercepting; establishing always further and more sharply the schizzes and breaks well below conditions of identity; and assembling desiring-machines that countersect everyone and group everyone with others."[99]

Once again, schizoanalysis made sense only given the particular definition of desire that Deleuze and Guattari posited at the beginning of their work. "The schizoanalytic argument is simple," they wrote: "desire is a machine, a synthesis of machines, a machinic arrangement—desiring machines."[100] If desire in its fullness and its productivity was the starting point of *Anti-Oedipus* and if this desire had been repressed by familialism—and helped, in this process, by psychoanalysis—then the purpose of schizoanalysis was not to resolve Oedipus but rather to "de-oedipalize the unconscious in order to reach the real problems": "Schizoanalysis proposes to reach those regions of the orphan unconscious—indeed, 'beyond all law'—where the problems of Oedipus can no longer be raised."[101] Deleuze and Guattari's argument here was not that a "de-oedipalized" desire would threaten society because it would reveal that people secretly all wished to sleep with their mothers. Rather, desire threatened society because it was, in its very nature, revolutionary: "And that does not at all mean that desire is something other than sexuality, but that sexuality and love do not live in the bedroom of Oedipus, they dream instead of wide-open spaces, and cause strange flows to circulate that do not let themselves by stocked within an established order. Desire does not 'want' revolution, it is revolutionary in its own right, as though involuntarily, by wanting what it wants."[102]

From a political perspective, this ability of desire to form different assemblages, unpredictable rhizomes, threatened the unity of class, race, gender, and identity more generally. As Deleuze and Guattari wrote, "The revolutionary unconscious investment is such that desire . . . cuts across the interest of the dominated, exploited classes, and causes flows to move that are capable of breaking apart both the segregations and their Oedipal applications. . . . No, I am not of your kind, I am the outsider and the deterritorialized."[103] Unlike Freudian and Lacanian psychoanalysis that Deleuze and Guattari characterized as "metaphysical," schizoanalysis would be strictly materialist. The point was not only to become "minoritarian" but to consciously remain so.[104]

Schizoanalysis was in its very nature political or "militant" as it sought to "demonstrate the existence of an unconscious libidinal investment of sociohistorical production, distinct from the conscious investments coexisting with it."[105] More precisely, schizoanalysis was able to "analyze the specific nature of the libidinal investments in the economic and political spheres, and thereby to show how, in the subject who desires, desire can be made to desire its own repression."[106] In this sense, schizoanalysis had both a diagnostic and a revolutionary potential: diagnostic in that it traced the conscious or unconscious repressions of desire; revolutionary in the sense that it freed this desire to disorganize social hierarchies, norms, identities, and authoritarianisms of all sorts. Schizoanalysis, in other words, helped to prevent "subject-groups" (*groupes-sujets*) from becoming "subjugated groups" (*groupes-assujettis*). As the Cold War, the repeated disappointments of the French Communist Party, and the "aborted revolution of May '68" had made clear, "subject-groups" always had the potential to turn into "subjugated groups" who desired their own repression.[107] "A revolutionary group" according to Deleuze and Guattari, remained a subjugated group even after it had seized power, "as long as this power itself refers to a form of force [*puissance*] that continues to enslave and crush desiring-production." By contrast, a subject-group was "a group whose libidinal investments are themselves revolutionary; it causes desire to penetrate into the social field, and subordinates the socius or the form of power to desiring-production."[108]

As Deleuze and Guattari explained in an interview in which they returned to the question of fascism: "like many others, we announce the development of a generalized fascism. . . . There is no reason why fascism would not develop." In this sense, "either the revolutionary machine"—or, we could say, schizoanalysis—will be able to take charge of desire . . . or else desire will remain manipulated by the forces of oppression and repression, and will threaten, even from within, the revolutionary machineries."[109] In opposition to fascism, schizoanalysis thus offered "lines of flight" because these "lines lead to desire, to the machines of desire, and to the organization of the social field of desire."[110] Like the Oedipus complex, schizoanalysis as a concept originated in the fields of psychiatry and psychoanalysis. But like the Oedipus complex, schizoanalysis did not simply operate on this limited terrain: in the work of Deleuze and Guattari, both had a much broader philosophical, social, and political significance. It was this political potential of schizoanalysis, a politics of desire modeled on institutional psychotherapy, that Guattari examined and tried to enact under the name of "institutional analysis."

Institutional Analysis and Anti-oedipal Politics

Long before he began writing *Anti-Oedipus*, Guattari had been thinking about how to apply the principles of institutional psychotherapy to the world of politics. In this sense, Guattari's philosophy was fundamentally shaped by his activism at La Borde and in various political groups that he created and participated in throughout the 1960s. As he put it, his idea was never to "generalize the experience of La Borde to the rest of society, since no such model was transportable. However, it seemed to me that subjectivity . . . was never self-evident, that it was produced under certain conditions, and that these conditions could be modified . . .

in order to orient them in a more creative direction."[111] La Borde had convinced Guattari that institutions could play a key role in producing these "more creative directions," as long as they were "disalienated" and "disalienating." For example, he asked, what would large urban centers, schools, hospitals, or prisons look like "if instead of conceiving them along a mode of empty repetition, we tried to reorient their goal towards a permanent internal re-creation?"[112] This was precisely the goal of "institutional analysis." Institutional analysis depended on the mobilization of a "totally different kind of unconscious," which Guattari called the "schizoanalytic unconscious": "It is not the unconscious of specialists, but a region everyone can have access to . . . it is open to social and economic interactions and directly engaged with major historical currents." Inspired by psychosis rather than neurosis "on which psychoanalysis was built," the schizoanalytic unconscious was "'machinic' because it was not necessarily centered around human subjectivity. Rather, it involved the most diverse material fluxes and social systems."[113] Like institutional psychotherapy, and like *Anti-Oedipus*, institutional analysis sought to create subject-groups (*groupes-sujets*). Guattari defined subject-groups as collectives structured around their own law, "agents of enunciation, pillars of desire [*supports de désir*]." He opposed these collective formations to "subjected-groups" (*groupes-assujettis*), who were paralyzed by hierarchies, mechanisms of exclusion, and oedipalization.[114]

Guattari claimed that he first put forth the possibility of an "institutional analysis" of the social and political fields as early as 1961, during a meeting of the GTPSI, the Groupe de travail de psychothérapie et sociothérapie institutionnelle (also known as "GT-Psy").[115] Formed in 1960, the GTPSI included the main practitioners of institutional psychotherapy: Tosquelles (who had originally lobbied for the creation of a "French Psychiatric Party" or PPF: Parti psychiatrique français), Jean Oury, Roger Gentis, Horace Torrubia, Jean Ayme, Yves Racine, Jean Colmin, Maurice Paillot, and Hélène Chaigneau. They were eventually joined by Guattari (who was the first nonpsychiatrist to be invited), Ginette Michaud, Claude Porcin, Henri Vermorel, Michel Baudry, Robert Million, Philippe Rappard, Jean-Claude Polack, Nicole Guillet, Gisela Pankow, and Jacques Schotte. The group met two to three times a year, over the course of a weekend, from 1960 to 1966. It provided a space to share papers, discuss new work (the recently published texts of Lévi-Strauss and Jakobson for example), and think about the theory and practice of institutional psychotherapy. The group's fourteen meetings included panels called "Fantasy and Institution," "Transference and Institution," "Superego and Institution," "The Position of the

Psychiatrist," "On Hierarchy," and "Money in the Psychiatric Hospital." As Tosquelles declared, "despite the heterogeneity of our working condition, it is the 'Institution' that determines the space of our action."[116]

According to Olivier Apprill, who has written a history of the GTPSI, what distinguished this group from other professional associations was its explicit investment in taking into account each member's "personal equation." This required each participant to "question their implication and their desire" and examine in depth what they meant when they assumed the "position of the psychiatrist."[117] The point was not simply to encourage each individual participant to adopt a self-critical attitude but also to enable the analysis of the group *as a whole*, of the collective as such, to use Oury's term. This process thus required a particular process of self-reflexivity, a "methodology that needed to constantly be tested."[118] As Oury summarized it, the basic principle of this "methodology" consisted in *ne pas laisser en passer une*—which we could translate as "not to miss an occasion" or "not to pass up an opportunity." This meant examining what fantasies, desires, and dynamics were at play at any given moment in group dynamics. Another way to put this would be to say that the goal of the GTPSI was to create autonomous "subject-groups" in Guattari's understanding of the term.[119]

When Guattari first brought up the idea of institutional analysis during one of the early GTPSI meetings in 1961, he received lukewarm support (*peu d'écho*) from the rest of the group, who could conceive only of a "timid extension of [institutional] analysis to the fields of psychiatry, and maybe, of pedagogy." For Guattari, however, unless institutional psychotherapy could reach the broader social and political worlds, it would soon face an "impasse." More specifically, Guattari argued, institutional analysis could play an important role in discerning the "phenomena of bureaucratization of militant organization," one of the main reasons why, in his mind, leftist politics felt so stranded during the 1960s.[120] It was in response to these questions raised at the GTPSI meetings that Guattari invented his concept of "transversality," which he first presented during a colloquium on psychodramas in September 1964. As its name indicates, the goal of transversality was to extend and to socialize the intersubjective notion of "transference," which, according to Guattari, had become "stuck . . . obligatory, predetermined, 'territorialized' on a specific role or stereotype" by mainstream psychoanalysis. Even worse, transference was the form of interiorization of bourgeois repression, the evidence that the Oedipus complex, familialism, and normative social integration were one.[121] In this sense, transversality could be compared to Tosquelles's notion of "burst transference" (*transfert éclaté*) or to Oury's "transferential constellation"—both slightly different terms used in institutional psychotherapy to describe the nature of transference in psychosis.

Guattari's notion of transversality, however, was somewhat more specific. Because Guattari found the concept of institutional transference "too vague," transversality was designed to establish a bridge between institutional psychotherapy and institutional analysis. Indeed, as Guattari presented it, transversality was opposed to "verticality" (of pyramidal structures, for example) but also to "horizontality" (the random juxtaposition of people with no relation to one another).[122] All groups, Guattari posited, had a particular "coefficient of transversality" in the sense that they were more or less blind to the power dynamics that governed them, more or less aware of the dangers of verticality and horizontality. This "coefficient of transversality" could, however, be altered at various levels of the institution. Transversality could thus help us overcome the "impasses of pure verticality and that of mere horizontality" in order to facilitate the emergence of subject-groups who could "enunciate" their own law.[123] "Transversality," as Guattari put it, was "the unconscious source of action in the group, going beyond the objective laws on which it is based, carrying the group's desire."[124]

Thus, changing the "coefficient of transversality" of an institution could, as Guattari saw it, produce "a different kind of dialogue: delusions and all other unconscious expressions which had, until then, kept the patient in a state of solitary confinement could now become a type of collective expression."[125] Furthermore, individual actors could move from an imaginary position to a symbolic one. Instead of having everyone "play their role," transversality implied, like the grid at La Borde, the contestation and redefinition of each role: "Such a reshuffling of ego ideals also changes the introjections of the superego, and makes it possible to set in motion a type of castration complex related to social demands different from those patients previously experienced in their familial, professional and other relationships. Accepting to be 'put on trial,' to be laid bare by the words of others, a certain type of reciprocal challenges, and humor, the elimination of hierarchical prerogatives, etc, all this will help to establish a new law for the group."[126] Institutional analysis, Guattari concluded, consisted in the "reorganization" (*remaniement*) of transversality. In this sense, the "bureaucratic self-mutilation of a subject-group" could indeed be prevented through the careful study of transversality.[127]

In the years that followed the GTPSI, Guattari tried to implement this idea of transversality through various political and intellectual vectors. In 1965, for instance, he redacted "nine theses" for a new party that he had just founded with some of his friends from La Borde, the Opposition de gauche. Guattari first presented his theses at the Eighth Congress of the Union des Étudiants Communistes (UEC) in Montreuil, in April 1965. By the 1960s, the UEC, the most important student union, originally created by the French Communist Party (PCF) after the war, had grown progressively impatient with the political and intellectual rigidity of the PCF. The increasingly radicalized students deplored the PCF's subservience to Moscow, its unrepentant Stalinism, its ambivalence toward and often condemnation of the anticolonial revolutions spreading throughout the Third World, and its moralism, especially on sexual issues. At the Montreuil Congress, these tensions finally exploded, and various more radical groups (Maoists, Trotskyists, "Italians" . . .)—including the Opposition de gauche—split from the main party line.[128] Guattari's text thus served as a manifesto for a new politics, one committed to the analysis of global capitalism but explicitly anticolonialist, thirdworldist, critical of centralism, and sexually progressive. Most important, Guattari's vision of leftist politics was premised on the simultaneous fight against social and psychic alienation—the "two legs of institutional psychotherapy," as Tosquelles had described them. As Guattari put it: "it is not enough for the working class to have a party and revolutionary unions. It needs to be structured along an organizational framework adapted to its level: committees, soviets, etc. through which it can express its deepest desires. This will also give avant-garde organizations the means to reorganize the true combativeness of different sectors, their level of awareness, their understanding of advanced watchwords, etc."[129] Revolutionary politics, in other words, needed to turn the masses into subject-groups capable of setting their own political agenda and enouncing their own law.[130]

To accompany and support these political projects, Guattari also established around the same time, in 1965, the FGERI (Fédération des groupes d'études et de recherches institutionnelles), a "federation" of groups that included psychiatrists, anthropologists, psychoanalysts, educators, urbanists, architects, economists, writers, filmmakers, and others, inspired by institutional analysis and committed to the principle of transversality. More broadly, the goal of the FGERI was to spread institutional analysis to the nonmedical and nonacademic world. The following year, as a complement to the FGERI, Guattari founded the CERFI (Centre d'étude, de recherche et de formation institutionnelles), an independent and self-managed research body (fig. 3.5).[131] One of the missions of the CERFI was to fundraise for the FGERI by procuring research contracts with private and public enterprises.[132] In order to advertise and to promote its research, the FGERI and the CERFI published a journal, Recherches, which ran from 1966 until 1983.[133]

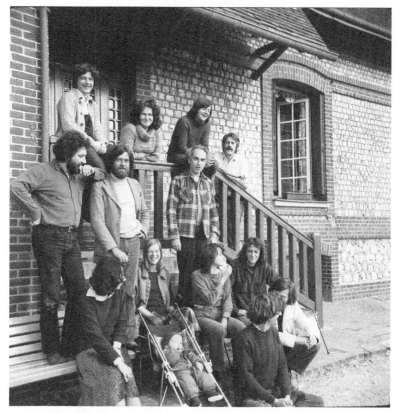

3.5 A CERFI meeting in the 1970s
© Public Domain, CC BY-SA 3.0

We can think of the FGERI, the CERFI, and *Recherches* as a triangle structured around La Borde and institutional psychotherapy, both from a theoretical and from a logistical standpoint. Jean Oury, for instance, relied on the structure of the CERFI to fund and organize many of the activities at La Borde.[134] Similarly, several issues of *Recherches* focused on questions of psychiatry and psychoanalysis.[135] From an institutional perspective, the members of the CERFI also went back and forth between Paris and La Borde. François Fourquet and Anne Querrien, for instance, recall how they were seduced by Guattari's intellectual and political aura when they were still students at Sciences Po. The first step when you joined the CERFI, they recounted, was to "read everything," especially Freud and Lacan, and then to head to La Borde to work as interns. As Fourquet put it, it was the summer of 1965 and "as other leftist students went to China or to Cuba, we headed to La Borde which in many ways was much further than China from the point of view of the unconscious." For Fourquet and the other students, La Borde represented a "house where the ego had exploded," and what remained of this explosion was much superior, much more interesting, politically and socially, than their "egoized selves."[136]

Aside from Fourquet and Querrien, the CERFI nucleus (the "mafia" as Guattari referred to it) included other students disillusioned by the more traditionally Marxist student unions and attracted to the possibilities offered by the unconscious: economists such as Liane Mozère and Hervé Maury, historians such as Lion Murard, philosophers like Michel Rostain, psychologists like Gérard Grass. The Tuesday CERFI meetings, however, attracted a much wider crowd including some of the most important names in French intellectual life during the 1960s and 1970s, who also often contributed articles to *Recherches*. These included many psychiatrists and psychoanalysts associated with Saint-Alban and La Borde, but also Gilles Deleuze, Guy Hocquenghem, Luce Irigaray, Jean Starobinski, René Schérer, Georges Perec, Antonio Negri, Jean Genet, Michel Foucault, and many others. The CERFI thus greatly contributed to the diffusion of institutional psychotherapy to a broader audience just as it placed the unconscious at the center of radical social, political, and intellectual discussions.

As the first editorial of *Recherches* stated, the goal of the FGERI was to invent mechanisms that would prevent the "ineffable-force-of-circumstances" (*l'ineffable-force-des-choses*) and the "inevitable-alienation-of-the-project" (*l'aliénation-inévitable-du-projet*) that haunted all collective ventures.[137] The editorial thus called for a return to theory but only as a "radical project of questioning": "Repetition is death. To use Marx or Freud following the mode of repetition is to give in to a kind of fatal sacralization."[138] To prevent the appearance of "concentrationisms"—the driving concern behind *Recherches*, the FGERI, and the CERFI—Guattari's article in this first issue, titled "Somewhat Philosophical Reflections on Institutional Psychotherapy," put forth many of his central concepts concerning institutional objects, group subjectivity, and group transference. As Guattari framed it, the key question for all collective enterprises was the following: "How can a group speak, in a given institution, at a given point in its history, without reinforcing the serial and alienating mechanisms that generally characterize collectivities in industrial societies?"[139] To tackle this problem, the FGERI designated a series of "working groups," all of which were listed at the end of each journal. Some focused on the "feminine condition" including access to abortion and contraception, others on health policies, urbanism and architecture, ethnology, pedagogy, literature and theater, among other topics.

Recherches was different from other scientific journals or specialized publications. As its second volume stated, the journal did not have an "editorial board to put forth a program or to select articles. There was no theory and no concepts to defend." Rather, *Recherches* was the product of a group committed to the analysis of institutions in which "everyone agreed to be constantly interpellated by other groups anchored in other sectors."[140] The "rules of the game" were that "everybody speak their own language without concessions, without shame, without all the social compromises that create the illusion of understanding when in fact they pull back people into their own system, their own 'truth.'"[141] In this sense, the editorial meetings for *Recherches* were similar to the weekly meetings of the CERFI: both were structured according to the guidelines of schizoanalysis. The gatherings—like the grid at La Borde—provided a forum to review the group's ongoing projects but also to examine each member's subjective implication in the work and the collective, a forum to express his or her desire and libido.

The most famous number of *Recherches* was perhaps a special issue edited by Guy Hocquenghem in March 1973, titled "Three Million Perverts: The Big Encyclopedia of Homosexualities." The government brought up Guattari, officially the publishing director, on charges of obscenity (*outrage aux bonnes moeurs*) and ordered him to destroy all existing copies of the journal. This, of course, only contributed to the publication's notoriety. At the time, Hocquenghem was a twenty-six-year-old writer, philosopher, and graduate of the École Normale Supérieure who had been involved in various Maoist groups throughout the 1960s, especially during May '68. Most important, Hocquenghem was one of the founders of the FHAR, the Front homosexuel d'action révolutionnaire, France's first gay liberation movement, which had sprung out of the women's group MLF (Mouvement de libération des femmes) in 1971. Hocquenghem soon stood out as the more or less official spokesperson for the FHAR, especially after his long interview with the *Nouvel observateur* in January 1972, titled "The Homosexual Revolution." Later that year, Hocquenghem published his best-known work, *Le désir homosexuel*. Deeply influenced by the theoretical framework of *Anti-Oedipus*, Hocquenghem offered his readers an unrelenting attack on psychoanalysis and familialism, a celebration of desire and of the "free plugging of organs," and, perhaps most important, he called for a revolution that would begin at the level of the sexual.[142] One way to interpret Hocquenghem's *Homosexual Desire* and his activism within the FHAR is thus as an example of what Guattari had tried to push for over many years: an explicitly "anti-oedipal" analysis of the social and political fields in which theory and praxis went hand in hand.

Félix Guattari, La Borde, and the Search for Anti-oedipal Politics 105

The CERFI was especially successful after 1970, when it came to the attention of Michel Conan, an urban planner hired by the Ministry of Infrastructure (Ministère de l'équipement) to head its research department. Appointed by Prime Minister Jacques Chaban-Delmas, who was eager to gain a better grasp of the social factors that had led to the May '68 explosion, Conan disposed of a generous budget (four to five million francs per year) to study a wide range of questions. These included city planning, architecture, health management, housing, local psychiatric care, schools, cultural development, and the "new cities" of Ivry, Marne-la-Vallée, Évry, and Melun-Sénart. Conan met with Guattari, who convinced him that the CERFI was the perfect consortium to conduct these studies, to carry out the research and produce written documents that the government could use. The CERFI thus signed a series of contracts with the Ministry of Infrastructure that allowed the group to take on long-term assignments and to pay their researchers actual salaries. By 1973, the CERFI included seventy-five salaried researchers whose base earnings were 1,500 francs per month.[143] It was in this context, for instance, that Michel Foucault conducted a CERFI research project on the "genealogy of collective infrastructure" (*généalogie des équipements collectifs*), parts of which were published in the *Recherches* issue of December 1973 edited by François Fourquet and Lion Murard.[144] As we will see in the next chapter, Foucault, along with several of his students—many of whom went on to become important intellectuals in their own right—was involved in several collaborative projects that fell under the umbrella of the CERFI.[145] The CERFI public funding slowly dwindled after the presidential election of Valéry Giscard d'Estaing in 1974 that brought a new wave of fiscal conservatism and marked the end of the state's desire to oversee social reform.

For Guattari, the FGERI, the CERFI, and *Recherches* constituted essential terrains to think through and test how the insights of institutional psychotherapy would apply to broader social, political, and intellectual domains. Guattari's various collective enterprises can also give us a good insight into the meaning of some of the most obscure—and most often misunderstood—concepts of *Anti-Oedipus*. Schizoanalysis, for instance, could not possibly mean that we should all strive to become psychotics and reject all norms if we consider how the term was applied or enacted in the context of these groups. Instead, I have argued that the schizoanalysis that Deleuze and Guattari advocated in *Anti-Oedipus* was closely connected to the "institutional analysis" that Guattari promoted through his political activism and his various collective endeavors. Both notions were solidly anchored in the praxis of institutional psychotherapy—the ethics, we could say—that Guattari had observed and exercised at La Borde and at Saint-Alban. From this perspective, *Anti-Oedipus* did not constitute a break with institutional psychotherapy in favor of antipsychiatry, as some critics have suggested. To be sure, Guattari pushed against and contested several of the key ideas upon which institutional psychotherapy was built, notably some of the central presuppositions of Freudian and Lacanian psychoanalysis, but his engagement with institutional psychotherapy was thorough and constant. Perhaps a better way to frame this would be to suggest that Guattari "deterritorialized" institutional psychotherapy to other fields (philosophy, politics, sexuality, but also urban planning, architecture, public health) and to other contexts (the Cold War), just as Fanon "deterritorialized" it by bringing it to North Africa. Guattari and Fanon did not depart from institutional psychotherapy but took its injunction to question everything all the time, quite literally.

CHAPTER 4

Michel Foucault, Psychiatry, Antipsychiatry, and Power

The question of psychiatry haunted Michel Foucault's work throughout his life. From his student days at the École Normale Supérieure where he first discovered psychiatry, psychology, and psychoanalysis, madness fascinated Foucault. In these early years, Foucault read extensively the psychiatric, psychological, and psychoanalytic texts of his time, in their Freudian, Lacanian, phenomenological, and existentialist versions. As an intern at Sainte-Anne, Paris's most important psychiatric hospital, and in the medical division of the Fresnes prison, he dabbled in experimental and clinical psychology and contemplated a career in either psychology or psychiatry. To that end, right after receiving his bachelor's degree in philosophy in 1948, he pursued a degree in psychology. His first teaching position in 1952 was as a professor of psychology at the University of Lille. Finally, all of Foucault's work until the mid-1960s revolved around the problem of the psyche, his preface and translation of Ludwig Binswanger's *Dream and Existence*, his first published book, *Maladie mentale et personnalité*, his article on the history of psychology from 1850 to 1950, his translation of the German neuropsychiatrist Viktor von Weizsäcker's *Der Gestaltkreis*, and, of course, his 1961 doctoral thesis *Folie et déraison*, which would eventually become *History of Madness*, followed by *The Birth of the Clinic: An Archaeology of Medical Perception* in 1963.

Throughout these years, Foucault was clearly aware of the psychiatric reform movements that had developed in France after the Second World War, including institutional psychotherapy, Saint-Alban, and later La Borde. It was, in fact, through Georges Daumézon, one of the most important theorists and promoters of institutional psychotherapy and one of the key figures in the Saint-Alban experiment, that Foucault first got interested in psychology and psychopathology. Daumézon hap-

108   CHAPTER FOUR

pened to be friends with Georges Gusdorf, the head tutor (*caïman*) at the École Normale, and he invited Foucault to attend patient presentations at Sainte-Anne while he was still a student.[1] In *Maladie mentale et personnalité* published in 1954, Foucault cited the 1952 issue of the journal *Esprit* on "The Misery of Psychiatry" to which Daumézon, Lucien Bonnafé, and François Tosquelles all contributed, calling it a "remarkable" achievement and praising these doctors' commitment to reforming medical assistance and psychiatric care.[2] And in 1964, several historians including Fernand Braudel and Jacques Le Goff associated with the *Annales* invited Bonnafé, Daumézon, and a few other psychiatrists to participate in a roundtable on the *History of Madness*.[3]

Toward the end of the 1960s, however, something changed, both at the level of Foucault's reception within the psychiatric community and at the level of Foucault's own relation to the psychiatric field. In December 1969, during the annual meeting of the journal *L'Évolution psychiatrique*, which, as we saw in chapter 1, positioned itself as a leader in the psychiatric avant-garde, Daumézon, Henri Ey, and others took apart Foucault for his "ideological conception" in *History of Madness*. After praising Foucault's early work, including his translations of Binswanger and Weizsäcker that had made him "almost one of ours [*un des nôtres*]," and regretting his absence at the colloquium, Ey proceeded to attack Foucault's thesis, which he described as "psychiatricidal." More specifically, Ey decried Foucault's explicit decision to consider mental illness the "marvelous manifestation of a divine Madness, or more exceptionally, as the very spark of poetic genius." As Ey reminded his public, mental illness was "'something other' than a cultural phenomenon."[4] Similarly, Jean Oury regularly criticized Foucault, despite their mutual friendship with Gilles Deleuze and Félix Guattari. As Oury put it, Foucault did "not understand anything about the structures of mental illness [*les structures aliénatoires*]."[5] As he explained in an interview when *History of Madness* was first published in 1961, Oury was the first to encourage the members of the newly formed GTPSI group to read the book as a collective. Much of it was very helpful and enlightening, he claimed, but what Oury found unbearable was the "use that was made" of the book: "In June 1968 . . . La Borde was invaded by a bunch of zealots who swore only by Foucault. . . . It was a basic and stupid antipsychiatry" that ended up serving as a justification for suppressing hospital beds in psychiatric hospitals.[6] As Oury and many psychiatrists deplored, after 1968, *History of Madness* became a central reference—a sort of Bible—for the antipsychiatric movements that flourished in France but also in Great Britain, Italy, and the United States during these years.

Foucault himself was not oblivious to this "second"—less academic and more explicitly political—reading of *History of Madness*, but his relation to antipsychiatry, as we will see, was complex.[7] As he put it in a 1974 interview in which he was asked whether *History of Madness* was political: "Yes, but only now. That is to say, when *History of Madness* was published in France, in 1961–1962, there was not a single journal or a single group with political interests that talked about it. You see. Nothing in Marxist publications, nothing in leftist journals, nothing." "What happened?" Foucault continued: "The political border shifted, and now, topics such as psychiatry, the confinement and medicalization of a population have become political problems."[8] Hence, while Foucault considered for many years writing a sequel to *History of Madness*, one that would extend his study into the present, by 1972 he deemed this project "of no interest." Instead, "a concrete political action in favor of prisoners made more sense" to him, a politics directly linked to collective struggles.[9]

Thus, throughout the 1970s, Foucault returned time and again to the question of psychiatry but with a different approach: in his 1973–74 lectures at the Collège de France, *Psychiatric Power*, followed by *Abnormal* in 1974–75, and in the first volume of *The History of Sexuality*. During this decade, he also followed institutional psychotherapy closely but in its second-generation version, primarily through Deleuze and Guattari. As we saw in the previous chapter, Foucault, along with some of his students, participated in some of the CERFI's collective research projects, on the "genealogy of collective infrastructure" (*généalogie des équipements collectifs*), on planification, urban policy, health, and education. Parts of these studies were published in the *Recherches* issue of December 1973 titled *Les équipements du pouvoir* to which François Fourquet, the manager of La Borde at the time, also contributed. Other parts appeared in a 1976 volume, *Généalogie des équipements de normalisation*, which included a text signed by Foucault, "The Hospital Institution in the Eighteenth Century." Others were included in the 1979 collective volume *Les machines à guérir (aux origines de l'hôpital moderne)*.[10] In other words, throughout the 1970s, Foucault collaborated with various figures directly involved with La Borde, figures who were also very much invested in Guattari's goal of implementing schizoanalysis at the political level and of fostering the development of "subject-groups" (*groupes-sujets* as opposed to *groupes-assujettis*). The GIP (Groupe d'information sur les prisons), which occupied a central role in Foucault's life and thought from 1971 to 1972, emerged out of similar political and theoretical concerns. And, in fact, Deleuze and Guattari attended several of the GIP meetings.

Foucault's vocabulary and theoretical framework were clearly not

Guattari's. Furthermore, it is quite certain that the later Foucault—the author of the *History of Sexuality* for instance—would have objected to Guattari's ideas on the plenitude of desire, the foundational role of the unconscious, or the possibility of liberation or disalienation through institutions, reformed as they may be. Yet Foucault was drawn to institutional psychotherapy as a prism to think through these new forms of "the political." This was especially evident in his preface to the English translation of *Anti-Oedipus*. Foucault celebrated *Anti-Oedipus* as a new type of scholarship, a different kind of theoretical work, which, given the growing disillusion with Marxism after May '68, could lead to a different form of political action, what Foucault called an "art" or an "ethics": "I think that *Anti-Oedipus* can best be read as an 'art' . . . Questions that are less concerned with *why* this or that than *how* to proceed. How does one introduce desire into thought, into discourse, into action? How can and must desire deploy its forces within the political domain and grow more intense in the process of overturning the established order? *Ars erotica, ars theoretica, ars politica.*"[11] Deleuze also regularly commented on his intellectual proximity to Foucault. As he put it, at the time of *Anti-Oedipus*, he and Guattari perceived Foucault as an "ally": "our method is not the same, but we seem to meet him on all sorts of points that seem basic, on paths that he has already mapped out."[12]

The goal of this chapter is to trace Foucault's shifting notions of the psychiatric, from the 1950s to the 1970s. Foucault, unlike the other figures in this book, was never directly involved in the practice of institutional psychotherapy, and he remained much more skeptical of the emancipatory potential of psychiatry throughout his life. Yet we can read him as a sort of "fellow traveler" to institutional psychotherapy, a fellow traveler who accompanied and followed its development but who ultimately chose a different road. More specifically, I want to suggest that Foucault's attention to psychiatric questions, to the asylum, but also to institutional psychotherapy and antipsychiatry ("institutional critique,"[13] as he preferred to call it) largely contributed to his critique of norms in the 1960s and shaped his new theory of power in the 1970s. Psychiatry, in other words, provided a template for Foucault to rethink the political along these theoretical but also activist lines and to study the mechanisms of what he would later call "disciplinary society" and "disciplinary power."

Before the *History of Madness*: The Early Years

Foucault arrived at the École Normale Supérieure in 1946, at the age of twenty. Over the next decade, he read widely in the psychological field but also practiced psychiatry at various institutions: hospitals, clinics, and prisons. It was these intellectual and practical encounters, especially in the context of the asylum, that led Foucault to articulate the critique of institutions, norms, and normalization that he first developed in *Maladie mentale et personnalité* and later in *History of Madness*, critiques that were, in some ways, close to those formulated by the first practitioners of institutional psychotherapy. Foucault's professor at the École, Georges Gusdorf, had been a student of Gaston Bachelard and Léon Brunschvicg, and he was passionate about psychology, a burgeoning and exciting discipline in postwar France that sought to demarcate itself from both psychiatry and philosophy. With Daumézon's guidance, Gusdorf organized various activities to introduce his students to questions of psychopathology: patient presentations at Sainte-Anne, internships at the psychiatric hospital of Fleury-les-Aubrais where Daumézon worked, but also a series of lectures at the École, by Daumézon himself and by some of the young and promising psychiatrists of his time, including Jacques Lacan, Julian de Ajuriaguerra, and Henri Ey.[14] Also at the École Normale, Foucault studied under Maurice Merleau-Ponty, whose seminars from 1947 to 1949 focused on the "unity of body and soul" in Malebranche, Maine de Biran, and Bergson, figures that remained important in Foucault's early work.[15] In 1949, after he was elected professor of Psychology at the Sorbonne, Merleau-Ponty turned to questions of language, phenomenology, and child psychology.[16] This theoretical corpus was central for Fanon, as we saw in chapter 2, but also for Foucault, who regularly attended these lectures as well as those of Daniel Lagache, who also tried to bring together clinical psychology, psychoanalysis, and phenomenology at the Sorbonne. It was Lagache who, in 1947, instituted psychology as a major in the university. This was the psychology bachelor's degree that Foucault obtained in 1949, alongside a diploma from the Institut de psychologie de Paris.[17]

Since Foucault did not write directly on Merleau-Ponty or Lagache, it is difficult to pinpoint what exactly drew him to phenomenology, psychology, and psychoanalysis during these years. However, from his notes at the École Normale, it seems that the question of psychic causality preoccupied him consistently. More precisely, these three fields appeared to offer Foucault a more complex framework to think through the self, to analyze the symptom, and to understand alienation—a framework that went beyond biological essentialism and neurological objectivism. Thus, Foucault read extensively in psychology and psychoanalysis, including Freud, Eugen Bleuler, Pierre Janet, Henri Bergson, Alfred Adler, Melanie Klein, Karen Horney, Karl Abraham, Sándor Ferenczi, and Lacan, in addition to many of the leading psychoanalytic journals of his time, such as the *Revue de psychanalyse* and the *Cahiers de psychopathologie*.[18] From these notes, we can observe Foucault's early interest in the structure of psychosis.

In the case of Henri Ey, for instance, Foucault pointed to the distinction between negative symptoms (dissociation, verbal incoherence) and positive symptoms (hallucinations, delirium, depersonalization) in autism. In the case of Lacan, he highlighted the question of psychic causality in madness and the "moment of deviation" (*moment de virage*) during the mirror stage. Similarly, we can also observe Foucault's close attention to certain figures—the criminal, the hysteric, the homosexual, the child—figures who accompanied him throughout his career. In relation to Freud's Dora, a case on which he commented expansively, Foucault asked whether the unconscious was "influenceable"—in other words, how did social and cultural factors affect psychic processes? In the context of Lagache's lectures, Foucault pointed to the problematic definition of "the normal," to the relationship between language and the unconscious, and to the uses of psychoanalysis for social life.[19] Presumably, these theoretical concerns also inspired Foucault to turn to Kurt Goldstein and to Henry Head, both of whom had tried to propose more holistic theories of mental processes.[20] We can also read Foucault's early interest in Marx and Marxism along those lines: it was primarily the psychological Marx that caught Foucault's eye, Ivan Pavlov and psychoanalysis in Russia but also Marx himself for his theory of alienation, the issue at the heart of institutional psychotherapy during the war.[21]

Foucault's interest in the psyche, however, was not simply theoretical. His notes also include several index cards on electroencephalograms (invented by the German psychiatrist Hans Berger in 1924) and the Rorschach test, which Lagache had introduced in France and which fascinated Foucault. Foucault was able to explore the limits of these theoretical hypotheses through the extensive clinical work that he undertook with Jacqueline and Georges Verdeaux, friends of his parents who regularly invited him to dinner while he was a student at the École Normale. Georges Verdeaux, who had written a thesis under the direction of Lacan, had set up with his wife an electroencephalogram laboratory at Sainte-Anne. They offered Foucault an internship in which he helped them measure cerebral waves, test skin resistance, and analyze respiration rhythms.[22] The laboratory was under the supervision of Jean Delay, one of the most important psychiatrists at the time, with whom Foucault kept up a long-lasting friendship. Delay directed the Institut de psychologie in Paris, presided over the first World Psychiatric Congress, held the chair of mental illness and brain sciences at the Sorbonne after 1946, and headed the department of psychiatry at Sainte-Anne from

Michel Foucault, Psychiatry, Antipsychiatry, and Power

1946 to 1970. He was one of the first doctors to experiment with neuroleptic drugs. Yet, despite his anchoring in pharmacology and clinical experimentation, he remained an advocate for the importance of the "human sciences" for the field of psychiatry.[23]

Through the Verdeaux couple, Foucault also worked at the prison of Fresnes, established in 1950 as France's main medical facility for inmates. Foucault performed a series of psychological tests on the prisoners to orient them within the criminal justice system. To be sure, this experience was formative for Foucault as it allowed him to enter a prison facility for the first time, but also as it brought to light with particular clarity the multiple links between criminology and psychiatry, links that Foucault would study in the years to come. This experience in clinical psychology encouraged Foucault to apply for a research grant from the Thiers Foundation, which he received in 1951. The following year, Foucault left the Foundation for a position as assistant professor of psychology at the University of Lille. As a professor and as the director of the Institut de psychologie de Lille, he continued to explore, in his teaching and in his own research, the themes that had occupied him as a student: anthropology, phenomenology, psychoanalysis, the unconscious, alienation, and *Erlebnis*, "the specific way in which reality is here for me."[24]

Finally, it was through Jacqueline Verdeaux, who had translated various German medical texts, that Foucault traveled to Switzerland to meet the psychiatrist Ludwig Binswanger. Foucault had first heard about Binswanger in Merleau-Ponty's lectures, and he found in Binswanger's notion of *Daseinanalyse* (a concept inspired by Martin Heidegger, whom Foucault was just beginning to read) a helpful bridge between psychology and philosophy. In addition, for Foucault, *Daseinanalyse* could also function as an alternative to Marxism and to Freudianism to think through the experience of alienation.[25] This was particularly clear in Foucault's 1954 long preface to Verdeaux's translation of Binswanger's *Dream and Existence*. As Foucault put it, Binswanger's anthropology was situated in "direct opposition to all forms of psychological positivism that try to reduce the significant content of man to the limited concept of *homo natura*," replacing it instead with "an ontological reflection that takes as its major theme the presence-to-being, existence, *Dasein*"—in other words, man in his milieu.[26] While psychiatry for Foucault tended to "consider illness as an objective process," and while "the Freudian method" remained insufficiently attentive to the notion of symbols, *Daseinanalyse* or "anthropology" as Foucault called it could provide a fuller and richer understanding of the self, of its psyche, but also of pathologies, which Binswanger perceived as different ways of inhabiting the world.

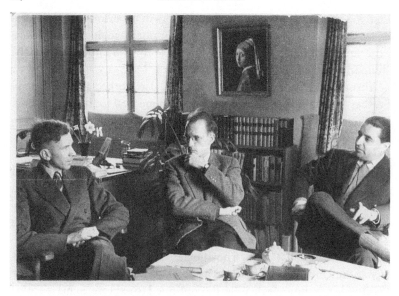

4.1 Michel Foucault (center) in Münsterlingen with Roland Kuhn (left) and Georges Verdeaux (right)
© Éditions de l'École des Hautes Études en Sciences Sociales (From *Foucault à Münsterlingen: À l'origine de l'Histoire de la folie*, ed. Jean-François Bert & Elisabetta Basso, 2015)

Once again, Foucault's intellectual work was accompanied by a "hands-on" application, as Foucault, along with Jacqueline Verdeaux, visited Binswanger and Roland Kuhn at the Münsterlingen asylum (fig. 4.1). Both Binswanger and Kuhn were known for trying to implement *Daseinanalyse* in their psychiatric practice. Furthermore, both had created a warm and familial environment free of all coercive treatments in their respective institutions, the Bellevue Sanatorium in Kreuzlingen for Binswanger and Münsterlingen for Kuhn.[27] Foucault met the two psychiatrists at Münsterlingen on March 2, 1954. His visit happened to coincide with Mardi Gras—*Fasnachtsumzug*—which the asylum celebrated with a long procession of a "carnival king" and a costume party at the end of the day. Foucault did not comment directly on this carnivalesque performance at Münsterlingen, but Jacqueline Verdeaux's photos give us a good sense of how the day proceeded.[28] Foucault, however, returned to the connection between madness and festivity in his later work, certainly in *History of Madness* but also in subsequent interviews. In 1963, for instance, he discussed a movie by the Italian filmmaker Mario Ruspoli, whose 1962 documentary *Regard sur la folie* filmed daily life—including the preparations for a party—at Saint-Alban during the years that Tosquelles worked there. As Foucault put it: "These days ... we try to reconstitute in psychiatric hospitals ways of life close, or as close as possible, to what you and I, what everybody calls 'normal.' And through a strange paradox, through a strange return, we organize for them, around them, with them, a parade, with dancing and masks, a whole carnival, that is, in the strict sense of the term, a new festival of the mad."[29] As this quote indicates, the encounter with the asylum—at Münsterlingen but also perhaps at Saint-Alban, where similar practices with explicit therapeutic goals were being played out—was essential in persuading Foucault that the notion of normality was ultimately arbitrary. As he commented in a 1982 interview, when he began working in the asylum, "he accepted these things [pharmacology, neurosurgery, institutionalization] as necessary, but ... after three months, I quit this job and went to Sweden, with a feeling of great unease; there, I began to write the history of these practices."[30] This would become *History of Madness*.

Before leaving for Sweden in October 1955, however, Foucault brought these various insights together in two pieces: an article on the history of psychology from 1850 to 1950 (published in 1957 but drafted by 1954) and his first book, published in 1954, *Maladie mentale et personnalité*. Both of these texts can be read in continuity with Foucault's early concerns around psychic causality, normativity, and institutions. Foucault wrote the essay on psychology for a history of European philosophy edited by Denis Huisman and Alfred Weber. As he put it, the history of psychology since the nineteenth century had been the history of the tension between a scientific method committed to "natural objectivity" and a philosophical discourse interested in man's constant contradictions that challenge the smoothness or regularity of a "positivist knowledge" template.[31] After surveying the different models of psychology (physico-chemical, organic, evolutionist, behaviorist, anthropological, and others), and emphasizing the seismic effect that Freudian psychoanalysis had on the discipline of psychology—"the greatest reversal of psychology ... through which causal analysis became the genesis of significations, evolution gave way to history, and the analysis of cultural context substituted for the recourse to nature"[32]—Foucault concluded that psychology was still unable to account for the contradictions of human existence. Perhaps, Foucault asked, the "future of psychology" should be to take seriously these contradictions, to keep examining man's conditions of existence and returning "to what was most human in man, that is, his history."[33] In other words, history and the historical construction of human experience constituted, for Foucault, a necessary tool for the understanding of the psyche and of the self.

Maladie mentale et personnalité was originally commissioned by Louis Althusser (who had, by then, replaced Gusdorf as *caïman* at the

École Normale Supérieure) for a collection at the Presses Universitaires de France (PUF) titled "Philosophical Initiation," directed by Jean Lacroix.[34] Lacroix, a contemporary of Georges Canguilhem at the École Normale Supérieure (as well as of Lagache and Merleau-Ponty), was a Catholic personalist philosopher who had been a founding member of the journal *Esprit* along with Emmanuel Mounier in the 1930s. *Esprit*, as we saw in previous chapters, had been at the forefront of the critique of psychiatry in the postwar years, from the December 1952 issue "The Misery of Psychiatry," which included many of the Saint-Alban doctors, to Fanon's essays "The North African Syndrome" and "The Lived Experience of the Black Man," both published in the journal around the same time. Lacroix, in fact, also played an important role in Fanon's philosophical trajectory in Lyon, and it was through Jean-Marie Domenach, also associated with *Esprit*, that Fanon found a publisher for *Black Skin, White Masks*. As Luca Paltrinieri has recently noted, many of Foucault's preparatory notes for *Maladie mentale et personnalité* cited the *Cahiers de psychopathologie*, another important journal in the genesis of institutional psychotherapy to which Daumézon, Bonnafé, and Henri Ey all contributed.[35] *Maladie mentale et personnalité*, in other words, was published in a particular context and in rather direct dialogue with the world of institutional psychotherapy.

We can thus read *Maladie mentale et personnalité* in three ways: first, as Foucault's attempt to bring together his various readings in psychology, psychoanalysis, and psychiatry from his student years, especially around the question of psychic causation; second, as a preview of *History of Madness*; third, and as I wish to argue here, as Foucault's own take on the issues that were at the heart of institutional psychotherapy—the link between psychic and social alienation, the relativity of norms especially in relation to definitions of illness and health, and the role of institutions in the constitution of the social and of the self. In Foucault's words, the main questions that structured his book were twofold: "Under what conditions can we speak of mental illness in the psychological domain?" and "What is the relationship between mental pathology and organic pathology?"[36] Alternatively, how is "mental illness" defined and what are its causes? From the beginning of the book, Foucault set up his argument against two other theses: Kurt Goldstein's holistic model, which, according to Foucault, was unable to discern the specificity of the psychic (if a reaction was "general," Foucault asked, then how do we know what caused it?); and the simple conflation of mental and organic pathologies.[37] As Foucault made clear, his interest lay in the particularity of psychic activity, in understanding what made it different from—but not completely autonomous from—other biological, social,

Michel Foucault, Psychiatry, Antipsychiatry, and Power

and cultural factors. Foucault developed his argument most forcefully in the conclusion and the last two chapters of *Maladie mentale et personnalité*, the sections that Foucault most significantly revised—or rather, rewrote—for the 1962 reprint of the book under its new title *Maladie mentale et psychologie*. These were also the chapters in which Foucault's engagement with institutional psychotherapy was most obvious. The fact that Foucault revised them so substantially after the publication of *History of Madness* in 1961 also raises questions about Foucault's own changing views on psychiatry and its possibilities but also on Marxism.

Chapter 5, "The Historical Sense of Alienation," began with an analysis quite close to the one that Foucault developed in *History of Madness* a few years after, one that traced the shifting meanings of madness from possession in antiquity and early Christianity, through the eighteenth century, to the birth of modern psychiatry with Philippe Pinel and Jean-Étienne Dominique Esquirol. As Foucault argued, it was the nineteenth century that invented the modern notion of alienation when it stripped away all rights from the mentally ill, when, in clear contradiction with its declarations of universal freedom and human rights for all, it excluded the mad from society and from the community of men. It is this "abstraction" that according to Foucault culminated in the process of confinement.[38] If psychic processes were never "autonomous" and thus had to be constantly related to social and historical factors, they could also not be *reduced* to external factors. Indeed, as Foucault explained in his sixth and final chapter, "The Psychology of Conflict," not all individuals who experienced contradictions with their environments—even when these conflicts were understood consciously at the psychological level—were mentally ill. Thus, Foucault defined madness as the confluence of two "contradictions": "social and historical conditions that ground psychological conflicts on the real contradictions of the milieu; and the psychological conditions that transform this conflictual content of an experience into a conflictual reaction."[39] This was Foucault's way of insisting on the complementarity of psychological and historical/sociological factors in the genesis of mental illness but also on their significant differences. It was in this context that Foucault turned to the work of the Russian physiologist Ivan Pavlov, as a "materialist" model in which social and psychic factors constantly interacted: a "unitary conception of the pathological" and a "materialist" psychiatry quite close, from Foucault's description, to what Tosquelles, Bonnafé, Daumézon and institutional psychotherapy more broadly called for.[40]

As Foucault put it, while alienation was certainly "real" (while it was not, in other words, a socially constructed or simply imagined condition), it needed to be understood primarily as an effect rather than a cause. Thus, Foucault referred to alienation as a "defense mechanism" for individuals who needed to "switch off" (*se mettre hors circuit*) when the conflict or contradiction with their social environment appeared too absolute or untenable. From this perspective, an individual was "alienated" not because he had become a "stranger to human nature, as the doctors and lawyers of the nineteenth century used to say," but rather because he could no longer "recognize himself in the conditions of existence that man himself had constituted." Given this definition, alienation was "no longer a psychological aberration" but was defined by a historical moment: "only this moment had made it possible."[41] Thus, instead of beginning with a preestablished definition of the "abnormal" as a "pure state" and defining illness as the pathological behavior of the abnormal and alienation as the alteration of personality resulting from this process, classical pathology needed to "reverse the order of things": begin with alienation as the original situation, to then understand illness, and finally arrive at the definition of the abnormal.[42] The sections appear particularly indebted to Georges Canguilhem, whose thesis, *The Normal and the Pathological*, dated from 1943, but also to several of the founding texts of institutional psychotherapy (Tosquelles and Bonnafé, for example), which all called for the reexamination of the distinction between normality and abnormality, as we saw in chapter 1.[43]

In opposition to these "abstractions," Foucault called for a "materialist" psychiatry—the same term that Deleuze and Guattari used in *Anti-Oedipus* as a synonym of schizoanalysis. For Foucault, psychiatry needed to avoid two fundamental errors: first, "conflating the morbid and psychological conflicts with the historical contradictions of a milieu and thus confusing social and mental alienation; second, wanting to reduce all illness to a disruption of the nervous system" in order to treat it from a purely physiological perspective.[44] Another way to put this would be to say that Foucault warned against an exclusively socially constructivist approach to mental illness but also against any biological and neurological essentialism. If, indeed, the source of illness was located "in a conflict within the human milieu and if illness constituted a generalized defense mechanism against this conflict, then therapeutic treatment needed to take on a new shape."[45] One possible version of this "new shape" for the discipline, Foucault acknowledged, was Freudian psychoanalysis. However, Foucault continued, psychoanalysis had remained caught in "abstractions": it created an "artificial milieu, intentionally cut off from normal and socially integrated forms of intersubjective relations"; it remained stuck on past traumas; and it avoided providing "real solutions," proposing instead to "liberate instincts" or to simply make patients "aware of their drives." Instead, Foucault sug-

Michel Foucault, Psychiatry, Antipsychiatry, and Power 119

gested, what psychiatry needed were "therapies that offered patients concrete means to overcome their situation of conflict, to modify their milieu, or to respond in a more adapted way to the contradictions of their conditions of existence." "There can be no possible cure," Foucault concluded, "when we undo the relationship between an individual and his milieu." In fact, "the only possible cure is one that can reconstruct new relationships between the patients and their milieu."[46] This, Foucault added in a footnote, was exactly what "certain doctors" were trying to do in their efforts to "reform medical assistance and psychiatric hospitals." As evidence, Foucault referenced that famous issue of *Esprit* on "The Misery of Psychiatry" from December 1952. As Foucault concluded in the last lines of his book, real psychology needed to "free itself from psychologism" if its goal was, like that of all human science, to "disalienate man."[47]

The *History of Madness* before and after 1968

From Foucault's interviews in later years, it seems that his departure to Sweden in October 1955 marked a break that was as much personal as it was intellectual. By the time he had finished drafting *History of Madness* in 1957, he appeared to have lost hope in the possibility that psychiatry and psychology would give up their objectivism, reform themselves, and provide any genuine "disalienation" for man. Foucault in fact removed most references to "disalienation" in the 1962 reprint of the book and radically changed the last two chapters and the conclusion, as if he had given up on alienation and disalienation as a theoretical framework. In the 1962 version of his text, Foucault was much more explicit about the historical role that psychology had played as a discourse and as a form of power-knowledge that produced and objectified madness. As he put it, it was ludicrous to expect psychology to reflect on its own conditions of existence: "psychology will never be able to tell the truth about madness because it is madness that holds the truth about psychology." "The psychology of madness," Foucault contended, "would no longer be the control of mental illness and thereby its possible disappearance, but the destruction of psychology itself," calling into question the relationship between reason and unreason.[48] By the early 1960s, Foucault was less interested in alienation as a phenomenological experience and more preoccupied with the historical construction of madness by an entire disciplinary apparatus that encompassed psychiatry, psychology, and psychoanalysis. According to his biographer, Didier Eribon, Foucault consistently refused to have the 1954 version of *Maladie mentale et personnalité* reprinted or translated into English, and he always referred to his "first book" as the *History of Madness*.[49] We can certainly point to intellectual reasons for why Foucault shifted in his understanding of the psyche-disciplines—notably, his reading of Nietzsche, which was foundational in his reassessment of discourse, genealogy, and especially power. But perhaps this disillusionment also had to do with the actual experience in psychiatric hospitals and prisons, institutions of confinement that, as he said, left him with "a feeling of great unease" and pushed him to write the "history of these practices." As he put it in a 1961 interview, after working in psychiatric clinics, including that of Jean Delay, he had become disappointed with the psychiatrists' "good conscience."[50]

Foucault continued to work in the psychiatric field in Sweden, in the medical collections of the library at the University of Uppsala but also alongside Arne Tiselius at the Svedberg laboratory. This was, however, his last venture into clinical experimentation. He devoted the last months of his Swedish stay to the composition of *History of Madness*, which he sent to Jean Hyppolite—who was by then director of the École Normale Supérieure—in December 1957. Foucault first thought of submitting his manuscript for a Swedish doctorate, but it failed to impress Stirn Lindroth, the local specialist in the history of science whom Foucault had contacted as a potential director. Hyppolite had been Foucault's philosophy teacher during his year of hypokhâgne at the Lycée Henri IV in 1945. He had also followed the publication of *Maladie mentale et personnalité* closely as many of its themes resonated with his own interests in psychiatry and alienation. As he put it in a conference in 1955, "I have become convinced that the study of madness—alienation in the profound sense of the term—is at the center of anthropology, the study of man. The asylum is a refuge for those whom we can no longer let live among other humans. It thus serves a means to indirectly understand our world and the problems that it constantly raises for normal men."[51] It was also Hyppolite who suggested that Foucault turn his manuscript into a French doctoral thesis. As a possible supervisor, Hyppolite recommended Canguilhem, who had just published an article on psychology, "What Is Psychology?," in which he attacked the discipline's inability to discern with precision its object of study.[52] Foucault, who had by then moved to Warsaw to head the Center for French Civilization at the university, thus sent Canguilhem the revised manuscript in December 1958. He defended his thesis at the Sorbonne in May 1961, before a committee presided over by Canguilhem that also included Lagache. The book was published as *Folie et déraison. Histoire de la folie à l'âge classique* that same year, by Plon, in the collection directed by the historian Philippe Ariès, "Civilisations et mentalités."

As several critics have pointed out, and as Foucault himself acknowledged, there were two readings of the *History of Madness*: before and after 1968. Before 1968, *History of Madness* was received primarily as a scholarly work that engaged questions of epistemology in the history of science, in the tradition of Léon Brunschvicg, Gaston Bachelard, and Canguilhem. After '68, it was essentially perceived as a manual for political activism, as a "toolbox" for anti-authoritarianism.[53] As Foucault put it in 1976:

> At the beginning, nobody was interested in my first book, except literary critics such as Barthes and Blanchot. But no psychiatrist, no sociologist, no leftist thinker. With *Birth of the Clinic*, it was even worse: a total silence. Madness and health were not yet noble political and theoretical problems at that time. What was noble was the rereading of Marx, psychoanalysis, semiology. I was very disappointed by this lack of interests, it is not a secret. . . . And then, in 1968, abruptly, the problems of health, of madness, of sexuality, of bodies, entered directly into the field of political concerns. The status of the mad all at once interested everybody. Suddenly, these books were overconsumed while they had been underconsumed during the previous period. After that time, I got back on track, with more serenity of spirit and with the certainty that I had not been mistaken.[54]

And indeed, *History of Madness* was essentially ignored by the psychiatric and medical fields when it was published in 1961. As Foucault suggests, literary critics—Roland Barthes, Maurice Blanchot, and most famously, Jacques Derrida—engaged with the work, as well as historians—Robert Mandrou, for example—but very few psychiatrists and psychoanalysts did.[55] This silence from the psychiatric world was especially difficult for Foucault, who, as we saw, had spent his student years and the 1950s immersed in this field, working in hospitals, reading extensively the medical literature, and wrestling with questions of theory and practice concerning madness.

Around the mid-1960s French psychiatrists finally began to pay attention to the *History of Madness*. But while Foucault's book shared many thematic and methodological continuities with his earlier work, the main thesis of *History of Madness* represented a much more radical blow against psychiatry as a discipline and as a profession. Foucault's original idea was to write a history of psychiatry, a project that had been commissioned by Colette Duhamel, a friend of Jacqueline Verdeaux who was an editor at the Éditions de la Table Ronde, a subdivision of Gallimard.[56] But as Foucault quickly realized and as he clarified in the 1961 preface to the book, *History of Madness* was a history not of psychiatry but of madness itself, of how the experience of madness shifted from the Middle Ages to the nineteenth century: "To write the history of madness will therefore mean conducting a structural study of the historical ensemble—notions, institutions, judicial and police measures, scientific concepts—which hold captive a madness whose wild state can never be reconstituted."[57] In other words, from this structural perspective, madness, whether it was considered from a religious, philosophical, or medical standpoint, could not exist without its opposite, non-madness, just as reason needed unreason. These terms, Foucault argued, were "confusedly implicated in each other, inseparable as they do not yet exist, and existing for each other, in relation to each other, in the exchange that separates them."[58] Methodologically, Foucault's enterprise of denaturalization (entering an "uncomfortable region," as he put it) meant abandoning all "concepts of psychopathology." That is, it meant treating madness as a social and historical notion rather than a medical, psychological, or biological self-evident reality.[59] To some extent, Foucault had foreshadowed much of this in his earlier work, especially in *Maladie mentale et personnalité*, but his phenomenological language of the 1950s still pointed to a certain anthropological "truth" or content to madness.

In *History of Madness*, Foucault famously distinguished three periods, three different articulations of reason and unreason: the Renaissance when madness was perceived as a form of knowledge, of special insight; the classical age (around the seventeenth and eighteenth centuries) with the creation of the General Hospital in 1657 and the *grand renfermement*, institutions of confinement designed to exclude madness from the rest of society; and finally, the modern positivist moment that began at the end of the eighteenth century with the birth of the asylum and the rise of scientific psychiatry, from William Tuke's York Retreat to Philippe Pinel liberating his patients from their chains at the Salpêtrière in 1794. Instead of presenting this history as one of progress, of better and more humane care for the mentally ill, Foucault stressed the continuities between these various forms of social control: "The positivist psychiatry of the nineteenth century, like our own, may no longer have used the knowledge and practices handed on from the previous age, but they secretly inherited the relationship that classical culture as a whole had set up with unreason. They were modified and displaced, and it was thought that madness was purely being studied from the point of view of an objective pathology; but despite those good intentions, the truth was that madness was still haunted by an ethical view of unreason, and the scandal of its animal nature."[60] Psychiatry, according to Foucault, continued to administer and exclude madness, but alienation was no lon-

Michel Foucault, Psychiatry, Antipsychiatry, and Power   123

ger considered simply a social ill; it had become psychologized. Thus, Tuke and Pinel, the two heroes of the more compassionate, modern, and scientific version of psychiatry, did not open the asylum to medical knowledge as it is often believed. Rather, they introduced a "new character"—*un personnage*: the psychiatrist, defined not by his medical expertise but by his ability to "take on the mantle of Father and Lord of Justice," "the almost magical practitioner of the cure" and "worker of miracle."[61] In other words, according to Foucault, it was not so much the mad who needed the psychiatrists to cure them as the psychiatrists who needed the mad to articulate and consolidate their power.

It was this construction of the psychiatrist as "character" or *personnage* that appeared to be at the root of the hostility with which *History of Madness* was finally received in French psychiatric circles. In October 1965, at the *Évolution psychiatrique* annual conference, Lucien Bonnafé delivered a talk titled "Personnage du psychiatre" in which he praised Foucault for highlighting the ways in which psychiatry had so often participated in oppression. This was, after all, as Bonnafé reminded his audience, what had driven institutional psychotherapy from its beginnings: the search for a more humane psychiatric practice in the aftermath of the genocide of World War II. Describing Foucault's 1961 book as a "gunshot" (*coup de pistolet*) for the psychiatric field, Bonnafé complimented its author for being overall correct.[62] To be sure, he continued, a "psychiatric revolution" had begun twenty years ago, one in which he but also Daumézon, Tosquelles, and others had played a central role. However, given that institutional psychotherapy remained marginal in most psychiatric centers in France, Bonnafé concluded that the revolution—like so many other revolutions—had been "betrayed" (*révolution trahie*). Henri Ey, however, who was also in the audience, engaged with Foucault much more harshly. He was especially upset by what he perceived as Foucault's interrogation of the "naturality" of madness: "No lyrical or metaphysical treaty—as eloquent as it is—will ever lead me to say that mental illness is a 'product of culture' . . . or an 'effect of mystification.'" Psychiatry, unlike politics, concerns itself not with "ideals" but with "scientific reality": "either psychiatry exists and the psychiatrist is not mad, or else psychiatry (myth or imposture) does not exist and the psychiatrist is mad." As Ey concluded, Foucault's "accusation of imposture was itself an imposture and this myth also needed to be demystified."[63]

Ey had been Foucault's teacher at Sainte-Anne, and he had helped him with his translation of Viktor von Weizsäcker's *Der Gestaltkreis* in the 1950s.[64] Yet he prolonged his attacks in December 1969 at another *Évolution psychiatrique* conference devoted, exclusively this time, to "The Ideological Conception of *The History of Madness* by Michel Foucault." Foucault was invited to attend the conference, but according to his biographers, he canceled at the last minute.[65] It was surprising, Ey claimed in his opening remarks, that *The History of Madness*, "which questioned the very concept of 'mental illness' and the raison d'être of our therapeutic work, that this book so radically opposed to the validity of Psychiatry, had not raised more violent reactions among Psychiatrists."[66] Perhaps, Ey, suggested, this lack of interest in Foucault was due to the longstanding undermining of psychiatry from inside the field itself (*travail de sape*). Yet Foucault's thesis was "psychiatricidal," and Ey and others felt compelled to respond. In the opening remarks to the colloquium, Jean Laboucarié, after recognizing that psychiatry was being contested in its methods, its intentions, and in its very object, framed the problem in the following terms: the question was to figure out whether psychiatry ought to follow "structuralist conceptions" and seek to deliver man from a society that alienated him or whether, on the contrary, while obviously "taking into account sociocultural factors that diversify mental illness," it was more important to "recognize the originality of the psychiatric fact."[67] In Ey's words, the main point of contention with Foucault was the "morality of the concept of mental illness. Either it is a natural pathological reality, an unhappy attenuation of man's responsibility—or else, it is a cultural artifact, a scandalous effect of social repression."[68]

Also present at this colloquium was Georges Daumézon, who had been Foucault's conduit to psychiatry when he was a student at the École Normale. Like Bonnafé, Daumézon welcomed Foucault's challenge, which he did not find "shocking" and which in many ways disseminated to a larger public what he and the other practitioners of institutional psychotherapy had been maintaining for years.[69] Daumézon, however, shared his colleagues' concern about Foucault's understanding of mental illness: "I became quickly uneasy with the constant confusion between Madness, the category of trivial language, I mean banal and quotidian, and the mental troubles that we are assigned to treat, the object of our profession, of our little knowledge, of our practice."[70] From the perspective of the history of science, Daumézon continued, the epistemological problem could have been framed differently, more rigorously: Foucault could have "considered what, for the predecessors of the eighteenth-century doctors, stumped the medical gaze when faced with mental trouble," and he could have "asked how the conceptual apparatus to encompass mental disorder finally developed."[71]

Despite his methodological and historical objections to the *History of Madness*, Daumézon celebrated Foucault's work enthusiastically. The real problem, however, was its diffusion, the fact that his thesis had been "taken up and magnified by so many readers and, more dangerously, by non-readers." Too many "young psychiatrists" today, Daumézon continued, were "impregnated with this deformed vision. Their daily practice is inflected by the torment that it imposes upon them. Their behavior with patients is dictated by the fear that they might become the medical prison guard depicted by Foucault."[72] The references to these "times of contestation" recurred in almost every intervention at the colloquium, as if Foucault's thesis had fueled the flames of May '68. In his presentation, the psychiatrist Henri Sztulman brought up a poster from May 1968 that showed a disjointed body and that declared: "Bourgeois medicine does not heal, it repairs workers" (fig. 4.2). Was the point of Foucault's book to claim, similarly, that "mental illness did not exist, that psychiatry was a myth," and that psychiatrists simply persisted in segregating, excluding, and oppressing the sick?[73] Or as Dr. Aubin in the audience put it, Foucault's book needed to be inscribed in a broader revolutionary current "in the footsteps of Marcuse," in the philosophical whirlwind that sought to destroy the concepts of Reason and Order. *History of Madness*, he claimed, reminded him of a student group—self-described as "situationists"—that, right before May '68, had called for the suppression of the university psychological service center (BAPU: Bureau d'aide psychologique universitaire) because it was the "typical instrument of a consumer society in the hands of psychiatrists."[74]

Foucault was conscious of how his book had served as a "toolbox" for many thinkers and activists around May '68 but also for antipsychiatry.[75] Yet, as he repeated in several interviews, he was not directly engaged with antipsychiatry in *History of Madness* for the simple reason that "when I wrote the book, in Poland, in 1958, antipsychiatry did not exist in Europe." Furthermore, Foucault did not conceive of this project as an attack on psychiatry as a whole since his argument stopped "at the very beginning of the nineteenth century" without even addressing the work of Esquirol and his followers. Rather, his book was meant as an experience—for him as author, but also for the reader—in our understanding of truth. In that sense, the experience itself was neither true nor false—it was always subjective as all experiences are, but it served as a form of political awakening.[76]

Foucault referred to the 1969 *Évolution psychiatrique* Toulouse conference as an attempt to "excommunicate" the *History of Madness*. "Even Bonnafé," he specified, "a Marxist psychiatrist who had favorably welcomed my book when it came out, condemned it in 1968 as an ideological work."[77] As Foucault continued, once again revealing his familiarity with institutional psychotherapy, Bonnafé was part of a movement

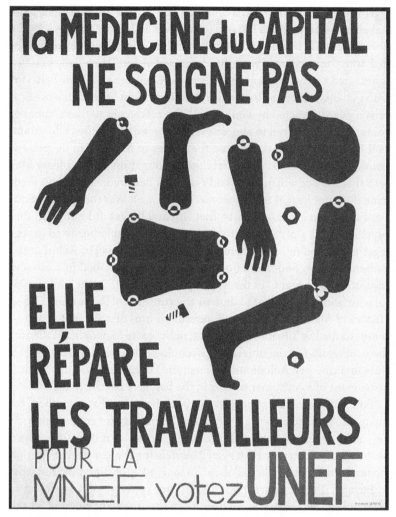

4.2 May '68 Poster: "Bourgeois Medicine Does Not Heal, It Repairs Workers"
© Beinecke Rare Book and Manuscript Library, Yale University

that "right before the war and especially after the war . . . had questioned psychiatric practice, a movement born within psychiatrists themselves. These young psychiatrists, after 1945, were engaged in analyses, reflections, and projects such that what would later be called 'antipsychiatry' could have probably emerged in France in the 1950s." Institutional psychotherapy, however, did not give birth to antipsychiatry, according to Foucault, for two reasons. First, many of these psychiatrists were either Marxists or "too close to Marxism." This led them to focus on the Soviet Union, Pavlov, reflexology, and a "materialist psychiatry" that

Michel Foucault, Psychiatry, Antipsychiatry, and Power   127

could only result in an "impasse," historically, theoretically, and scientif-
ically. Second, these psychiatrists retracted their more radical critiques
because of a "professional defense" (*defense syndicale*). It was at this
point, in the 1960s, that their rejection of antipsychiatry took a more
"aggressive turn" and that the *History of Madness* was "blacklisted as if
it was the devil's gospel." "In certain milieus," Foucault concluded, "*The
History of Madness* is still referred to with incredible disgust."[78] Interestingly, however, in this passage, Foucault failed to mention his own
interest in Pavlov, alienation, and the possibility of a "materialist psychiatry" in his early work. By the time this interview was published in
1980, Foucault had left those questions far behind.

Foucault and Antipsychiatry

What, then, happened with the *History of Madness* in 1968 and how did
it come to provide a "toolbox" for antipsychiatry, first abroad and later
in France? Part of the answer lies in the trajectory of the English translation of *History of Madness* and its diffusion. Foucault had agreed to
abridge his book for the 10/18 *poche* collection at Plon in 1963. This was
the version that circulated widely in France throughout the 1960s until
the thesis was finally republished in its entirety by Gallimard in 1971.[79]
It is also this shortened version—less academic and hence more seemingly polemical—that was translated into English by Richard Howard
in 1965 under the title *Madness and Civilization: A History of Insanity in
the Age of Reason*. Two years later, in 1967, the British publishing house
Tavistock, associated with the Tavistock Clinic and the Tavistock Institute for Human Relations, two of the main centers of British psychotherapy, reissued the condensed work in a collection called "Studies in
Existentialism and Phenomenology" directed by the Scottish psychiatrist and psychoanalyst Ronald Laing. Laing's friend and colleague, the
South African psychiatrist David Cooper, had just published earlier that
year with the same press *Psychiatry and Anti-Psychiatry*. As the first to
officially coin the term "antipsychiatry," Cooper wrote an enthusiastic
introduction to Foucault's book.[80] As Laing put it in his reader's report,
Madness and Civilization was an "exceptional book of very high caliber,
brilliantly written, intellectually rigorous, and with a thesis that thoroughly sheds the assumptions of traditional psychiatry."[81] Laing continued his praise of Foucault in a review for the popular magazine *New
Statesman* in June 1967. After celebrating the brilliance, the intensity,
and the verbal momentum of *Madness and Civilization*, Laing explained
that despite being a work of history, the book was "full of contemporary
relevance." It was surprising, Laing suggested, that Foucault had ended

his study at the beginning of the nineteenth century and that he "appears to have no axe to grind in contemporary psychiatric controversy." Perhaps "reticence, tact or lack of time . . . deterred him," perhaps "he was too clever to fall into a trap, he was not sufficiently wise fully to see," but in either case, "we can surmise that if Foucault continues to survive the torrent of his own intellect he will be one of the writers to whom we shall in our life time continue to turn with a somewhat terrified delight, to be instructed when we are not too dazzled."[82]

And indeed, Laing and Cooper brought Foucault right into the heart of the psychiatric controversies in which they themselves were fully immersed. In his review, Laing referred to the "moral coercion" of nineteenth-century psychiatry that replaced physical restraint as a "more effective technique of terrorism." Similarly, he highlighted the continuities between the modern doctor and the "guardian, keeper, jailer" of patients during the time of the "great confinement." With modern science came "a ferociously benevolent technology of personal control and domination," and "victory belonged to those who could control the power structures of society."[83] This was not Foucault's vocabulary, but it certainly was Laing and Cooper's. As Laing put it in his 1964 preface to the second edition of his first book, *The Divided Self*, psychiatry could be "on the side of transcendence, of genuine freedom, and of true human growth," but it could "so easily be a technique of brainwashing, of inducing behavior that is adjusted, by (preferably) non-injurious torture."[84]

In 1965, Laing and Cooper had moved to Kingsley Hall, a clinic for schizophrenics in the East End of London funded by the Philadelphia Association. It seems that Laing and Cooper were unaware of institutional psychotherapy, even though Kingsley Hall also had an open-door, no-restraint policy and patients and doctors lived together in communal space. Laing and Cooper's inspiration came primarily from Maxwell Jones's therapeutic community. Much less psychoanalytically inclined—and certainly much less Lacanian—than institutional psychotherapists, the doctors at Kingsley Hall were primarily existentialists. For them, the psychotic delusion was a "voyage" rather than a form of suffering, a breakthrough rather than a breakdown. As they saw it, psychosis resulted not from a brain pathology but rather from social and familial oppression. In this sense, psychosis was an act of rebellion against repressive normativity that needed to be applauded. Thus, British antipsychiatry was quite different from French institutional psychotherapy, especially that of Tosquelles, Bonnafé, or Oury. Kingsley Hall soon became a pilgrimage site for the counterculture, for hippies yearning for communal living and drug-induced "voyages," for anarchists seeking nonauthoritarian and self-managed social spaces, but also for artists who distinguished in madness a certain form of truth and authenticity.[85] In July 1967, right after Tavistock republished *Madness and Civilization*, Cooper organized a large congress, "Dialectics of Liberation," in London's Roundhouse that several important philosophers (for example, Herbert Marcuse) and activists (Stokely Carmichael, for instance) attended. Throughout the congress, Cooper and Laing praised Foucault's work as a guideline for antipsychiatry and ultimately for social and psychic emancipation.[86]

British antipsychiatry spread rapidly in France, carried by the revolutionary wave of May '68, but also by the second generation of institutional psychotherapy gathered around Guattari, the CERFI, and the journal *Recherches*. In October 1967, the FGERI, the research group founded by Guattari in 1965, invited Laing and Cooper to a colloquium on "childhood alienation" (*l'enfance aliénée*) organized by the psychoanalyst Maud Mannoni. The conference brought together British antipsychiatrists, Lacanians (including Lacan himself but also Françoise Dolto, Edmond Ortigues, and others), and French institutional psychotherapists (including Jean Ayme, Jean Oury, and François Tosquelles).[87] Foucault's name was repeatedly invoked throughout the colloquium, including in Mannoni's introductory remarks in which she claimed that they had all learned from Foucault that "mental illness had become 'alienated madness,' alienated in a psychology that it had itself made possible."[88] More broadly, Mannoni provided one of the important vectors between Foucault and the world of antipsychiatry. Mannoni had visited Laing at Kingsley Hall after hearing about his radical experiments through Donald Winnicott. Upon her return to France, in September 1969, she founded an experimental school for autistic children in Bonneuil, a suburb of Paris. Bonneuil followed many of the basic principles of institutional psychotherapy as practiced at La Borde. As Mannoni put it, the school's goal was the "continual questioning of institutional frameworks" to prevent authoritarian forms of government.[89] Her notion of "burst institution" (*institution éclatée*) was comparable to Tosquelles's concept of "burst transference" (*transfert éclaté*) or to Oury's "transferential constellation." Moreover, Mannoni, like Oury, inscribed her work in close allegiance to that of Lacan, especially in relation to the role of the symbolic.

However, Mannoni was much more adamant about aligning herself with antipsychiatry, which she perceived as a rejection of medicine rather than a supplement. This was especially clear in her 1970 book, *The Psychiatrist, His "Mad," and Psychoanalysis* (dedicated to Lacan), in which she thanked Laing and Cooper, her "hosts at Kingsley Hall."

While institutional psychotherapy still thought it could "act" upon a patient (through drugs or group therapy for instance), Mannoni argued that in antipsychiatry, the "cure" did not necessitate any therapeutic intervention. It required only "the freedom to let this process develop."[90] The point was not to "reform the institution" but rather to "radically question the economic and political structures that had given birth to alienating institutions."[91] As she put it, the true difference lay in the distinction between psychiatry and antipsychiatry. To support her book's claims, Mannoni relied heavily on Foucault, on *History of Madness* but also *Birth of the Clinic* and *Maladie mentale et psychologie*.

Antipsychiatry also made its way into the French academic and activist world in the late 1960s–early 1970s, through a series of translations, including Cooper's *Psychiatry and Anti-Psychiatry* in 1970, Erving Goffman's *Asylums* in 1968, and Thomas Szasz's *The Myth of Mental Illness* in 1975.[92] According to Didier Eribon, Foucault supported the translation of Szasz's work. He also invited Cooper to give a few lectures at the Collège de France in 1976. Finally, he engaged him in a public debate organized by Jean-Pierre Faye for the magazine *Change* following the campaign to free Vladimir Borisov, a Soviet dissident who had been committed to a psychiatric hospital in Leningrad.[93] Similarly, Foucault was directly involved with Italian antipsychiatry (later known as *psichiatria democratica*), especially through its main protagonist, Franco Basaglia, who had taken over the asylum at Gorizia in 1961. Foucault's *History of Madness* had provided an important theoretical framework for the Gorizian team, who read and commented on the book as soon as it was translated into Italian in 1963.[94] Foucault collaborated with several of these Italian psychiatrists and contributed a piece to *Crimini di pace*, a 1973 manifesto in solidarity with Basaglia who was in trouble with the Italian authorities.[95]

The critique of psychiatry, however, did not come only from abroad. Foucault worked closely with many of the French scholars who perfected this critique from within, especially at the University of Paris VIII, "Vincennes," where Foucault began teaching (for the first time, in philosophy and not in psychology) in December 1968. It was at Vincennes that Foucault met Robert Castel, who had been hired in the sociology department. Castel had pushed for the translation of Goffman's *Asylums* at the Éditions de Minuit in the prestigious collection "Le sens commun" directed by Pierre Bourdieu, Castel's colleague from the Centre de sociologie européenne.[96] Goffman's work, originally published in English in 1961, was based on the sociological fieldwork that the author had conducted at Saint Elizabeth's psychiatric hospital in Washington DC. In his introduction to the French translation, Castel cele-

Michel Foucault, Psychiatry, Antipsychiatry, and Power   131

brated Goffman for his methodological prowess, his ability to write a history from the patients' perspective without any trace of sentimentalism, morality, or metaphysical suppositions.[97] For Castel, Goffman had succeeded in giving agency to the patients in a context in which they suffered from a double alienation: psychic alienation (i.e., madness) and what he called *asilation*, "the process of adapting to a claustral universe" and "passive repetition."[98] Goffman had famously characterized the asylum as a "total institution," and according to Castel, this "totalitarian" experiment could help us better understand society and norms as a whole.[99]

Castel, however, also used his preface to attack French psychiatry, and in particular, institutional psychotherapy, for remaining wedded to the psychiatric paradigm, to what Castel called "the psychiatric discourse," despite all its talk of reform. Castel thus distinguished two models of institutional psychotherapy. The first included Tosquelles, Daumézon, Le Guillant, Paul Sivadon, and Paumelle, whose writings appeared "very close to [Goffman's] sociological formulation of the problem"—in other words, close to the understanding of the hospital as a "total institution." The significant difference, Castel continued, was that institutional psychotherapy still thought of itself as providing a "therapeutic care." Goffman and this first generation of institutional psychotherapy shared, according to Castel, a "logical filiation rather than a direct influence."[100] The second group, however, the "more recent theorists of this current, especially those influenced by the hypotheses of psychoanalysis, group psycho-sociology, and structural linguistics," had "tended to reinterpret the institutional determinisms from a more strictly psychosociological perspective. This group represents the most modern version of what I have called the 'psychiatric discourse.'"[101] Here of course, Castel was referring to La Borde, and as an example, he cited Oury's treatment of the institution as a symbolic form akin to language: "The current proliferation of meetings . . . only institutionalizes this perception of the hospital as a therapeutic environment."[102]

Castel pursued his critique of psychoanalysis and psychiatry in *Le psychanalysme* (published by Maspero in 1973 in a collection that included works by Laing and Guattari) and *L'ordre psychiatrique* (published by Éditions de Minuit in 1977, also in Bourdieu's collection "Le sens commun").[103] Both works drew heavily on Foucault's *History of Madness*, which Castel characterized "as a cut-off point in medical ethnocentricity."[104] Both books were immensely controversial in psychoanalytic and psychiatric circles, including those of institutional psychotherapy. As Castel maintained, institutional psychotherapy was merely an attempt to "sublimate the structures of the totalitarian institution," and it was hence complicit in the oppressive power structures of psychiatry and psychoanalysis.[105] Foucault's relationship to Castel was one of the reasons why he became so closely associated with antipsychiatry in the minds of many. This was especially true when Foucault published a glowing review of *L'ordre psychiatrique* in *Le nouvel observateur*.[106] Specifically, Foucault picked up on Castel's severe assessment of the *psychiatrie de secteur*, one of the main pillars of institutional psychotherapy. For Castel, institutional psychotherapy constituted not a "revolution," as its proponents argued, but rather the *aggiornamento* of psychiatry: "We must take seriously the new strategies that they have defined (the hospital sector, institutional psychotherapy, listening to the patient, serving the 'user,' etc.) . . . : they are ambitious strategies. But let us realize that such specialists do not possess papal infallibility when they decree that we have entered a totally new era. If *each one of the dimensions* of the complex of problems relating to mental health has been profoundly shaken up (or is in the process of transformation), *their interrelationship* continues fairly adequately to circumscribe almost everything in this field."[107] As Foucault asked in his review, was the *secteur* simply "another way, more subtle, to transform mental health into public hygiene, present everywhere and always ready to intervene?"[108] Later that year, Foucault referred to Castel's book once again as evidence that "from the outset, the goal of psychiatry was to serve as a tool for social order."[109]

Finally, Castel played a role in convincing Foucault to get involved in the world of antipsychiatric activism. Specifically, a handful of activists — mainly medical students who belonged to various Maoist political groups — approached Castel in 1971 to create the GIA (Groupe information asiles). Their idea was to model the GIA on the GIP (Groupe d'information sur les prisons), founded in February 1971. Foucault had been one of the most important figures behind the GIP, and so Castel discussed the project with him and invited him to attend one of the GIA meetings, which were held on Monday evenings at the Jussieu campus.[110] Like the GIP, the GIA did not aim simply to raise consciousness or to propose political reforms. Rather, both groups presented themselves as experiments in collective thought. Their strategy was to mobilize "specific" intellectuals (lawyers, doctors, social workers, etc.) and to give voice to the victims of these total institutions, whether it be the prison or the asylum.[111] In this sense, the GIP was similar to the CERFI, even though it did not share its interest in the libidinal.[112] As the GIA "charter of patients" declared: "This charter does not seek the improvement of psychiatry but rather the complete destruction of the medical-police apparatus. This charter is part of the struggle to conquer, first of all, the most elementary democratic rights that have been taken away

Michel Foucault, Psychiatry, Antipsychiatry, and Power   133

from all workers that psychiatry has been able to isolate."[113] In order
to reach this goal, the GIA aimed to "destroy the carceral institution,"
to "break the isolation of the patient who is considered assisted, unac-
countable, and mad" and to "break the isolation caused by silence."[114]

To "break the isolation caused by silence," the GIA, like the GIP,
distributed a series of questionnaires to hospital patients. One set of
questions, for instance, focused on the operations of ergotherapy within
hospitals. The questionnaire asked patients what kind of work they performed, for whom, for how many hours, with whom.[115] As the GIA argued, even antipsychiatry had not been able to let go of the idea that
being cured was "an individual affair." This also applied to institutional
psychotherapy, which, for the GIA, was simply the "reverse side of the
asylum": "two facets of the same enemy: the psychiatric apparatus in
its entirety."[116] Instead of advocating new reforms, the GIA wanted to
fight against "the terrorism of the law"; to set up "defense committees
for patients"; to end "the terrorism of knowledge"; to "depsychiatrize
madness" and to "deprivatize madness."[117] The GIA promoted these
goals in its meetings but also in a series of pamphlets and publications,
including their journal *Tankonalasanté* (Aslongaswehavehealth), which
ran from 1973 to 1976, and their newsletter *Psychiatrisés en lutte* after 1975
(figs. 4.3 and 4.4). Both publications took up many of the themes raised
by Foucault, especially in drawing our attention to the close nexus between psychiatry and bourgeois power, a power consolidated and ce-
mented by school, church, and family.[118]

The GIA was not the only group that turned to Foucault in the aftermath of May '68 to formulate an attack against psychiatry and institutional psychotherapy. We can also mention AERLIP (Association pour
l'étude et la rédaction du livre des institutions psychiatriques), which
ran a monthly newsletter from February 1976 to December 1978; the
Cahiers pour la folie, also in the 1970s; the GIS (Groupe information
santé) in May 1972; Partisans whose journal *Garde-fous* appeared in 1974
and which in 1975 published with Maspero a book titled *Garde-fous:
Arrêtez de vous serrer les coudes*.[119] The first lines of this book, written
by François Gantheret and Jean-Marie Brohm, appeared to reference
Foucault quite directly: "Not so long ago, the mad were still locked up
together with the prostitutes, the unemployed, the thieves, and other
underworld characters. In other words, they were confined with all
those who were not considered 'normal' according to the values up-
held by class society, with all those who upset the norms of private
property and the institutions of moral conformity."[120] These groups'
newsletters, publications, and pamphlets essentially developed this condemnation of psychiatry as a tool of bourgeois normalization. And, like

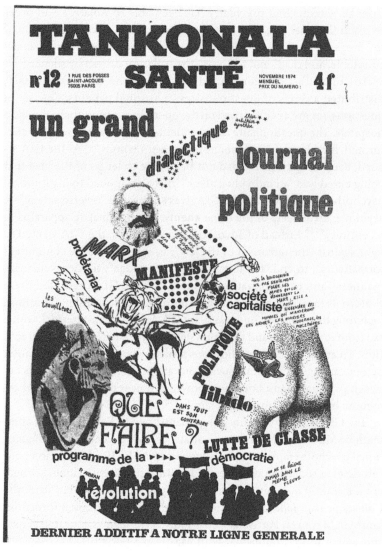

4.3 *Tankonalasanté*, November 1974
© Groupe Information Santé (GIS)

Castel, these activist circles were also vehemently critical of institutional psychotherapy, especially of La Borde, whose glory days were in the late 1960s. Thus, in the 1976 winter issue of *Garde-fous*, Bertrand Mary published a long and heated diatribe against La Borde and the CERFI. Mary based his attack primarily on the close reading of the March 1975 issue of the journal *Recherches* coordinated by François Fourquet and Lion Murard, "Histoire de la psychiatrie de secteur ou le secteur impos-

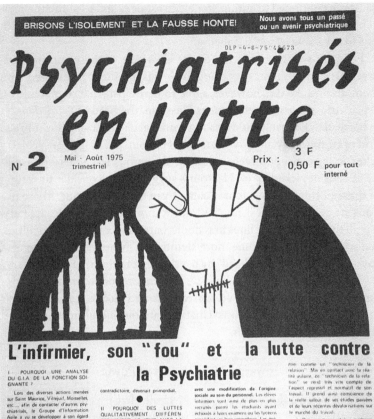

4.4 *Psychiatrisés en lutte*, May–August 1975
© Bibliothèque Nationale de France

sible?" According to Mary, despite *Recherches*'s hagiographic presentation, La Borde and the CERFI remained enamored with power, a "nice version" of psychiatry (*"psychiatrie sympa"*) that was perfectly adapted to the shape of power under the Fifth Republic. Once again, Mary relied on Foucault (and Szasz) to illustrate the growth of medical oppression since the eighteenth century.[121] After all, Mary contended, doctors at

136   CHAPTER FOUR

La Borde continued to administer electroshocks and to numb their patients with narcoleptics. In this sense, they remained strictly in line with
psychiatry's role of social policing.

Foucault was clearly aware of the existence of these various antipsychiatric movements even though he was not directly involved with
them. In 1974, he did, however, agree to participate in a roundtable on
psychiatric expertise with Jacques Hassoun, the head of *Garde-fous*.[122]
In particular, Foucault and Hassoun converged in decrying the imbrication of criminology and psychiatry. As Hassoun put it, "all of psychiatry
relies on the concepts of rehabilitation, dangerousness, and responsibility." Foucault picked up on Hassoun's suggestion to consider the origin
of these notions: "They do not come from law or medicine. These notions are neither juridical, nor psychiatric, nor medical, but disciplinary.
It is all these little disciplines in schools, barracks, correctional facilities,
factories, that have become more significant." More recently, they had
come to be "doubly sacralized" by psychiatry and the legal apparatus.[123]
It was this turn to the disciplinary, a turn that required a new theory of
power, that preoccupied Foucault from around 1968 to 1975. And it was
through psychiatry and antipsychiatry that Foucault ultimately arrived
at this new theory of power.

Toward a New Theory of Power

Foucault often acknowledged the key role that psychiatry and antipsychiatry played in his process of rethinking power after 1968. As he
put it in a 1975 interview:

> More generally, I would say that the antipsychiatry of Laing and Coo-
> per, between 1955 and 1960, marked the beginning of this critical and
> political analysis of power phenomena. I think that until 1970–75,
> analyses of power, analyses that were critical, at the same time theo-
> retical and practical, essentially focused on the notion of repression.
> The point was to denounce repressive power, to make it visible, to
> fight against it. But after the transformations brought about in 1968,
> we had to consider power from another register. We could no longer
> pose the problem in such terms. We had to pursue this theoretical
> and political analysis of power, but in another way.[124]

Throughout the 1960s, Foucault considered writing a sequel to *History
of Madness* for Pierre Nora's series at Julliard, one that would carry his
analysis through the nineteenth century. He also contemplated a history of hysteria for which he signed a book contract with Flammarion

Michel Foucault, Psychiatry, Antipsychiatry, and Power 137

in 1964.[125] Neither of these projects concretized. Later, Foucault pondered the possibility of coming to terms with this strange reception of *History of Madness* in a new preface for the 1972 Gallimard reprint of his book. As he put it, his idea was to "try to justify it for what it was, and reinsert it, insofar as such a thing might be possible, into what is going on today." But Foucault claimed that he "loathed the idea." Instead, he cut the original 1961 preface that he deemed too phenomenological and replaced it with a short notice. From the moment a book is produced, Foucault wrote, it is instantly "caught in an incessant game of repetitions": "its doubles, both near and far, start to multiply; each reading gives it, for an instant, an impalpable and unique body; fragments of it pass into circulation and are passed off as the whole thing, purporting to contain the book in its entirety, and the book itself sometimes ends up taking refuge in such summaries; commentaries double the text still further, creating even more discourses where, it is claimed, the book is itself at last, avowing all that it refused to say, delivering itself from all that which it so loudly pretended to be."[126] Given the multiple appropriations and reappropriations, readings and misreadings of *History of Madness* that we have traced, it is difficult not to think that Foucault had this particular context in mind when he refused to draft a sequel or to rewrite the preface in the early 1970s.

Interestingly, Foucault several times connected this sort of "exhaustion" concerning the *History of Madness* to his new work in the 1970s: his Collège de France lectures, *Discipline and Punish*, but also his activism, by which he meant the politicization of everyday life. Thus, in 1972, he reported that even though the second volume of *History of Madness* was "of no interest" to him, a "concrete political action in favor of prisoners" was much more appealing.[127] Here, of course, Foucault had in mind the GIP, which would last until December of that year. As Daniel Defert framed it, Foucault conceived of his participation in the GIP "directly in line" with the *History of Madness*.[128] The nexus between psychiatry, antipsychiatry, and prison activism but also the link between *History of Madness, Discipline and Punish*, and the Collège de France lectures during these years was power. In 1977, Foucault confessed that even though the *History of Madness* was all about power, he had had "trouble formulating this" at the time he wrote it. Part of the problem, Foucault explained, was that it was not clear from "which side—right or left—we needed to consider the problem of power." On the right, power was essentially thought of in juridical terms (sovereignty or the constitution, for example). On the left, it was reduced to the "state apparatuses." Only after 1968 and thanks to "the grassroots struggles of everyday life" was Foucault able to apprehend "the concrete [nature] of power." This activism revealed an "incredible fecundity" in its analyses of power, in its ability to study phenomena that had, until then, remained outside of the analytics of power. "Psychiatric confinement, the mental normalization of individuals, penal institutions" remained marginal if we considered them from a purely economic perspective, but they were essential to understand the "machinery of power."[129]

In other words, the new theory of power that Foucault was able to put forth after 1968 had at least two characteristics: it drew an intimate link between intellectual work and political activism ("power-knowledge," to use Foucault's terms), and it considered power as productive and generative rather than restrictive. To be sure, power relations were always historically determined, but they could also be reinterpreted and reappropriated with enough creative energy. This was, after all, the point of the GIP: not to seize power, not to conform or adapt to power, but rather to explode the terms that framed the debate, terms often deemed obvious, natural, or self-evident. In the case of the criminal justice system, these terms included the notions of guilt and innocence.[130] As Foucault put it in August 1971, once again highlighting the intimate link between psychiatry and the criminal justice system:

> Over the past few years, a movement known as antipsychiatry has developed in Italy around Basaglia and in England. Of course, these people developed their movement from their ideas and their experiences as psychiatrists, but they saw in [the *History of Madness*] a sort of historical justification. In this sense, they reassumed it, they took it over, to a certain extent they identified with it, and all of a sudden, this historical book started to have a sort of practical outcome. So let's say that I am a little jealous and that now I would like to do my own thing. Instead of writing a book about the history of justice that would later be taken up by others who question justice in their practice, I would like to begin by the practical questioning of the very category of justice and then, if I am still alive and, gosh, not in prison, well I'll write that book![131]

That book would be *Discipline and Punish*, which Foucault finished writing in August 1974 and which appeared in bookstores in February 1975, a self-avowed "history of the present" and a radically new theory of power: disciplinary power.[132]

Foucault laid out much of the groundwork for *Discipline and Punish*, including the exploration of the ties between psychiatry, prisons, and power, in his Collège de France lectures, especially in his 1973–74 course "Psychiatric Power." From his first lesson on November 7, 1973, Foucault inscribed *Psychiatric Power* in continuity with *History of Madness*. More specifically, Foucault explained, he was interested in using the course as a platform to reflect on some of the conceptual limits of *History of Madness*, especially in the last chapter on asylum power. The first problem, according to Foucault, was that *History of Madness* took representation as its object of study, "the perception of madness," a "history of mentality, of thought." Alternatively, Foucault argued, it was "possible to make a radically different analysis" if instead of beginning with this kind of representational core, one started with an "apparatus [*dispositif*] of power."[133] Power was not something that "one possessed" or that "emanated from someone" but rather something that could exist only in a "system of differences," in "dispersion, relays, networks, reciprocal supports, differences of potential, discrepancies, etc."[134] Power, Foucault claimed, needed to be understood as a "discursive practice," as what gave rise to a "game of truth."[135] The three other flaws—"three rusty locks"—that hampered the *History of Madness* stemmed from Foucault's ignorance of antipsychiatry. First, Foucault regretted his apprehension of violence as mere physical power, as an "unregulated, passionate power, an unbridled power." What was essential, rather, was to perceive how power always had its ultimate point of application in the body. As such, its application was "absolutely irregular."[136] Second, Foucault turned to the notion of institution that usually implied regularity and rules. What was more important, he maintained, was "the practical dispositions of power, the characteristic networks, currents, relays, points of support, and differences of potential that characterize a form of power, which are . . . constitutive of, precisely, both the individual and the group."[137] Third and final, Foucault lamented comparing the asylum to a family model. Neither the family nor the state apparatus could serve as a model for power because power was much too diffuse: "Rather, therefore, than speak of violence, I would prefer to speak of a microphysics of power; rather than speak of the institution, I would much prefer to try to see what tactics are put to work in these forces which confront each other; rather than speak of the family model or 'State apparatus,' I would like to see the strategy of these relations of power and confrontations which unfold within psychiatric practice."[138] Foucault's argument in all four cases was that if power was indeed a "game," a "microphysics," an uneven balance whose content could shift, it was also, always, up for grabs. This vision of power thus implied spaces for resistance if resistance was understood not as "taking over" but as "resignifying" or "reappropriating."

This was, as Foucault argued later in his course, the true genius of antipsychiatry. Indeed, antipsychiatry had begun with what Foucault called "institutional critique": the point was not to counterpoise a "supposedly true psychiatric discourse" to the existing regime, but to highlight, on the one hand, "the violence of the medical power exercised within [the institution], and on the other, the effects of incomprehension that right from the start distorted the supposed truth of medical discourse."[139] To illustrate this double critique, Foucault distinguished "two forms of the criticism of the asylum institution": the movement that led to sectorization in the 1930s ("diversification of ways of taking into care, projects for post-cure supervision, and, especially, the appearance of free services illustrated by an 'open service' . . . at Sainte-Anne") and "Saint-Alban" where doctors proposed to "reexamine how the psychiatric hospital works in order to turn it into a genuinely therapeutic organization." For Foucault, it was "this current [that] began to question the nature of the psychiatrist's relationships with patients."[140]

Even though this first critique was absolutely necessary, Foucault encouraged his audience to move beyond the framework of the institution and to think of power instead as "disciplinary."[141] In this sense, the "microphysics of asylum power" consisted in the "game between the mad person's body and the psychiatrist's body above it, dominating it, standing over it and, at the same time, absorbing it."[142] If psychiatry was indeed a game, antipsychiatry meant the manipulation of this game, the refusal to submit to the doctor's will. This was especially visible, Foucault suggested, in two famous accounts of madness: King George III, the ruler of the United Kingdom who developed dementia in the early nineteenth century, and Mary Barnes, the heroine of Kingsley Hall, whose memoir was translated into French in 1973.[143] As Foucault argued, even Mary Barnes, who was celebrated by Laing, Cooper, and their colleagues as the psychotic artist *cause célèbre* of their movement, managed to turn around, to manipulate, the discourse of her own doctors by covering herself in her feces. It is in this sense that Foucault referred to hysterics as the "true militants of antipsychiatry." Hysterics had essentially understood the rules of the "asylum game" and had learned to manipulate them. Hysterics exacerbated "the most precise and well-determined symptoms" but never allowed psychiatrists to "fix [their] illness in reality." They showed, repeatedly, that there was "no organic substratum" to their ailment. Hysteria, Foucault argued, was thus an "effective way of defending oneself from dementia; the only way not to be demented in a nineteenth century hospital." "By means of simulation," hysterics resisted "madness being fixed in reality."[144]

Foucault returned to this definition of antipsychiatry in a talk delivered in Montreal on May 9, 1973, right after he had ended his Collège de France lectures on psychiatric power. Foucault's paper was part of a conference titled "Should Psychiatrists be Committed?" that had been organized by Henri Ellenberger, the psychiatrist and historian of psychiatry. After apologizing for being "neither a psychiatrist nor an antipsychiatrist" (his "two flaws," as he put it), Foucault proceeded to map the field of antipsychiatry not in the singular, but in the plural: *antipsychiatries* in their diversity and complexity.[145] Before the nineteenth century, Foucault explained, the hospital functioned as a space to observe truth and to exercise a direct action on illness.[146] After the nineteenth century, however, when madness came to be understood as a deviation from normal behavior, the hospital became the "site of confrontation between the passion and the disturbed will of the patient and the passion and orthodox will of the doctor and the hospital staff."[147] Given this framework, the most profound impasse of psychiatry and the birth of antipsychiatry were simultaneous. Both occurred when Jean-Martin Charcot realized that his patients' great crises of hysteria on public display at the Salpêtrière were, in fact, fabricated. The hospital could no longer function as the arena for the instantiation of reason and madness. Rather, it became the site of the production of "obscure relations of power."[148] From this moment, antipsychiatry could emerge, if we understood by antipsychiatry everything "that challenges the role of the psychiatrist as the person previously designated to produce the truth of an illness within the realm of the hospital."[149]

From this perspective, there could be as many antipsychiatries as there were ways to shift the power relation between doctor and patient. Foucault proceeded to list the various forms that antipsychiatry had taken: psychosurgery and psychopharmacology, both of which sought to "mask" the organic support of madness, i.e., its symptom; psychoanalysis, which, on the contrary, sought to exacerbate the symptom; Laing and Cooper, for whom madness was not something that patients had to admit, to show, to manifest when pressed by the doctor, but rather the ultimate goal for the patient, the only true experience. Laing and Cooper thus sought to produce a demedicalized space for madness to express itself, to annihilate all power relations between doctors and patients. Finally, Foucault ended with a fourth version of antipsychiatry, the one he confessed feeling closest to: that of Basaglia and that of Guattari. Here, he argued, the point was not to elude or to bracket power relations but rather to understand that power had "shaped the entire existence of the patient, that it shaped his madness." For this version of antipsychiatry, the task was thus not to yearn for an escape, for total freedom or liberation. Rather, its task—its political work—was to bring to light these power relations, to unmask them, untangle them, and fight against them one by one.[150] This was precisely the kind of political work that Foucault had tried to enact through his participation in the GIP and the CERFI, both conceived as "subject-groups," to use Guattari's language. It was also the version of power that guided Foucault's remaining lectures at the Collège de France and the last books of his life.

EPILOGUE

The Hospital as a Laboratory of Political Invention

I began thinking about this book in 2013, as anti-austerity movements triggered by the 2008 subprime mortgage crisis and the Emergency Economic Stabilization Act that followed (also known as the "bank bailout") were spreading throughout the world. I finished writing it in the spring of 2020 during the generalized lockdown brought by the COVID-19 pandemic. In the midst, I witnessed the election of Donald Trump, Brexit, the so-called "migrant crises" in Europe and in the United States, the rise of an unabashed white nationalism, and the ascent of the extreme right in more countries than I could have imagined. These political contexts were central to the genesis, the conception, and the production of this book. More specifically, the problems of occupation, concentrationism, encampment, and alienation—themes that had been so central to the founders of institutional psychotherapy—still appeared to haunt our present. Despite their differences, movements such as Occupy in the US, Los Indignados in Spain, the Indignant Citizens in Greece, Tahrir Square in Egypt, Gezi Park in Istanbul, or Nuit Debout in France all insisted on the importance of taking over public space, mobilizing crowds, and calling assemblies as a way to begin assessing—and combatting—the effects of neoliberalism or political authoritarianism.[1]

The physical occupation of squares in the 2010s led to a broader reflection on psychic occupation, to a critique of privatization and what the French have called *la pensée unique*, the idea that economic metrics should govern all social, intellectual, and political life. If neoliberalism was indeed a normative order of reason and a governing rationality as thinkers such as Michel Foucault, Wendy Brown, or Michel Feher have suggested, then disoccupation required a different understanding of the political: new conducts, alternative life forms, a transformation at the level of subjectivity.[2] As many of these movements experimented with popular sovereignty and radical democracy on a practical terrain, as they defined and fought over who could speak, how to speak, what to demand, who to demand it from, and much more, they also contributed to a renewal of the theoretical conversation around the "common." For various of the participants in these public assemblies, if privatization was one of the dominant features of neoliberalism, then the common could offer an alternative political horizon. The common could serve as a weapon against capitalist forms of property but also against a more traditional version of state communism that still elevated state ownership of the means of production as its ultimate goal. The common opened up a new democratic imaginary premised on self-management, on nonhierarchal practices, on a new set of institutions. To that end, the experience of institutional psychotherapy could be helpful.

This was the argument that political theorists Pierre Dardot and Christian Laval put forth in their 2014 book *Commun*.[3] For these two authors, the common could offer a solution to the impasses of neoliberalism, but only if it was understood correctly. First, they clarified, the common was not an entity or a "thing" that could be appropriated but rather a political principle.[4] Second, the common did not emerge spontaneously through the simple juxtaposition of bodies or desires in a public space.[5] Third, the common was not a "ready-made universal model or a formulaic schema that could be transposed to any situation." Rather, it needed to be articulated in relation to what they called the "logic of institutionalization."[6] Indeed, for Dardot and Laval, the common's political potential came from the fact that it could be conceived and reconceived constantly through what the authors designated as an "emancipatory instituent praxis." This referred to a set of concrete political acts designed to prevent institutional inertia, ossification, or petrification — or, to use the authors' terms, to avoid the collapse of the "instituent within the instituted."[7] Instituent praxis, according to Dardot and Laval, "from the very beginning, consciously anticipates the need to modify and reinvent the institution that it has posited."[8] In other words, institutions were necessary in the long run but they were always temporary. Whereas liberal democratic theory presumed the existence of a rational subject endowed with a sovereign will from the outset (a subject who could decide, choose, declare, or proclaim), the instituent praxis in the common "produced its own subject by the very fact of its activity." More exactly, Dardot and Laval contended, "instituent praxis was the self-production of a collective subject in and through the continuous co-production of the rules of law."[9]

Dardot and Laval's considerations on the political were indebted to the work of the French-Greek philosopher Cornelius Castoriadis, but the example they turned to in order to "flesh out more fully" the operations of this "instituent praxis" that could lead to a radically democratic form of autonomy was institutional psychotherapy. The goal of institutional psychotherapy as Tosquelles, Oury, Guattari (and, I would add to this list, Fanon) conceived it was neither to impose institutions that had been previously determined by laws nor to officialize those that existed already. Rather, institutional psychotherapy strove for the "permanent reinvention of the institutions by the group that created them to counteract their potential inertia."[10] In this process, institutional psychotherapy foregrounded the role of the unconscious in all group formations but also the collective dimension of all subjective development. The unconscious was not an "add-on" or a supplement to the social theory but rather the basis of the transferential process, the vector through which individuals and collectives could explore fantasies, conflicts, and desires. Ultimately, the unconscious was the means by which the group could avoid closing on itself.

As I have argued in this book, theory and practice were intimately linked for the advocates of institutional psychotherapy. The various activities of the hospital—whether it be the club, the meetings, the ergotherapy stations, the publications, the cultural events—all sought to bring to light unconscious processes, crystallize transferential relations, channel clashes, aggressions, and wishes, all in the hope of facilitating the development of a more autonomous collective. As the doctors in this book insisted, their aim was to allow patients to be as free as possible of immediate assistance (*les responsabiliser* to use a recurring term), to lean on themselves, make their own decisions, and learn to articulate their own demands. The collective in institutional psychotherapy, just like the common in Dardot and Laval's text, needed to be produced at all times: it needed to be *instituted*.

In this sense, we could say that the public square for the anti-austerity movements and the hospital for institutional psychotherapy both functioned as laboratories of political invention. The goal was not to strive for doctrinal coherence or theoretical purity. Instead, both experiments can provide us with a set of practical tools—some successful, some less so—to erode hierarchy, domination, and forms of authoritarianism in group life and ultimately to envision a different political imaginary. In this process, institutions are crucial even if they are transitional, improvised, tentative, and always open to change. Today, as the COVID-19 quarantine has brought about a new form of confinement—and new types of psychic occupation—the reflection on the common has reemerged around the issues of health care, housing, education, employment, and many other topics.[11] Perhaps more than ever, the CERFI's incentive

146 EPILOGUE

to think through "collective infrastructures" (*équipements collectifs*) and to craft institutional alternatives to the state appears of dire necessity given the incompetence of the government's reaction and managing of the crisis.

As I intimated in the introduction, the specific context of the Second World War and the reality of fascism were integral to the development of institutional psychotherapy. It was the war—the Spanish Civil War, the Nazi Occupation of France, and the Resistance—that brought together to Saint-Alban the particular cast of characters, the physicians, staff, philosophers, artists, poets, who set up institutional psychotherapy. Many of the protagonists in this book were inspired by political experiences in their youth in which they were first encouraged to articulate another common, whether it be the POUM for Tosquelles or the Popular Front and the *auberges de jeunesse* for Oury and Guattari. As the founders of institutional psychotherapy saw it, fascism did indeed constitute the other side of these radically democratic leftist projects, not an external threat but a continual internal menace. Fascism in their work came to designate the possibility that any group will embrace concentrationism or le *tout-pouvoir*, to use Tosquelles's term. Several of the thinkers in this book used the term fascism hyperbolically, and it is clear that the fascism of the Franco regime and of the Third Reich was not the same as the "fascism in our heads" that Foucault and Guattari invoked during the 1970s, nor is it identical to neoliberalism or the extreme right of today. Yet without reproducing this ahistorical understanding of fascism, it is still possible to claim that institutional psychotherapy can offer us some useful tools to diagnose our present.

More specifically, by bringing the unconscious (individual and collective) to the political conversation, institutional psychotherapy can help us move beyond the liberal and the Marxist dismissal of "fascism" understood broadly as a pathology and a failure of rationality for the former and as false consciousness for the latter. Much of the political commentary in the aftermath of the Donald Trump election in 2016 still revolved around the supposedly contradictory motivations of the Trump electors, who had clearly "voted against their interests." Political analysis remained caught, in other words, in the "what's the matter with Kansas" paradigm, to invoke Thomas Frank's 2004 bestseller.[12] From the perspective of institutional psychotherapy, the "matter with Kansas" was not false consciousness or ideological dupery but rather these voters' desires, their *desire* for authoritarianism, for redemptive violence, for domination and a return to a mythic past. We can simply recall the many videos of the Trump rallies that preceded the 2016 election to realize the importance of the libidinal, the fantasmatic, the burst of energy, violence, and emotion that no rational argument of liberalism could ever counter or appease.

As I have tried to suggest here, this book can be read in at least two ways. On the one hand, it is an intellectual history of a group of doctors and thinkers who came together in a particular historical moment because of their political commitments but also because of their dissatisfaction with mainstream psychiatry. Each of these thinkers is interesting on his own, but the focus of the book is the conversation, at times obvious and at times surprising, among them. As I indicated in the introduction, we should think of figures in this book as a constellation within which unexpected relationships between characters, contexts, and ideas—often seemingly fragmentary or tangential—can emerge. In this way, the story that I trace here also seeks to reframe the intellectual history of a strain of what has come to be known as "French theory," not only by explaining the influence of psychiatry in its development, but also by showing the deep political and affective commitments that infused and shaped it. The prism of psychiatry allows us to depart from the usual treatment of these postwar thinkers within a structuralist/poststructuralist divide or by reference to the reception of phenomenology and existentialism in France. Many of the thinkers in this study were conversant in these philosophical traditions, but constructing this particular constellation around institutional psychotherapy can bring to light other seemingly disparate ideas, places, and peoples.

This is especially the case with Fanon, whose conspicuous absence in the genealogy of institutional psychotherapy is significant. My goal has not been to "replace" Guattari by rediscovering Fanon as the *true* theorist of this radical psychiatric tradition or to write a redemptive history designed to restore to Fanon the agency he deserves. Rather, my point is to show how Fanon, Guattari, Tosquelles, Oury, Foucault, and others partake of a shared history more complex and more relevant than the scholarship that incessantly divides "French" and "Francophone" thinkers from each other. A constellation allows us to observe what happens when the starring roles in a particular intellectual trajectory shift or when the nation no longer serves as the privileged grid of interpretation. Through the lens of institutional psychotherapy "French theory" was certainly not as "French" as we may think.

There is, however, a second way to read this book, as a contribution to critical theory, as an exercise in what Gary Wilder has called "thinking *with*" these authors. For Wilder, this type of critical history requires moving beyond simple contextualization in order to listen "carefully to

148 EPILOGUE

what their analysis of that world might teach us about ours."[13] Wilder refers to Dominick LaCapra's notion of a "dialogic history" whereby the historian enters into a "critical dialogue with texts that are allowed, in some sense, to speak back."[14] *Disalienation* was also conceived as a dialogical conversation between texts and contexts but also between past and present. When I have presented preliminary versions of these chapters over the past few years, one of the questions I inevitably get is "How successful was institutional psychotherapy?" In other words, was institutional psychotherapy an estimable theory and what normative lessons can we derive from it, either for psychiatry or for politics? In both cases, the answer is not exactly straightforward.

Within the field of psychiatry, institutional psychotherapy is quickly disappearing. The clinics and hospitals that functioned as epicenters of institutional psychotherapy are struggling financially, politically, and intellectually, if they have not given up on institutional psychotherapy altogether, as at Saint-Alban (where the hospital was renamed Centre hospitalier François Tosquelles). As a discipline, psychiatry appears to be moving more decidedly toward neuroscience, pharmacology, and cognitive behavior therapies, rather than toward the revalorization of the unconscious. Nonetheless, some of the more radical medical insights of institutional psychotherapy have been incorporated into the structure of French health care, notably the *secteur*, which allows patients to be treated close to their homes and communities. Furthermore, several young psychiatrists and psychoanalysts in France and abroad have returned to institutional psychotherapy to find concrete practices that will help alter psychic dynamics sufficiently to allow patients to imagine themselves anew and begin to heal.

More broadly, however, institutional psychotherapy fought to make possible a new form of self-knowledge by dismantling the regulatory system that governed the lives of the hospital community—and not just the patients—and replacing them with others. The radical reorganization of the asylum sought to disalienate alienation but never once and for all. To produce a collective was to produce its conditions of possibility, to work through the effects of transference, countertransference, resistances, and power, with constant vigilance—or, to recall Oury's words, *ne pas laisser en passer une* (not to miss an occasion). As I have indicated before, relying on psychosis as a model for political and social transformative critique was not a seamless or self-evident process, and the protagonists of this book often argued about the implications of shifting institutional psychotherapy into philosophy and politics, about turning to fascism and psychosis to interpret social and political phenomena more generally.

Furthermore, I have also noted how despite their explicit commitments to emancipatory politics, each one of these theorists had important limitations, notably around questions of gender and race. However, if we consider the ways in which Fanon transformed institutional psychotherapy to study colonialism or the ways in which Deleuze and Guattari provided a template for Guy Hocquenghem to develop a manifesto for the homosexual liberation front, then perhaps institutional psychotherapy already gives us the tools to disrupt the more normative understandings of race, sexuality, and gender that may have limited some of its practitioners' visions. In this sense, this study is neither a hagiography nor a repudiation of institutional psychotherapy. Rather, it is an attempt to *think with it*, to turn it on its head when necessary, to confront its blind spots and follow its ethical injunction to always be on the lookout for theoretical dogmatism and political inertia. As such, this book is an endeavor to take seriously the unconscious in politics, to remember the social dimension of the unconscious, and, I hope, to open up perspectives for other political imaginaries and new commons.

ACKNOWLEDGMENTS

This book is, in many ways, a product of chance. I never planned to write a history of institutional psychotherapy, but as I met some of its protagonists, followed a fascinating archival trail, and came to realize how relevant the insights of institutional psychotherapy could be to diagnose and make sense of our political present, my research slowly congealed into this book. I owe a huge thank you to Julian Bourg, who first made me aware of the existence of institutional psychotherapy in his excellent monograph *From Revolution to Ethics*. When I began working on this project, Julian also mailed me an entire box of research—printouts of obscure articles and difficult-to-locate works—that he no longer needed. This kind of generosity makes academic work as a collective enterprise so delightful and rewarding.

The first iteration of this project was a paper on Tosquelles that I wrote for a workshop on camps at the New School organized by Federico Finchelstein and Ann Stoler. Soon after, I presented a fuller version at a fantastically stimulating conference on history and psychoanalysis during the postwar period orchestrated by Michal Shapira at Columbia University. Several conference participants shaped this project foundationally at its very early stages and remained important interlocutors, especially Dagmar Herzog, Ben Kafka, George Makari, Sam Moyn, Daniel Pick, Eli Zaretsky, Matt Ffytche, and the late John Forrester.

My interest in Tosquelles led me to the Fundación Andreu Nin in Barcelona, where Maria Teresa Carbonell, the widow of Wilebaldo Solano, kindly shared with me her knowledge of the POUM. From there, I traveled to Reus, Tosquelles's hometown, where I learned more about institutional psychotherapy from Elisabet Vilella and Antonio Labad at the Institut Pere Mata. I also visited the psychiatric hospital of Saint-Alban (now renamed the Centre hospitalier François Tosquelles) and spent some time at La Borde, where I was incredibly lucky to meet and interview Jean Oury before he passed away. Being able to participate in daily life at La Borde, to interact with patients, walk with them, eat with them, accompany them in the ergotherapy stations, linger in the library, and observe the doctors and staff was absolutely essential for the development of this project.

These research trips were made possible with the generous help of travel grants from the Society for the Humanities and the Institute for Social Sciences at Cornell, and from the Humanities War and Peace Initiative at Columbia. In addition, I am grateful for two longer leaves that gave me the time and space to conceive and write much of the book. These were funded by the Society for the Humanities (where the yearly theme, "occupation," clearly had a profound impact); the National Endowment for the Humanities; the Remarque Institute at NYU; and the Institute for Advanced Study.

The libraries and archival collections at the Pere Mata, Saint-Alban, and La Borde—still largely unexplored—would delight any scholar interested in the history of psychiatry, and I am so thankful to have had access to these institutions. The Archives départementales de Tarn-et-Garonne also had very useful information on Spanish refugee camps. In Paris, the Fonds Michel Foucault at the Bibliothèque Nationale de France and the Fonds Jean Delay at the Bibliothèque littéraire Jacques Doucet provided the basis for my fourth chapter. Finally, anyone who has been at the IMEC (Institut mémoires de l'édition contemporaine) knows that it is simply the most magical and wonderful place to work. I could not have written this book without their amazing collections (on Bonnafé, Deligny, Foucault, Pankow, and of course on Guattari, Fanon, and Foucault), and I am grateful to the archivists, the librarians, and the staff (especially the chef!) who made my various stays there so pleasant and productive.

Throughout my research, I was also extremely fortunate to talk to several other people who were—or still are—directly involved with institutional psychotherapy. At another terrific conference at the Fundació Antoni Tàpies in Barcelona organized by Joana Masó and Carles Guerra, I met Jean-Claude Polack, who shared many stories about La Borde during a fascinating bus ride to and from Reus. Also at this conference, Martine Deyres introduced me to her beautiful movies on Oury and on Saint-Alban, and Christophe Boulanger made me realize how central art was to the project of institutional psychotherapy. Sophie Legrain, who has done a majestic work publishing some of the main texts of institutional psychotherapy at the Editions d'une, was also tremendously helpful in mapping out this world. In Paris, Anne Querrien was willing to talk to me about her years at the CERFI and in Guattari's orbit. Patrick Chemla welcomed me to his clinic in Reims, the Centre de jour Antonin Artaud, and recounted his own involvement with radical psychiatry.

Several other people were extremely helpful in sharing their knowledge of the various thinkers in this book and in guiding me through the history of institutional psychotherapy: Valentin Schaepelynck, who shares so many of my theoretical obsessions and who has become a friend; Laure Murat, with whom I always want to keep talking; Stuart Elden, who graciously agreed to help me with my chapter on Foucault; Étienne Balibar, who commented extensively on this chapter at the Columbia Theory Seminar; Robert Young, whom I met on that occasion and who helped me clarify several of my claims, especially on Fanon; Aurélie Vialette, who steered me through the history of labor movements in Spain; Meredith Tenhoor, who encouraged me to think through the architectural dimensions of institutional analysis and taught me about the CERFI; and Dagmar Herzog, whose own work on Cold War psychoanalysis has been so valuable and whose support, over many years now, has been constant.

As I wrote these chapters, I also benefited greatly from the intelligence, the generosity, and the engagement of the many audiences where I tested out the central ideas of this book: the Casa Italiana at NYU, the New School, the Instituto de Investigaciones Históricas at the UNAM, the Richardson Research Seminar in the History of Psychiatry at Cornell Weill Medical College, the New York Group in European Intellectual and Cultural History, the Department of Rhetoric at the University of California at Berkeley, the Cornell Comparative History Colloquium, the Center for 21st Century Studies at the University of Wisconsin, Milwaukee, the Night of Philosophy at the Brooklyn Public Library, the "Big Ideas Courses" at Bard College, the University of Paris VIII, the Society for French Historical Studies, the Committee on Globalization and Social Change at CUNY, the Institute for Cultural Inquiry in Berlin, the Global 1968 Conference at Stanford University, the Princeton School of Architecture, the Boston Psychoanalytic Circle, the Harvard History of Science Seminar, the NYC History of Science Lecture Series, and, at Columbia, the Maison Française and the "Beyond France," Literary Theory, and Critique & Praxis seminars. I am especially grateful to my hosts and, for their queries and remarks, to Eram Alam, David Bates, Judy Coffin, Ed Cohen, Madeleine Dobie, Kevin Duong, Dan Edelstein, Carolyn Eichner, Kennan Ferguson, John Foot, Pierre Force,

David Forgacs, Jack Frost, Jane Gallop, Matthew Jones, Regina Kunzel, Liz Marcus, Sarah Marks, Robert Paxton, Hannah Proctor, Andres Rios Molina, Bruce Robbins, and Gary Wilder.

My editor at the University of Chicago Press, Priya Nelson, who embraced this book from the beginning, has been amazing to work with. Along with Dylan Montanari, Tristan Bates, my excellent copy editor Susan Tarcov, and Karen Darling, who took over the project in the last stages, Priya pushed it through the various stages of publishing seamlessly. She secured two great reader reports and organized an incredibly valuable workshop with the editorial board of the Chicago Studies in Practices of Meaning series. I am grateful to William Mazzarella, Jennifer Cole, Jan Goldstein, Bill Sewell, and Kaushik Sunder Rajan for their insightful comments and questions, and I feel very privileged to be included in this outstanding series. I am immensely indebted also to Giuseppe Penone for his stunning drawing for the cover—an image in memory of Jean Oury, who likened psychosis to an uprooted tree, but also a tribute to the rhizomatic connections between thinkers, groups, and ideas in this project.

Parts of this book appeared in earlier abridged versions. Sections of chapter 1 were published under the title "François Tosquelles and the Psychiatric Revolution in Postwar France" in *Constellations* 23, no. 2 (June 2016); fragments of chapter 2 in "Frantz Fanon, Institutional Psychotherapy, and the Decolonization of Psychiatry" in the *Journal of the History of Ideas* 81, no. 2 (April 2020) and in "Fanon and Institutional Psychotherapy" in *Frantz Fanon's Psychotherapeutic Approaches to Clinical Work: Practicing Internationally with Marginalized Communities*, ed. Lou Turner and Helen Neville (New York: Routledge, 2019). I thank these publications for allowing me to reprint some of this material here and the editors and readers, especially my brilliant friends and co-conspirers, Stefanos Geroulanos and Judith Surkis, for working through the arguments thoroughly with me. In addition, two online interviews, one with Todd Meyers for *Somatosphere* and the other with Katie Joice and Sarah Marks for *Hidden Persuaders*, were also tremendously useful to sharpen my claims and delimit the contours of the project.

I began working on this book at Cornell and finished it at Columbia, and it was profoundly shaped by these two institutions, my colleagues, and my fantastic students in both places. In Ithaca, the Mellon Sawyer Seminar on "Political Will" allowed me to ponder many of these ideas with Elizabeth Anker, Jason Frank, Jill Frank, Rayna Kalas, Mitchel Lasser, Tracy McNulty, Aziz Rana, and Neil Saccamano. In New York, my beloved writing group—Susan Pedersen, Stephanie McCurry, Carrie Elkins, and Karuna Mantena—gave me the impetus to finish the epilogue in the midst of the pandemic. This book, like everything I do, is the result of sustained conversations with friends whose brilliance and generosity never cease to impress me. Thank you especially to Jason Frank for co-teaching a wonderfully lively course on "Revolution" in which we thought about the common and the collective together; to Stefanos Geroulanos with whom I can always plot conferences, adventures, and joint projects; to Carolyn Dean, who was one of the Press's readers and who has been a mentor and a dear friend for many years now; to Miriam Ticktin, who discussed every idea here on our lovely drives between Brooklyn and Princeton; to Judith Surkis, Todd Shepard, and Sandrine Sanos, cherished friends who make French history the best field to work in; and to Stephanie McCurry, who is a constant source of awe and inspiration. For the joy of common intellectual invention and shared lives, I am also grateful to Tanya Agathocleous, Bruno Bosteels, Zahid Chaudhary, George Chauncey, Thomas Dodman, Tarek el-Ariss, David Eng, Eric Fassin, Michel Feher, Antonio Feros, Paul Friedland, Rossana Fuentes-Berain, Ron Gregg, Itsie Hull, Jerry Johnson, Maria Ospina, Simon Parra, Judith Peraino, Bruno Perreau, Simone Pinet, Teemu Ruskola, Emmanuelle Saada, Francesca Trivellato, and Claudia Verhoeven.

Finally, I want to thank my parents, Sandra Fuentes-Berain and Henri Robcis, for their unwavering love and support, Sebastien Robcis, Darrell Blakely, and Nathan Geddie, for being the best, Gloria Deitcher for her enduring care and affection, and Yael Kropsky, my amazing co-parent, for raising with me such a smart, awesome, and feisty kid. Mila Robcis, Lucia Navarro-Toscano, and Minka, the latest (and most adorable) addition to our household, open new horizons and brighten my life in more ways than I could have imagined. This book is dedicated, with gratitude and devotion, to Caterina Toscano who was very much at the origin of this project when she encouraged me to keep working on "my Catalan doctor." She has never left my mind or my heart since then.

NOTES

All translations are my own, unless otherwise noted.

Introduction

1. See Isabelle von Bueltzingsloewen, *L'hécatombe des fous: La famine dans les hôpitaux psychiatriques français sous l'Occupation* (Paris: Aubier, 2007), 101; Max Lafont, *L'extermination douce: La mort de 40,000 malades mentaux dans les hôpitaux psychiatriques en France sous le Régime de Vichy* (Ligné: Editions de l'Arefppi, 1987).

2. The term "institutional psychotherapy" was first coined in an article written by Georges Daumézon and Philippe Koechlin titled "La psychothérapie institutionnelle française," published in the *Anais portugueses de psiquiatria* in 1952. For some general histories of institutional psychotherapy, see Jean Ayme, "Essai sur l'histoire de la psychothérapie institutionnelle," *Actualités de la psychothérapie institutionnelle* (1985); Pierre Chanoit, *La psychothérapie institutionnelle* (Paris: Presses Universitaires de France, 1995); Jean-Marc Dutrenit, *Sociologie, travail social et psychiatrie: Le berceau lozérien de la psychothérapie institutionnelle* (Paris: Études vivantes, 1981); Patrick Faugeras, ed., *L'ombre portée de François Tosquelles* (Ramonville Saint-Agne: Érès, 2007); Joseph Mornet, *Psychothérapie institutionnelle: Histoire & actualité* (Nîmes: Champ Social Editions, 2007); Jean Oury, *La psychothérapie institutionnelle de Saint-Alban à la Borde* (Paris: Editions d'une, 2016).

3. Jean Oury, "La psychothérapie institutionnelle de Saint-Alban à La Borde," conférence à Poitiers, 1970. Archives IMEC, Fonds Lucien Bonnafé, LBF 70 St Alban 95. ["La psychothérapie institutionnelle, c'est peut-être la mise en place de moyens de toute espèce pour lutter, chaque jour, contre tout ce qui peut faire reverser l'ensemble du collectif vers une structure concentrationnaire ou ségrégative."]

4. For a history of psychiatry in the first part of the twentieth century (especially the tension between biology and culture), see Anne Harrington, *Mind Fixers: Psychiatry's Troubled Search for the Biology of Mental Illness* (New York: W. W. Norton, 2019); Edward Shorter, *A History of Psychiatry: From the Era of the Asylum to the Age of Prozac* (New York: John Wiley, 1997); Andrew Scull, *Madness in Civilization: A Cultural History of Insanity, from the Bible to Freud, from the Madhouse to Modern Medicine* (Princeton: Princeton University Press, 2015); Mark S. Micale and Roy Porter, *Discovering the History*

158 NOTES TO PAGES 5–13

of Psychiatry (New York: Oxford University Press, 1994); Katja Guenther, *Localization and Its Discontents: A Genealogy of Psychoanalysis and the Neuro Disciplines* (Chicago: University of Chicago Press, 2015); Orna Ophir, *Psychosis, Psychoanalysis and Psychiatry in Postwar USA: On the Borderland of Madness* (London: Routledge, 2015). And in the case of France more specifically, see Daniel Widlöcher, "Psychanalyse et psychiatrie française. 50 ans d'histoire," *Topique* 88, no. 3 (2004): 7–16; Jacques Hochmann, *Histoire de la psychiatrie* (Paris: Presses Universitaires de France, 2015).

5. See for example Lacan's manifesto against behaviorism and communication in ego psychology in his 1953 "return to Freud," "The Function and Field of Speech and Language in Psychoanalysis," in Jacques Lacan, *Ecrits: The First Complete Edition in English*, trans. Bruce Fink (New York: W.W. Norton, 2006), 197–268.

6. For a helpful introduction to these other currents, see Jacques Hochmann, *Les antipsychiatries: Une histoire* (Paris: Odile Jacob, 2015); Michael E. Staub, *Madness Is Civilization: When the Diagnosis Was Social, 1948–1980* (Chicago: University of Chicago Press, 2011); Mathieu Bellahsen, *La santé mentale vers un bonheur sous contrôle* (Paris: La Fabrique, 2014).

7. Cited in Homi Bhabha's preface to Frantz Fanon, *The Wretched of the Earth* (2004), xxxvii.

8. Fernand Deligny, *Œuvres*, ed. Sandra Alvarez de Toledo (Paris: L'Arachnéen, 2007); Igor Krtolica, "La 'tentative' des Cévennes. Deligny et la question de l'institution," *Chimères* 72, no. 1 (2010): 73–97.

9. Michel Foucault, preface to Gilles Deleuze and Félix Guattari, *Anti-Oedipus: Capitalism and Schizophrenia* (Minneapolis: University of Minnesota Press, 1983), xiii.

10. See among others, Jan Goldstein, *The Post-Revolutionary Self: Politics and Psyche in France, 1750–1850* (Cambridge: Harvard University Press, 2005); Fernando Vidal, *The Sciences of the Soul: The Early Modern Origins of Psychology* (Chicago: University of Chicago Press, 2011); Jerrold E. Seigel, *The Idea of the Self: Thought and Experience in Western Europe since the Seventeenth Century* (New York: Cambridge University Press, 2005); George Makari, *Soul Machine: The Invention of the Modern Mind* (New York: W. W. Norton, 2015); Nikolas S. Rose, *Inventing Our Selves: Psychology, Power, and Personhood* (Cambridge, UK: Cambridge University Press, 1996).

11. Dagmar Herzog, *Unlearning Eugenics: Sexuality, Reproduction, and Disability in Post-Nazi Europe* (Madison: University of Wisconsin Press, 2018), 12.

12. In Deleuze and Guattari, *Anti-Oedipus*, xii.

13. On the dangers of metaphorizing fascism, see for example Samuel Moyn, "The Trouble with Comparisons," *New York Review of Books*, NYR Daily, May 19, 2020, https://www.nybooks.com/daily/2020/05/19/the-trouble-with-comparisons/.

14. See for example Joy Damousi and Mariano Ben Plotkin, *Psychoanalysis and Politics: Histories of Psychoanalysis under Conditions of Restricted Political Freedom* (New York: Oxford University Press, 2012); Eli Zaretsky, *Political Freud: A History* (New York: Columbia University Press, 2015); Martin Jay, *The Dialectical Imagination: A History of the Frankfurt School and the Institute of Social Research, 1923–1950* (Boston: Little Brown, 1973).

15. See Dominick LaCapra, "History, Language, and Reading: Waiting for Crillon," *American Historical Review* 100, no. 3 (1995): 799–828.

16. Walter Benjamin, *The Origin of German Tragic Drama* (London: Verso, 2003). On this idea of constellations and intellectual history, I am indebted to the work of Gary Wilder and Susan Buck-Morss. See Gary Wilder, *Freedom Time: Negritude, Decolonization, and the Future of the World* (Durham: Duke University Press, 2015); Susan Buck-

NOTES TO PAGES 15–18   159

Morss, *Hegel, Haiti, and Universal History* (Pittsburgh: University of Pittsburgh Press, 2009). See also David Kazanjian's critique of regionalism and his theory of appositional reading (which he opposes to analogy, causality, contrast, or comparison), in *The Brink of Freedom: Improvising Life in the Nineteenth-Century Atlantic World* (Durham, NC: Duke University Press, 2016).

Chapter 1

1. Marius Bonnet, "Le témoignage d'un infirmier," *Esprit* 197, no. 12 (1952): 816.

2. Bruno Coince, "Malades, médecins, infirmiers . . . 'Qui guérissait qui?,'" *Midi libre*, Dec. 3, 1991, Archives IMEC, Fonds Lucien Bonnafé, LBF 70 St Alban 95.

3. Bonnet, "Le témoignage d'un infirmier."

4. "Histoire de Saint-Alban," Archives IMEC, Fonds Lucien Bonnafé, LBF 70 St Alban 95.

5. Freud was especially clear on the challenges that psychotic patients posed to the framework of psychoanalysis in his interpretation of Daniel Paul Schreber's delusions. See Sigmund Freud, *The Schreber Case*, trans. Andrew Webber (New York: Penguin Books, 2003). See also Thomas G. Dalzell, *Freud's Schreber between Psychiatry and Psychoanalysis: On Subjective Disposition to Psychosis* (London: Karnac Books, 2011); Nicolas Gougoulis, "Freud et les psychiatres," *Topique* 88, no. 3 (2004): 17–35.

6. On the idea of "double alienation," see Jean Oury, Félix Guattari, and François Tosquelles, *Pratique de l'institutionnel et politique* (Vigneux: Matrice, 1985), 93; François Tosquelles, "L'effervescence saint-albanaise," *L'Information psychiatrique* 63, no. 8 (1987): 961; François Tosquelles, *L'enseignement de la folie* (Paris: Dunod, 2014), 233–38.

7. François Tosquelles, "Francesc Tosquelles," *Primera Plana* (1984), 18. ["A los 10 años ya sabía lo que haría: llevar a Freud al manicomio, hacer llegar el psicoanálisis a los internados. Ahora bien, luego entendí que sin Marx un psiquiatra no es nada. Marx habla de los problemas del hombre social y Freud habla de la psicopatología del hombre, de por qué está condenado a sufrir. Sin ellos no se entiende nada del hombre, luego no se entiende nada de los locos. Esto no lo quieren entender todos estos psiquiatras biologistas que se creen que van a arreglar el mundo con una pastilla."]

8. Jesus de Felipe-Redondo, "Worker Resistance to 'Social' Reform and the Rise of Anarchism in Spain, 1880–1920," *Critical Historical Studies* 1, no. 2 (2014): 256.

9. See, amongst others, Chris Ealham, *Class, Culture, and Conflict in Barcelona, 1898–1937* (London: Routledge, 2005); Josep Termes, *Història del moviment anarquista a Espanya (1870–1980)* (Barcelona: Avenç, 2011); Frank Mintz, *Anarchism and Workers' Self-Management in Revolutionary Spain* (Oakland, CA: AK Press, 2013); Aurélie Vialette, *Intellectual Philanthropy: The Seduction of the Masses* (West Lafayette, IN: Purdue University Press, 2018). Tosquelles discusses the importance of culture as a vehicle for socialist ideas in Catalonia and mentions, for instance, the Paul Casals "worker concerts," in Tosquelles, *L'enseignement de la folie*, 53.

10. On the POUM, see Víctor Alba and Stephen Schwartz, *Spanish Marxism versus Soviet Communism: A History of the P.O.U.M.* (New Brunswick, NJ: Transaction Books, 1988); Michel Christ, *Le POUM: Histoire d'un parti révolutionnaire espagnol (1935–1952)* (Paris: L'Harmattan, 2005); Wilebaldo Solano, *El POUM en la historia: Andreu Nin y la revolución española* (Madrid: Los Libros de Catarata, 1999). George Orwell also provided a detailed account of the POUM in *Homage to Catalonia* (London: Secker and Warburg, 1938).

11. Alba and Schwartz, *Spanish Marxism Versus Soviet Communism*, 94–95.

160 NOTES TO PAGES 18–22

12. Ibid., 57.

13. Paul Preston, *The Spanish Civil War: Reaction, Revolution and Revenge* (New York: W. W. Norton, 2007), 254.

14. Some of this information concerning Tosquelles's participation in the POUM comes from my conversations with Maria Teresa Carbonell, the widow of Wilebaldo Solano, a close friend of Tosquelles, a historian of the POUM, and the founder of the Andreu Nin Foundation.

15. François Pain, Jean-Claude Polack, and Danielle Sivadon, dirs., *Francesc Tosquelles: Une politique de la folie* (1989). See also François Tosquelles, *Fonction poétique et psychothérapie: Une lecture de "In memoriam" de Gabriel Ferrater* (Ramonville Saint-Agne: Erès, 2003), 167–184; François Tosquelles, "La guerre d'Espagne," *VST—Vie sociale et traitements* (1987): 37. Tosquelles discusses the importance of Catalan workers' self-management in *L'enseignement de la folie*, 172–73.

16. Josep M. Comelles, "Forgotten Paths: Culture and Ethnicity in Catalan Mental Health Policies (1900–39)," *History of Psychiatry* 21, no. 4 (2010): 407.

17. Ibid., 412.

18. Félix Martí Ibáñez, *Obra. Diez meses de labor en Sanidad y Asistencia Social* (Barcelona: Ediciones Tierra y Libertad, 1937), 33. Cited in Comelles, "Forgotten Paths," 415.

19. For more on Mira, see http://www.miraylopez.com and Annette Mülberger and Ana Maria Jacó-Vilela, "Es mejor morir de pie que vivir de rodillas: Emilio Mira y López y la revolucion nacional," *Dynamis* 27 (2006): 309–32. On the history of psychiatry and psychoanalysis in Spain during this period, see Anne-Cécile Druet, "La psychiatrie espagnole et la psychanalyse des années 1910 à la guerre civile. De la presse médicale au discours social," *El Argonauta Español* 8 (2001); Thomas F. Glick, "The Naked Science: Psychoanalysis in Spain, 1914–1948," *Comparative Studies in Society and History of European Ideas* 24 (1982): 533–71.

20. Tosquelles discusses this in *Le vécu de la fin du monde dans la folie: Le témoignage de Gérard de Nerval* (Grenoble: Jérôme Millon, 2012).

21. Tosquelles, *L'enseignement de la folie*, 41–53.

22. Faugeras, *L'ombre portée de François Tosquelles*, 147.

23. Albert Londres, *Chez les fous* (Paris: Albin Michel, 1925), cited in Hochmann, *Les antipsychiatries*, 111. Cursorily defined, moral treatment designated those methods that "engaged or operated directly upon the intellect and emotions, as opposed to the traditional methods of bleeding and purging applied directly to the lunatic's body." Jan Goldstein, *Console and Classify: The French Psychiatric Profession in the Nineteenth Century* (Chicago: University of Chicago Press, 2001), 65.

24. Tosquelles mentions a reading group formed by Mira at the Pere Mata with Villaseca and other doctors in which they read Lacan's thesis, which Tosquelles describes as a "lever" (*levier*). In François Tosquelles, "François Tosquelles par lui-même," *L'âne: Le magazine freudien*, no. 13 (Nov.–Dec. 1983): 5.

25. Pain, Polack, and Sivadon, "Francesc Tosquelles."

26. Jean Ayme, for instance, recounts how Tosquelles printed Lacan's thesis at the Saint-Alban printer and sold copies for 50 French Francs. In Faugeras, *L'ombre portée de François Tosquelles*, 95.

27. Hermann Simon, *Une thérapeutique plus active à l'hôpital* (Berlin: Walter de Gruyter, 1929), 13–14. Translated by François Tosquelles and André Chaurand. Archives Saint-Alban. For more on Simon, see Angela Grütter, *Hermann Simon: Die Entwicklung der Arbeits- und Beschäftigungstherapie in der Anstaltspsychiatrie: Eine biographische Betrachtung* (Herzogenrath: Murken-Altrogge, 1995).

NOTES TO PAGES 22–24

28. Simon, *Une thérapeutique plus active à l'hôpital*, 51.

29. Ibid., 149.

30. Ibid., 16.

31. Ibid., 160.

32. Oury, Guattari, and Tosquelles, *Pratique de l'institutionnel et politique*, 158–59. The Saint-Alban group appeared unaware of—or at least failed to mention—Simon's complicated political convictions. Based on his letters and diaries, by June 1929, Simon was already a proponent of eugenics. By 1946, however, he claimed to be horrified by the mass murder of the cognitively disabled under National Socialism. Like many other conservative German doctors during the interwar period, Simon was a harsh critic of the Weimar Republic, and he welcomed Hitler's seizure of power as the best antidote against communism. According to B. Walter, Simon's commitment to psychiatric reform was driven less by humanitarian concerns than by his attempt to redefine the medical profession and to improve welfare care. See "Hermann Simon—Psychiatriereformer, Sozialdarwinist, Nationalsozialist?," *Der Nervenarzt* 73, no. 11 (2002): 1047–54.

33. François Tosquelles, *Le travail thérapeutique à l'hôpital psychiatrique* (Paris: Editions du Scarabée, 1967), 28.

34. Ibid., 31.

35. Ibid., 36.

36. Ibid., 37.

37. Ibid., 41.

38. For a detailed account of the French battles between psychiatry, psychology, and psychoanalysis, see Elisabeth Roudinesco, *La bataille de cent ans: Histoire de la psychanalyse en France*, vol. 1 (Paris: Ramsay, 1982); Annick Ohayon, *Psychologie et psychanalyse en France: L'impossible rencontre, 1919–1969* (Paris: La Découverte, 2006).

39. On Lacan and psychiatry, see Jacques Sédat, "Lacan et la psychiatrie," *Topique* 88, no. 3 (2004): 37–46; Elisabeth Roudinesco, *Jacques Lacan: Esquisse d'une vie, histoire d'un système de pensée* (Paris: Fayard, 1993); Carolyn J. Dean, *The Self and Its Pleasures: Bataille, Lacan, and the History of the Decentered Subject* (Ithaca: Cornell University Press, 1992), 43–57. On Ey, see Robert Michel Palem, *Henri Ey et la philosophie: Les racines et référents philosophiques et anthropologiques d'Henri Ey* (Paris: L'Harmattan, 2013).

40. Jacques Lacan, *De la psychose paranoïaque dans ses rapports avec la personnalité* (Paris: Seuil, 1975), 15.

41. Ibid. "[La psychose paranoïaque] représente-t-elle le développement d'une personnalité, et alors traduit-elle une anomalie constitutionnelle, ou une déformation réactionnelle? Ou bien la psychose est-elle une maladie autonome, qui remanie la personnalité en brisant le cours de son développement?"]

42. Ibid., 346. ["Il est absurde de rapporter aucun de ces phénomènes à un fait d'automatisme spécifiquement neurologique. Nous démontrons qu'ils relèvent, les uns d'altérations communes de la conscience causées occasionnellement par des troubles organiques généraux, les autres de structures conceptuelles qui tiennent dans notre doctrine à la phénoménologie même de la psychose."]

43. Ibid., 311.

44. Ibid., 323. ["1) les situations de l'histoire infantile du sujet; 2) les structures conceptuelles que relève son délire; 3) les pulsions et les intentions que traduit son comportement social."]

45. Ibid., 41 and 129. For a helpful introduction to the subject as theorized by Freud and Lacan, see Kaja Silverman, *The Subject of Semiotics* (New York: Oxford University Press, 1983), 126–93.

162 NOTES TO PAGES 24-28

46. See Dean, *Self and Its Pleasures*; Michael S. Roth, *Knowing and History: Appropriations of Hegel in Twentieth-Century France* (Ithaca: Cornell University Press, 1988).

47. Roudinesco, *Jacques Lacan*, 78.

48. Roudinesco, *La bataille de cent ans*, 416.

49. Jacques Lacan, *Ecrits*, 58. [Jacques Lacan, *Écrits* (Paris: Seuil, 1966), 73.]

50. *Ecrits*, 75-81. [*Écrits*, 93-100.]

51. *Ecrits*, 65-66. [*Écrits*, 81-82.]

52. *Ecrits*, 72. [*Écrits*, 90.]

53. See for example Oury, Guattari, and Tosquelles, *Pratique de l'institutionnel et politique*, 146.

54. François Tosquelles, Lucien Bonnafé, and André Chaurand, "Note sur l'originalité du pathologique d'après la psychanalyse et sur la valeur du complexe comme perspective structurale dans l'existence pathologique," *Annales médico-psychologiques* 2 (1946): 61. ["C'est dans l'œuvre de Lacan que nous trouverons les thèses les plus aptes à dégager les aspects structuraux de l'existence pathologique, tels que peut les mettre en évidence la perspective psychanalytique."]

55. Ibid., 62. ["Il conditionne l'attitude du malade devant son propre vécu morbide et devant sa situation de malade dans la société."]

56. Ibid. ["Cette conception du complexe a permis à Lacan de préciser le concept d'identification. Celui-ci dépasse l'assimilation globale d'une imago vue de façon statique, il inclut le potentiel impliqué dans le développement par l'imago."]

57. Tosquelles, *L'enseignement de la folie*, 214. ["comme le démontre la thèse de Lacan, il faut envisager le phénomène de la folie dans sa totalité phénoménale, qui se manifeste déjà dans la personnalité."]

58. Pain, Polack, and Sivadon, "Francesc Tosquelles." See also Tosquelles, *L'enseignement de la folie*, 206-7; Tosquelles, "La guerre d'Espagne," 38.

59. See Edgar Jones, "War and the Practice of Psychotherapy: The UK Experience, 1939-1960," *Medical History* 48 (2004): 493-510; Maxwell Jones, *Social Psychiatry: A Study of Therapeutic Communities* (London: Tavistock, 1952); Henry Victor Dicks, *Fifty Years of the Tavistock Clinic* (London: Routledge, 1970); Teri Chettiar, "Democratizing Mental Health: Motherhood, Therapeutic Community and the Emergence of the Psychiatric Family at the Cassel Hospital in Post–Second World War Britain," *History of the Human Sciences* 25, no. 5 (2012): 107-22.

60. Comelles, "Forgotten Paths," 417. See also Mira's account in Emilio Mira y López, *Psychiatry in War* (New York: Norton, 1943).

61. Tosquelles cited in Comelles, "Forgotten Paths," 418.

62. Pelai Pagès i Blanch, *War and Revolution in Catalonia, 1936-1939* (Leiden: Brill, 2013).

63. For a good overview of the historiography of the Spanish camps in France, see Scott Soo, *The Routes to Exile: France and the Spanish Civil War Refugees, 1939-2009* (Manchester: Manchester University Press, 2013). See also Denis Peschanski, *La France des camps: L'internement, 1938-1946* (Paris: Gallimard, 2002); Geneviève Dreyfus-Armand, *L'exil des républicains espagnols en France: De la Guerre civile à la mort de Franco* (Paris: Albin Michel, 1999); Geneviève Dreyfus-Armand and Émile Temime, *Les camps sur la plage: Un exil espagnol* (Paris: Autrement, 1995); Anne Grynberg, *Les camps de la honte: Les internés juifs des camps français 1939-1944* (Paris: La Découverte, 1999).

64. On Septfonds, see Jean-Claude Fau, "Le camp des réfugiés espagnols de Septfonds (Tarn-et-Garonne) 1939-1940," in *Les camps du Sud-Ouest de la France, 1939-1944: Exclusion, internement et déportation*, ed. Monique-Lise Cohen and Éric Malo (Toulouse:

NOTES TO PAGES 29–34   163

Privat, 1994); Geneviève Dreyfus-Armand, *Septfonds, 1939–1944 dans l'archipel des camps français* (Perpignan: Le Revenant, 2019).

65. Dreyfus-Armand, *L'exil des républicains espagnols en France*, 60–61.

66. Archives de l'Association des amis de Septfonds.

67. Archives départementales de Tarn-et-Garonne: 4M vrac4 (État sanitaire des réfugiés espagnols).

68. Soo, *Routes to Exile*, 63.

69. Cited in ibid., 62–64.

70. Cited in Dreyfus-Armand and Temime, *Les camps sur la plage*, 87. ["La neurasthénie faisait des ravages parmi nous. Les maniaques et les obsédés étaient nombreux. Le manque d'alimentation affaiblissait nos têtes, et le désespoir faisait chavirer nos raisons."]

71. Tosquelles cited in Dreyfus-Armand, *Septfonds*, 90.

72. Pain, Polack, and Sivadon, "Francesc Tosquelles." On this period of Tosquelles's life, see also his daughter's memoir, Marie-Rose Ourabah, *À l'ombre des poiriers: Hélène et François Tosquelles, un secret de famille* (Saint-Denis: Édilivre, 2014).

73. Testimony of Henri Salès from Caussade (formerly detained at Septfonds) collected by the Museum of the Resistance and Deportation in Montauban, cited in Dreyfus-Armand, *Septfonds*, 92.

74. Tosquelles, *L'enseignement de la folie*, 109; Faugeras, *L'ombre portée de François Tosquelles*, 128.

75. Tosquelles, *L'enseignement de la folie*, 110.

76. See Jacques Tosquellas, "Courriers Tosquelles-Balvet," *Sud/Nord* 19, no. 1 (2003): 171–84.

77. See Alice Ricardi von Platen, *L'extermination des malades mentaux dans l'Allemagne nazie* (Toulouse: Erès, 2001); Robert N. Proctor, *Racial Hygiene: Medicine under the Nazis* (Cambridge: Harvard University Press, 1988); Herzog, *Unlearning Eugenics*.

78. See Bueltzingsloewen, *L'hécatombe des fous*, 101; Lafont, *L'extermination douce*. For a refutation of this thesis that Vichy had a secret plan to exterminate psychiatric patients, see Pierre Bailly-Salin, "The Mentally Ill under Nazi Occupation in France," *International Journal of Mental Health* 35, no. 4 (2006–7): 11–25.

79. Martine Deyres, *Les heures heureuses* (Marseille: Les Films du tambour de soie, 2019).

80. As Peter Lieb and Robert O. Paxton have shown, the Germans, in fact, never had quite enough troops to actually control all of the French territory: "Maintenir l'ordre en France occupée. Combien de divisions?," *Vingtième Siècle. Revue d'histoire* 112, no. 4 (2011): 115–26.

81. Tosquelles, *L'enseignement de la folie*, 117. According to Bonnafé, Balvet was a *catholique de gauche* who welcomed Pétain's arrival to power but later became an active member of the Resistance (Archives IMEC, Fonds Lucien Bonnafé, LBF 70 St Alban 95).

82. Cited in Deyres, *Les heures heureuses*. ["Docteur Toscalès, aurait une influence des plus néfastes sur tout le personnel de cet hôpital. Tendances nettement révolutionnaires et anti-nationales. Bon praticien; a toute la confiance et l'estime du docteur Balvet, médecin directeur de l'asile. Reconstitution C.G.T. et menées anti-nationales voire même communistes. Gasc-Pic-Bonnet-Kayzac-Constant. Tous ces hommes, employés à l'asile de St-Alban, auraient une action des plus louches parmi le personnel."] (Renseignements Généraux, Mende, April 29, 1942).

83. Lafont, *L'extermination douce*, 146. ["L'occupation a joué un rôle d'une importance extrême dans cette initiation du Je vers le nous de l'équipe soignante. Il y a eu sous l'oc-

164 NOTES TO PAGES 34–36

cupation une expérience de fraternité qui est essentielle, et pas seulement à St. Alban."]
For an account of Saint-Alban during the war (between fiction and memoir), see Didier
Daeninckx, *Caché dans la maison des fous* (Paris: Gallimard, 2017).

84. See "L'esprit de secteur: Entretien avec Lucien Bonnafé," http://ancien.serpsy
.org/histoire/bonnafe1.html. On French communists' role during the Resistance, see
Stéphane Courtois, *Le PCF dans la guerre: De Gaulle, la Résistance, Staline* (Paris: Ramsay, 1980); Jean-Pierre Rioux, Antoine Prost, and Jean-Pierre Azéma, *Le Parti communiste
français des années sombres, 1938–1941* (Paris: Seuil, 1986).

85. This biography of Bonnafé comes from Armand Olivennes's introduction to Lucien Bonnafé, *Désaliéner?: folie(s) et société(s)* (Toulouse: Presses universitaires du Mirail,
1991), and from the Lucien Bonnafé archives at the IMEC. For more on the Balvet/
Bonnafé relationship, see Paul Balvet, "L'ambre du musée," *L'Information psychiatrique*
54, no. 8 (1978): 861–64. See also the testimony of Marie Bonnafé (Lucien's wife) in
Deyres, *Les heures heureuses*.

86. On Éluard at Saint-Alban, see Dominique Mabin and Renée Mabin, "Art, folie et
surréalisme à l'hôpital psychiatrique de Saint-Alban-sur-Limagnole pendant la guerre
de 1939–1945," *ASTU* (2015), https://melusine-surrealisme.fr/wp/?p=1775#_ftn12. See
also Jean-Charles Gateau, *Paul Éluard ou le frère voyant, 1895–1952* (Paris: Robert Laffont, 1988).

87. Archives IMEC, Fonds Lucien Bonnafé, LBF 70 St Alban 95 (+ autres dates):
Dossier: Saint-Alban et la Résistance: Proscrits et patriotes. ["Nous partions à Saint-Flour, le bourg voisin, dans la voiture gazogène de l'hôpital pour rendre visite à Amarger, un résistant qui avait sa propre imprimerie; nous emportions avec nous du papier
Canson ou Ingres pour qu'Amarger imprime des éditions de luxe destinées aux mécènes
de la Résistance."]

88. Archives IMEC, Fonds Lucien Bonnafé, LBF 70 St Alban 95: "Désaliénisme et
histoire des idées, 26 mai 1995." ["De cette vision surréaliste restaurant le sujet souffrant
de troubles relationnels comme sujet humain, Éluard fut le plus constant porte-parole;
le thème de résistance aux proscriptions de la différence, et d'éloge des similitudes, est
présent partout: 'Je suis la ressemblance. Tu es la ressemblance'; 'Le surréalisme travaille
à réduire les différences qui existent entre les hommes, et, pour cela, il refuse de servir un
ordre absurde.' Il est riche de sens que, quand il fallut que 'la poésie prenne le maquis,' ce
fut en partageant la vie d'un hôpital psychiatrique que s'accomplirent amour des différences et dénonciation d'un ordre absurde, avec le regard sur les vivants: 'ma souffrance
est souillée,' et sur les morts: 'Ce cimetière est un lieu sans raison.'"]

89. Georges Canguilhem, *Résistance, philosophie biologique et histoire des sciences,
1940–1965*, ed. Camille Limoges (Paris: Librairie philosophique J. Vrin, 2015), 16 and
183. See also Elisabeth Roudinesco, *Philosophes dans la tourmente* (Paris: Points, 2011);
Dominique Lecourt, *Georges Canguilhem* (Paris: PUF, 2016); Giuseppe Bianco, "La réaction au bergsonisme: Transformations de la philosophie française de Politzer à Deleuze,"
Université Charles de Gaulle—Lille 3, 2009; Stuart Elden, *Canguilhem* (Cambridge, UK:
Polity, 2019).

90. Paul Arrighi, *Silvio Trentin: Un Européen en résistance, 1919–1943* (Portet-sur-Garonne: Loubatières, 2007).

91. Bonnafé, *Désaliéner?*, 213.

92. Lucien Bonnafé, "Rencontres autour de François Tosquelles," *L'Évolution psychiatrique* 60 (Jul.–Aug. 1965): 662.

93. Lucien Bonnafé, André Chaurand, and François Tosquelles, "Structure et sens de
l'événement morbide," *Annales médico-psychologiques* 1 (1945): par175–76. ["En clinique

psychiatrique, le malade se donne d'emblée comme une 'forme de vie' différente, mais les travaux de méthodologie médicale s'orientent dans la même voie. Canguilhem a souligné récemment, dans une étude sur le normal et le pathologique, sans faire appel aux notions de la clinique psychiatrique, que l'événement morbide n'est pas un simple prolongement quantitativement varié de l'état physiologique, il est une autre 'forme de vie.'"]

94. Archives IMEC, Fonds Lucien Bonnafé, LBF 70 St Alban 95, "Journées de Saint-Alban." ["Ce qui est advenu à Saint-Alban n'est vraiment intelligible que si l'on le comprend comme produit de la radicalité dans la résistance à l'inhumanité aliéniste ou asilaire. . . . Ce qui est advenu à Saint Alban n'est bien intelligible qu'en le situant dans la Résistance à l'occupation nazie et à la collaboration. . . . C'est maintenant résistance à l'ignorantisme que de rappeler quelle fut la fonction, dans 'ce qui est advenu, ' du regard surréaliste sur la folie, que représenta notre fraternité avec Éluard. Ce ne l'est pas moins que de rappeler notre participation au travail de 'nouvel esprit scientifique' dépisteur de méconnaissances et ouvreur de connaissances, en rupture avec l'étroitesse scientiste, que représenta notre fraternité avec Georges Canguilhem."]

95. Archives IMEC, Fonds Lucien Bonnafé, LBF 70 St Alban 95: Handwritten notes. ["Tout ce qui tend à soumettre le sujet à une puissance étrangère à lui-même. À l'intoxiquer de 'c'est plus fort que moi.' À le soumettre à une directrice de conscience, à une interdiction de penser."]

96. Coince, "Malades, médecins, infirmiers," *Midi libre*, Dec. 3, 1991, Archives IMEC, Fonds Lucien Bonnafé, LBF 70 St Alban 95 (+ other dates). ["C'est là que j'ai changé. Dans ce camp de concentration, je me suis rappelé l'asile et j'ai comparé ma condition de prisonnier à celle des malades mentaux."]

97. Jean Oury, "La psychothérapie institutionnelle de Saint-Alban à La Borde," conférence à Poitiers, 1970. Archives IMEC, Fonds Lucien Bonnafé, LBF 70 St Alban 95. ["La psychothérapie institutionnelle, c'est peut-être la mise en place de moyens de toute espèce pour lutter, chaque jour, contre tout ce qui peut faire reverser l'ensemble du collectif vers une structure concentrationnaire ou ségrégative."]

98. Bonnafé, *Désaliéner*, 212. ["société à vocations multiples: il y a la recherche incessante, ancrée dans la pratique quotidienne, d'une nouvelle clinique, fondée sur l'insoumission au modèle 'clinicoïde' dominant, signifiant clairement l'effacement du sujet derrière le symptôme. Il y a l'approfondissement incessant de la critique constructive de l'institution instituée comme lieu de ségrégation avec, dans le même mouvement, à la fois le travail pour instituer dans ce lieu voué à produire un système de rapports suraliénant des rapports désaliénants, à la fois le développement de pratiques désenclavées, hors les murs, à l'enseigne d'une 'géo-psychiatrie.'"]

99. Tosquelles, *L'enseignement de la folie*, 213. ["La spéculation psychologique et psychopathologique doit avoir pour but la vérité pratique."]

100. Archives IMEC, Fonds Lucien Bonnafé, LBF 67: Manifeste de la Société du Gévaudan, July 1941. ["On peut aller plus loin. Est-ce que ce sont des malades? Est-ce que la conception de 'maladie' épuise tout le sens de l'aliénation mentale?"]

101. Tosquelles, *L'enseignement de la folie*, 214. ["On peut dire que la folie n'a pas de commencement. Malgré l'utilité des troubles générateurs, comme le démontre la thèse de Lacan, il faut envisager le phénomène de la folie dans sa totalité phénoménale, qui se manifeste déjà dans la personnalité."]

102. Ibid., 216. ["La folie n'a pas son début dans un trouble générateur; elle est un phénomène historique et dialectique. Les investigations génétiques de la personnalité d'un malade sont des investigations unilatérales; elles ne saisissent pas l'ensemble du fait historique."]

166 NOTES TO PAGES 39–41

103. Balvet, "L'ambre du musée," 861.

104. Cited in Lafont, *L'extermination douce*, 131. ["Nous n'avons en psychiatrie aucune doctrine générale d'assistance. . . . L'asile d'aliénés a changé de nom, la réalité est restée."]

105. Cited in ibid., 132.

106. Coince, "Malades, médecins, infirmiers.'" *Midi libre*, Dec. 3, 1991, Archives IMEC, Fonds Lucien Bonnafé, LBF 70 St Alban 95. ["on a abattu des murs d'enceinte. Ainsi, il n'y avait plus de frontière entre l'hôpital et la commune de Saint-Alban. . . . Après la guerre, la Libération du territoire a aussi libéré l'asile."]

107. Cited in Lucile Johnes, "Désaliénisme à l'hôpital psychiatrique de Saint-Alban-sur-Limagnole: L'accueil de la folie dans un hôpital public de Lozère de la fin de la deuxième guerre mondiale au début des années 1970," Université de Lettres Paul Valéry, 2010, 39.

108. Cited in ibid., 35. ["lorsqu'on ne peut plus camisoler ou enfermer purement et simplement un malade, on est obligé de penser à prévoir ses réactions, et de ce fait, pénétrer les mécanismes de sa maladie."]

109. Georges Daumézon, "Le poids des structures," *Esprit* 197 (Dec. 1952): 944.

110. Louis Le Guillant and Lucien Bonnafé, "Le condition du malade à l'hôpital psychiatrique," *Esprit* 197(Dec. 1952): 868. ["Les aliénés sont (aux yeux de la classe dominante) les noirs, les indigènes, les juifs, les prolétaires des autres malades."]

111. François Tosquelles, "La société vécue par les malades psychiques," *Esprit* 197 (Dec. 1952): 901. ["Chez la plupart de nos malades, les actes, les délires ou les confidences traduisent facilement des conflits intimes toujours intersociaux, et plus précisément familiaux, conflits dont il est parfois possible de mettre à jour la filière ou les emboitements successifs, qui nous mènent toujours à des situations typiques de l'enfance, semblables à celles qui ont été décrites par les psychanalystes. L'hôpital jouerait au point de vue thérapeutique un rôle analogue à celui du psychanalyste. Il serait l'objet d'investissements successifs de ces conflits; et la dialectique de la guérison passerait, pour ainsi dire, dans ce laminoir de transferts et de projections que la structure de l'hôpital pourrait permettre."]

112. François Tosquelles, "L'effervescence saint-albanaise," 960. ["C'est dans ces collectifs que surgit, avec les échanges sociaux concrets, toute une autre dynamique des 'éléments psychiques' en jeu à saisir. Il s'agit des collectifs des 'ensembles,' qui fonctionnent toujours en systèmes ouverts et incidents dans le temps et l'espace."]

113. "Symposium sur le psychothérapie collective," *L'Évolution psychiatrique* 3 (1952): 535. ["C'est cette vie interne qu'il importe de saisir comme constituant le milieu inter-social de cure: l'ensemble de malades, ses groupements, ses inter-relations avec le personnel soignant, avec le personnel administratif et les médecins aussi."]

114. Ibid., 542. ["Le Club est en grande partie l'expression automatique de l'ensemble de l'hôpital, du fait que bien qu'ayant pour ainsi dire un grand nombre d'activités propres, ces activités transcendent à la vie des quartiers."]

115. Jean Lafeuillade, "Mémoire de stage: Structures et problèmes de l'hôpital psychiatrique moderne, exemple de l'hôpital psychiatrique de Saint-Alban (Lozère)," Dec. 1968, p. 16. Archives St. Alban.

116. Coince, "Malades, médecins, infirmiers," *Midi libre*, Dec. 3, 1991, Archives IMEC, Fonds Lucien Bonnafé, LBF 70 St Alban 95. ["Quand le bureau du club se réunissait, il analysait les idées émises dans les commissions. Et lorsqu'un malade, sans prévenir, confiait l'un de ses problèmes, l'ordre du jour était abandonné et tout le monde l'écoutait. Commençait alors le dialogue psychothérapique. Mais je peux prendre un autre cas: par exemple, quand un patient déclarait, concernant les fournitures de la bibliothèque, "qu'on n'aurait jamais dû acheter tel livre," un médecin lui demandait s'il avait lu dans ce

NOTES TO PAGES 41–47

livre un passage qui l'avait gêné. Et de nouveau, ça discutait. Vous voyez, à Saint-Alban, tout était prétexte à un dialogue et pas seulement dans ce genre de réunion. Ailleurs, également, dans la vie de tous les jours. Le jardinier, le cuisinier, la secrétaire, l'infirmier, l'électricien . . . tous les employés intervenaient dans le système de la psychothérapie. Si le jardinier proposait une idée, un malade pouvait lui répondre qu'elle était mauvaise. Au fond, quand je repense à cette période, j'en viens à me poser la question suivante: à Saint-Alban, qui guérissait qui?"]

117. Tosquelles's editorials from *Trait d'union* were collected in François Tosquelles, *"Trait-d'union" journal de Saint-Alban: éditoriaux, articles, notes (1950–1962)* (Paris: Éditions d'une, 2015).

118. Archives Saint-Alban. ["un intérêt d'ordre thérapeutique actif qui dépasse sa valeur proprement documentaire, littéraire ou d'information générale et locale. Lire le journal est un acte typiquement social . . . , c'est sortir de soi pour écouter la voix des autres et s'intéresser à leurs joies et à leur peines. Beaucoup de vous ont perdu le goût, le courage ou l'initiative, du fait même de la fatigue ou des chagrins, ou n'aiment plus entrer en contact avec d'autres personnes. Vous vous isolez trop; vous vivez ensemble, mais le plus souvent chacun dans sa coquille. *Trait-d'union* entre vous, et entre vous et le monde, entre vos pavillons, entre vous et le personnel."]

119. Jean Lafeuillade, "Mémoire de stage: Structures et problèmes de l'hôpital psychiatrique moderne, exemple de l'Hôpital Psychiatrique de Saint-Alban (Lozère)," Dec. 1968, p. 18. Archives Saint-Alban.

120. Tosquelles cited in Johnes, "Désaliénisme à l'hôpital psychiatrique de Saint-Alban-sur-Limagnole," 43.

121. Christophe Boulanger et al., *Trait d'union: Les chemins de l'art brut à Saint-Alban-sur-Limagnole* (Lille: Musée d'art moderne Lille, 2007).

122. Jean Dubuffet, *L'art brut préféré aux arts culturels* (Paris: Galerie René Drouin, 1949).

123. Daniel Abadie, ed., *Dubuffet: Catalogue de l'exposition "Jean Dubuffet" présentée à l'occasion du centenaire de la naissance de l'artiste, Centre Pompidou, 2001* (Paris: Centre Pompidou, 2001); Julien Dieudonné and Marianne Jakobi, *Dubuffet* (Paris: Perrin, 2007).

124. Cited in Deyres, *Les heures heureuses*. On Forestier, see https://www.artbrut.ch /en_GB/author/forestier-auguste.

125. In Deyres, *Les heures heureuses*. See also Jean Oury, *Essai sur la création esthétique* (Paris: Hermann, 2008); Henning Schmidgen, "Jean Oury et la conation esthétique. Un parcours entre Sartre, Goldstein et Lacan," *Revue germanique internationale* 30 (2019); Christophe Boulanger, "La conation esthétique de Jean Oury," in *Le Collectif à venir* (Toulouse: ERES, 2018), 101–14.

126. Rencontres de Saint-Alban, June 20–21, 1986. Archives Pere Mata in Reus.

127. Dutrenit, *Sociologie, travail social et psychiatrie*, 15.

128. Pain, Polack, and Sivadon, "Francesc Tosquelles." ["Abattre les murs, enlever les barreaux, supprimer les serrures. Ce n'est pas suffisant. Il faut analyser, mais surtout combattre les pouvoirs, les hiérarchies, les habitudes, les féodalités locales, les corporatismes. Rien ne va jamais de soi, tout est prétexte à réunions. Chacun doit être consulté, chacun peut décider. Non simple souci de démocratie, mais conquête progressive de la parole, apprentissage réciproque du respect. Les malades doivent avoir prise sur leurs conditions de séjour et de soins, sur les droits d'échanges, d'expression et de circulation."]

129. Ibid. ["Troisième principe, de révolution permanente: le travail n'est jamais terminé, qui transforme un établissement de soins en institution, une équipe soignante en

168 NOTES TO PAGES 48–52

collectif. C'est l'élaboration constante des moyens matériels et sociaux, des conditions conscientes et inconscientes d'une psychothérapie. Et celle-ci n'est pas le fait des seuls médecins ou spécialistes, mais d'un agencement complexe où les malades eux-mêmes ont un rôle primordial."]

Chapter 2

1. Frantz Fanon, *Toward the African Revolution: Political Essays*, trans. Haakon Chevalier (New York: Grove Press, 1967), 53. [Frantz Fanon, *Œuvres* (Paris: La Découverte, 2011), 734.]

2. In her biography, Alice Cherki recounts how Fanon first became involved with the FLN through various members of the editorial board of the journal *Consciences maghrébines*. Cherki, *Frantz Fanon: portrait* (Paris: Seuil, 2000), 113–16.

3. Fanon, *Toward the African Revolution*, 53.

4. Cited in Homi K. Bhabha's forward to Frantz Fanon, *The Wretched of the Earth*, trans. Richard Philcox (New York: Grove Press, 2004), xxxvii.

5. Frantz Fanon, *Alienation and Freedom*, ed. Jean Khalfa and Robert Young, trans. Steve Corcoran (London: Bloomsbury, 2018), 497. [Frantz Fanon, *Écrits sur l'aliénation et la liberté*, ed. by Jean Khalfa and Robert Young (Paris: La Découverte, 2015), 419.]

6. In addition to the introductory essays by Jean Khalfa and Robert Young in Fanon, *Alienation and Freedom*, see Cherki, *Frantz Fanon*; Richard C. Keller, "Clinician and Revolutionary: Frantz Fanon, Biography, and the History of Colonial Medicine," *Bulletin of the History of Medicine* 81 (2007): 823–41; David Macey, *Frantz Fanon: A Biography* (London: Verso, 2012); Hussein Abdilahi Bulhan, *Frantz Fanon and the Psychology of Oppression* (New York: Plenum Press, 1985); Claudine Ranzanajao and Jacques Postel, "La vie et l'œuvre psychiatrique de Frantz Fanon," *Sud/Nord* 22, no. 1 (2007): 147–74; Achille Mbembe, *Politiques de l'inimitié* (Paris: La Découverte, 2016); Jean Khalfa, "Fanon and Psychiatry," *Nottingham French Studies* 54, no. 1 (2015): 52–71; Françoise Vergès, "Creole Skin, Black Mask: Fanon and Disavowal," *Critical Inquiry* 23, no. 3 (1997): 578–95; Nigel C. Gibson and Roberto Beneduce, *Decolonizing Madness: The Psychiatric Writings of Frantz Fanon* (New York: Palgrave Macmillan, 2014); Frantz Fanon, *Frantz Fanon par les textes de l'époque* (Paris: Les Petits Matins, 2012); David S. Marriott, *Whither Fanon?: Studies in the Blackness of Being* (Stanford: Stanford University Press, 2018); Gavin Arnall, *Subterranean Fanon: An Underground Theory of Radical Change* (New York: Columbia University Press, 2020).

7. Macey, *Frantz Fanon*, 208–9.

8. Ranzanajao and Postel, "La vie et l'œuvre psychiatrique de Frantz Fanon," 148.

9. François Tosquelles, "Frantz Fanon à Saint-Alban," *Sud/Nord* 22, no. 1 (2007):

10. ["caricature . . . du cartésianisme analytique, fleuron de son efficacité sur l'objet anatomo-physiopathologique qui fonde la médecine en général et s'émiette en spécialisations sans fin ni mesure. Lyon avait produit . . . des 'Abrégés médico-chirurgicaux' dont deux volumes voués à la psychiatrie et à la formation professionnelle des psychiatres. Un chapitre par maladie. L'enchaînement bien connu: diagnostic, pronostic, traitement . . . TRAITEMENT: INTERNEMENT."]

10. It is likely that Fanon encountered the work of Lacan through Merleau-Ponty, who referenced it frequently in his 1950s courses on psychology and pedagogy, but it is also possible that he first read him through the Saint-Alban doctors, who cited Lacan extensively in *L'Évolution psychiatrique*, as we saw in chapter 1. On the importance of phenomenology for Fanon, see Hourya Bentouhami, "L'emprise du corps: Fanon à l'aune de

NOTES TO PAGES 52–57

la phénoménologie de Merleau-Ponty," *Cahiers Philosophiques* 3, no. 138 (2014): 34–46; David Macey, "Fanon, Phenomenology, Race," *Radical Philosophy* 95 (May/June 1999): 8–14; Gayle Salamon, "'The Place Where Life Hides Away': Merleau-Ponty, Fanon, and the Location of Bodily Being," *differences* 17, no. 2 (2006): 96–112. A list of the books in Fanon's library with his notes is available in Fanon, *Alienation and Freedom*, 719–78 [*Écrits sur l'aliénation et la liberté*, 587–654].

11. Fanon, *Alienation and Freedom*, 206. [*Écrits sur l'aliénation et la liberté*, 170.] Some translations are modified.

12. Fanon, *Alienation and Freedom*, 224. [*Écrits sur l'aliénation et la liberté*, 187.]

13. Fanon, *Alienation and Freedom*, 247. [*Écrits sur l'aliénation et la liberté*, 206.]

14. Fanon, *Alienation and Freedom*, 254. [*Écrits sur l'aliénation et la liberté*, 213.]

15. Fanon, *Alienation and Freedom*, 258. [*Écrits sur l'aliénation et la liberté*, 216.] For more on Goldstein's holism, see Stefanos Geroulanos and Todd Meyers, *The Human Body in the Age of Catastrophe: Brittleness, Integration, Science, and the Great War* (Chicago: University of Chicago Press, 2018).

16. Fanon, *Alienation and Freedom*, 262. [*Écrits sur l'aliénation et la liberté*, 220.]

17. Fanon, *Alienation and Freedom*, 264. [*Écrits sur l'aliénation et la liberté*, 221–22.]

18. Fanon, *Alienation and Freedom*, 265. [*Écrits sur l'aliénation et la liberté*, 222.]

19. Fanon, *Toward the African Revolution*, 8. [*Œuvres*, 696.]

20. Fanon, *Toward the African Revolution*, 6. [*Œuvres*, 694.]

21. Fanon, *Toward the African Revolution*, 7. [*Œuvres*, 694.]

22. Fanon, *Toward the African Revolution*, 13. [*Œuvres*, 700.]

23. Fanon, *Toward the African Revolution*, 15. [*Œuvres*, 702.]

24. On the Fourth Republic and decolonization, see Frederick Cooper, *Citizenship between Empire and Nation: Remaking France and French Africa, 1945–1960* (Princeton: Princeton University Press, 2014); Wilder, *Freedom Time*.

25. Alice Cherki recounts that Fanon was able to publish in *Esprit* at such a young age through one of his professors, Michel Colin, who happened to be the brother-in-law of Jean-Marie Domenach, the editor-in-chief of the journal at that time. Cherki, *Frantz Fanon*, 31.

26. Macey, *Frantz Fanon*, 153.

27. Ibid., 136–37.

28. Frantz Fanon, *Black Skin, White Masks*, trans. Richard Philcox (New York: Grove Press, 2008), xiv. [*Œuvres*, 66.]

29. Fanon, *Black Skin, White Masks*, xvi. [*Œuvres*, 67.]

30. Fanon, *Black Skin, White Masks*, xv. [*Œuvres*, 66.]

31. Fanon, *Black Skin, White Masks*, xv. [*Œuvres*, 66.]

32. Fanon, *Black Skin, White Masks*, 92. [*Œuvres*, 155.]

33. Fanon, *Black Skin, White Masks*, 73. [*Œuvres*, 137.]

34. Fanon, *Black Skin, White Masks*, 95. [*Œuvres*, 158.] On Sartre's *Anti-Semite and Jew*, see Jonathan Judaken, *Jean-Paul Sartre and the Jewish Question: Anti-Antisemitism and the Politics of the French Intellectual* (Lincoln: University of Nebraska Press, 2006).

35. Fanon, *Black Skin, White Masks*, 199. [*Œuvres*, 245.]

36. Fanon, *Black Skin, White Masks*, chap. 2. As many commentators have noted, Fanon was remarkably ungenerous in his reading of Capécia. For a more nuanced approach to the intersections of race and gender in her novels, see Myriam Cottias and Madeleine Dobie, *Relire Mayotte Capécia: Une femme des Antilles dans l'espace colonial français* (Paris: Armand Colin, 2012).

37. Fanon, *Black Skin, White Masks*, xiv. [*Œuvres*, 65.]

170 NOTES TO PAGES 57–61

38. Fanon, *Black Skin, White Masks*, 202. [*Œuvres*, 248.]

39. Much of the recent work on *négritude* has in fact emphasized its deep interest in the question of time, temporality, and hybridity, thus challenging Fanon's claim that *négritude* was simply an unsophisticated return to the past. See Wilder, *Freedom Time*; Souleymane Bachir Diagne, "La Négritude comme mouvement et comme devenir," *Rue Descartes* 83, no. 4 (2014): 50–61; Natalie Melas, "Untimeliness, or Négritude and the Poetics of Contramodernity," *South Atlantic Quarterly* 108, no. 3 (2009): 563–80. And for a *rapprochement* between Fanon and Césaire, see Gary Wilder, "Race, Reason, Impasse: Césaire, Fanon, and the Legacy of Emancipation," *Radical History Review* 90 (Fall 2004): 31–61.

40. Fanon, *Black Skin, White Masks*, 112. [*Œuvres*, 171.] On the triangulation of Sartre, Fanon, and *négritude*, see also Ranjana Khanna, *Dark Continents: Psychoanalysis and Colonialism* (Durham, NC: Duke University Press, 2003), 138–42; Paige Arthur, *Unfinished Projects: Decolonization and the Philosophy of Jean-Paul Sartre* (London: Verso, 2010), 30–41.

41. Fanon, *Black Skin, White Masks*, 114. [*Œuvres*, 172.]

42. Fanon, *Black Skin, White Masks*, 201. [*Œuvres*, 247.]

43. Fanon, *Black Skin, White Masks*, 205. [*Œuvres*, 250.]

44. Fanon, *Black Skin, White Masks*, xvii. [*Œuvres*, 68.] Octave Mannoni, *Psychologie de la colonisation* (Paris: Seuil, 1950). Translated in English as Octave Mannoni, *Prospero and Caliban: The Psychology of Colonization* (Ann Arbor: University of Michigan Press, 1990).

45. See Jennifer Cole, *Forget Colonialism?: Sacrifice and the Art of Memory in Madagascar* (Berkeley: University of California Press, 2001).

46. Fanon, *Black Skin, White Masks*, 65. [*Œuvres*, 130.]

47. Fanon, *Black Skin, White Masks*, 66. [*Œuvres*, 130.]

48. Fanon, *Black Skin, White Masks*, 74. [*Œuvres*, 138.]

49. Fanon, *Black Skin, White Masks*, 66. [*Œuvres*, 131.]

50. Fanon, *Black Skin, White Masks*, 68. [*Œuvres*, 132.]

51. Fanon, *Black Skin, White Masks*, 72. [*Œuvres*, 136.] On Mannoni and Fanon, see also Jock McCulloch, *Colonial Psychiatry and "the African Mind"* (Cambridge: Cambridge University Press, 1995); Bulhan, *Frantz Fanon and the Psychology of Oppression*; Claire Mestre and Marie-Rose Moro, "L'intime et le politique: Projet pour une ethnopsychanalyse critique," *L'Autre* 13, no. 3 (2012/13): 263–72; Macey, *Frantz Fanon*; Christopher Lane, "Psychoanalysis and Colonialism Redux: Why Mannoni's 'Prospero Complex' Still Haunts Us," *Journal of Modern Literature* 25, nos. 3/4 (2002): 127–50.

52. Macey, *Frantz Fanon*, 139.

53. Ranzanajao and Postel, "La vie et l'œuvre psychiatrique de Frantz Fanon," 149.

54. For more on Fanon and psychiatry in Martinique, see Didier Tristram, "Frantz Fanon, le 'chaînon manquant' de la psychiatrie martiniquaise," *Sud/Nord* 22, no. 1 (2007): 39–43.

55. François Tosquelles, "Frantz Fanon et la psychothérapie institutionnelle," *Sud/Nord* 22, no. 1 (2007): 75–76; Tosquelles, "Frantz Fanon à Saint-Alban."

56. Archives IMEC, Fonds Frantz Fanon, FNN1.17 and FNN1.18. These editorials have been reprinted in Fanon, *Alienation and Freedom*, 279–84. [*Écrits sur l'aliénation et la liberté*, 234–37.]

57. "On Some Cases Treated with the Bini Method" (July 1953), in *Alienation and Freedom*, 285–90. [*Écrits sur l'aliénation et la liberté*, 238–42.] For a historical perspective on these techniques, including in institutional psychotherapy, see Hervé Guillemain,

"Les effets secondaires de la technique. Patients et institutions psychiatriques au temps de l'électrochoc, de la psychochirurgie et des neuroleptiques retard (années 1940–1970)," *Revue d'histoire moderne & contemporaine* 67-1, no. 1 (2020): 72–98.

58. Tosquelles, "Frantz Fanon à Saint-Alban," 11–12. ["Saint-Alban constituait le lieu d'une hypothèse. . . . Un lieu 'ouvert' par dedans et pas dehors. . . . L'hypothèse posée à Saint-Alban rassemblait des êtres humains, fous ou pas fous, pour qu'ils puissent puiser dans leurs propres possibilités la matière mobile articulable et réarticulable dont ils sont constitués . . . par l'histoire . . . Certains appelleraient cela processus de guérison."]

59. See Fanon's letter to Maurice Despinoy from June 1953, at the Archives IMEC, Fonds Frantz Fanon, FNN2.4, reprinted in Fanon, *Alienation and Freedom*, 277. [*Écrits sur l'aliénation et la liberté*, 233.]

60. Ranzanajao and Postel, "La vie et l'œuvre psychiatrique de Frantz Fanon," 151–52.

61. Macey, *Frantz Fanon*, 206–7; Cherki, *Frantz Fanon*, 39.

62. Richard C. Keller, *Colonial Madness: Psychiatry in French North Africa* (Chicago: University of Chicago Press, 2007), 48. The literature on psychiatry and colonialism is rich and helpful in situating Fanon in a wider context but also in pointing to the specificity of his project. See, among others, Megan Vaughan, *Curing Their Ills: Colonial Power and African Illness* (Stanford: Stanford University Press, 1991); Matthew M. Heaton, *Black Skin, White Coats: Nigerian Psychiatrists, Decolonization, and the Globalization of Psychiatry* (Athens: Ohio University Press, 2013); Warwick Anderson, Deborah Jenson, and Richard C. Keller, *Unconscious Dominions: Psychoanalysis, Colonial Trauma, and Global Sovereignties* (Durham, NC: Duke University Press, 2011); Sloan Mahone and Megan Vaughan, *Psychiatry and Empire* (Basingstoke, UK: Palgrave Macmillan, 2007); Dagmar Herzog, *Cold War Freud: Psychoanalysis in an Age of Catastrophes* (Cambridge: Cambridge University Press, 2017); Erik Linstrum, *Ruling Minds: Psychology in the British Empire* (Cambridge: Harvard University Press, 2016); Jonathan Sadowsky, *Imperial Bedlam: Institutions of Madness in Colonial Southwest Nigeria* (Berkeley: University of California Press, 1999); McCulloch, *Colonial Psychiatry and "the African Mind."*

63. On Porot and the Algiers School, in addition to Keller, Macey, Gibson and Beneduce, and Cherki, see Jean-Michel Bégué, "French Psychiatry in Algeria (1830–1962): From Colonial to Transcultural," *History of Psychiatry* 7 (1996): 533–48; Françoise Vergès, "Chains of Madness, Chains of Colonialism," in *The Fact of Blackness: Fanon and Visual Representation*, ed. Alan Read (London: Institute of Contemporary Arts, 1996); Robert Berthelier, *L'homme maghrébin dans la littérature psychiatrique* (Paris: L'Harmattan, 1994).

64. "Ethnopsychiatric Considerations" in Fanon, *Alienation and Freedom*, 406. [*Écrits sur l'aliénation et la liberté*, 343.] Fanon pursued his critique de l'École d'Alger in the last chapter of *The Wretched of the Earth*, "Colonial War and Mental Disorders" (181–233). [*Œuvres*, 625–72.]

65. Cherki, *Frantz Fanon*, 93. For patient testimonies, see the film by Abdenour Zahzah and Bachir Ridouh, dirs., *Frantz Fanon, mémoire d'asile*, Centre national de la cinématographie, Paris, 2008. See also Idriss Terranti, "Fanon vu de Blida," *Sud/Nord* 22, no. 1 (2007): 89–95; Numa Murard, "Psychothérapie institutionnelle à Blida," *Tumultes* 31, no. 2 (2008): 31–45.

66. Fanon, *Toward the African Revolution*, 49. [*Œuvres*, 730.] According to Nigel Gibson, Raymond Lacaton was arrested and tortured in 1956 because he was suspected of collaborating with the FLN and he left Algeria soon after. In Gibson and Beneduce, *Decolonizing Madness*, 25 and 175.

67. Fanon, *Alienation and Freedom*, 350. [*Écrits sur l'aliénation et la liberté*, 295.]

172 NOTES TO PAGES 64–69

68. For more on the doctors and interns, see Macey, *Frantz Fanon*, 214–15; Cherki, *Frantz Fanon*, 92.

69. Joseph and Juliette Pradin recall their extensive training as nurses at Saint-Alban in 1953, first in general medicine and then in psychiatry, with Tosquelles and Fanon. In Deyres, *Les heures heureuses.*

70. Testimonies of Mohamed Belgrade and Ahmed Ahmane in Zahzah and Ridouh, *Frantz Fanon, mémoire d'asile.*

71. Fanon, *Alienation and Freedom*, 331. [*Écrits sur l'aliénation et la liberté*, 278.]

72. The Algerian artist Farès Boukhatem, who was treated by Fanon, recalled Fanon's interest in his patients' art. See "Farés époque Fanon," in *El Moudjahid*, December 16, 1987, viii.

73. Archives IMEC, Fonds Frantz Fanon, FNN1.20, FNN1.21, FNN1.22. Some of the editorials are reprinted in Fanon, *Alienation and Freedom*, 311–48. [*Écrits sur l'aliénation et la liberté*, 260–93.]

74. Fanon, *Alienation and Freedom*, 325. [*Écrits sur l'aliénation et la liberté*, 273.]

75. Fanon, *Alienation and Freedom*, 346. [*Écrits sur l'aliénation et la liberté*, 291.] Translation modified.

76. "Le phénomène de l'agitation en milieu psychiatrique" in Fanon, *Alienation and Freedom*, 442. [*Écrits sur l'aliénation et la liberté*, 373.]

77. Fanon, *Alienation and Freedom*, 440. [*Écrits sur l'aliénation et la liberté*, 371.]

78. Fanon, *Alienation and Freedom*, 357. [*Écrits sur l'aliénation et la liberté*, 300.]

79. Fanon, *Alienation and Freedom* [*Écrits sur l'aliénation et la liberté*, 300.]

80. Fanon, *Alienation and Freedom*, 358. [*Écrits sur l'aliénation et la liberté*, 301.] Translation modified.

81. Fanon, *Alienation and Freedom*, 362–63. [*Écrits sur l'aliénation et la liberté*, 305.]

82. Fanon, *Alienation and Freedom*, 361. [*Écrits sur l'aliénation et la liberté*, 304.]

83. Fanon, *Alienation and Freedom*, 362. [*Écrits sur l'aliénation et la liberté*, 305.] Translation modified.

84. Fanon, *Alienation and Freedom*, 362–63. [*Écrits sur l'aliénation et la liberté*, 305.] In this sense, Nigel Gibson and Roberto Beneduce tribute Fanon for having inaugurated what we would refer to today as "critical ethnopsychiatry" (*Decolonizing Madness*, 21).

85. Fanon, *Alienation and Freedom*, 363. [*Écrits sur l'aliénation et la liberté*, 306.]

86. Fanon, *Alienation and Freedom*, 371. [*Écrits sur l'aliénation et la liberté*, 313.] On institutional psychotherapy in Blida, see also the accounts of Cherki, *Frantz Fanon*, 98–109; Zahzah and Ridouh, "Frantz Fanon, mémoire d'asile."

87. Cherki, *Frantz Fanon*, 164. See also the testimony of Youcef Yousfi at the Archives IMEC, Fonds Frantz Fanon, FNN 7.2, témoignages. For a provocative reading of these case studies in relation to Fanon's theory of violence, see Emma Kuby, "'Our Actions Never Cease to Haunt Us': Frantz Fanon, Jean-Paul Sartre, and the Violence of the Algerian War," *Historical Reflections* 41, no. 3 (2015): 59–78.

88. Fanon, *Wretched of the Earth*, 182–83. [*Œuvres*, 626.]

89. On the relationship between Fanon and Maspero, see their correspondence in Fanon, *Alienation and Freedom*, 675–93. [*Écrits sur l'aliénation et la liberté*, 549–64.] On Maspero's political activism, see Bruno Guichard, Julien Hage, and Alain Léger, *François Maspero et les paysages humains* (Lyon: La fosse aux ours, 2009); François Dosse, "François Maspero: La joie de lire: 1932–," in *Les hommes de l'ombre: Portraits d'éditeurs* (Paris: Perrin, 2014); Julien Hage, "François Maspero: Éditeur partisan," *Contretemps* 13 (2005): 100–107. Maspero published several French antipsychiatric books during the 1970s, including the work of Roger Gentis, for example.

NOTES TO PAGES 69–75   173

90. Marie-Jeanne Manuellan has written an account of her collaboration with Fanon at the Archives IMEC, Fonds Frantz Fanon, FNN 7.2, témoignages. Some of it was published in Marie-Jeanne Manuellan, *Sous la dictée de Fanon* (Paris: L'Amourier, 2017).

91. "Day Hospitalization in Psychiatry: Value and Limits," in Fanon, *Alienation and Freedom*. [*Écrits sur l'aliénation et la liberté*, 398.]

92. Fanon, *Alienation and Freedom*, 493. [*Écrits sur l'aliénation et la liberté*, 416.]

93. "Day Hospitalization in Psychiatry: Value and Limits, Part 2: Doctrinal Considerations" in Fanon, *Alienation and Freedom*, 497. [*Écrits sur l'aliénation et la liberté*, 419.]

94. Fanon, *Alienation and Freedom*, 498. [*Écrits sur l'aliénation et la liberté*, 420.] Translation modified.

95. Fanon, *Wretched of the Earth*, 31. [*Œuvres*, 478.]

96. See Fanon, *Wretched of the Earth*, 50–51. [*Œuvres*, 495–86.] Fanon's apology for violence has been, of course, the subject of much debate. Violence, in his work, has a redemptive function, to be sure, but not one necessarily tied to illiberal or fascist politics as many commentators have argued. Rather, if we consider it within the framework of institutional psychotherapy, violence can be seen as a form of collective agency for the people to govern themselves by their own rules. In this sense, I would compare Fanon's theory of violence to the radical democratic genealogy of that Kevin Duong traces in *The Virtues of Violence: Democracy against Disintegration in Modern France* (New York: Oxford University Press, 2020).

97. Jean-Paul Sartre, preface to Fanon, *Wretched of the Earth*, xlv. The discrepancy between these two audiences is evident in Sartre's preface, which was ultimately written for a French public, even if Sartre's point was to tell Europe that it was "done for" and that the Third World would pave the way for the Revolution. On Sartre and thirdworldism, see Arthur, *Unfinished Projects* and Yoav Di-Capua, *No Exit: Arab Existentialism, Jean-Paul Sartre, and Decolonization* (Chicago: The University of Chicago Press, 2018).

98. Fanon, *Wretched of the Earth*, 238. [*Œuvres*, 675.]

99. Fanon, *Wretched of the Earth*, 236. [*Œuvres*, 674.]

100. Fanon, *Wretched of the Earth*, 236 and 239. [*Œuvres*, 674–75.]

101. Fanon, *Wretched of the Earth*, 55. [*Œuvres*, 500.]

102. Fanon, *Wretched of the Earth*, 158–59. [*Œuvres*, 601.]

103. Fanon, *Wretched of the Earth*, 151. [*Œuvres*, 594.]

104. Fanon, *Wretched of the Earth*, 174. [*Œuvres*, xxx.]

105. Fanon, *Wretched of the Earth*, 175. [*Œuvres*, 617.]

106. Fanon, *Wretched of the Earth*, 177. [*Œuvres*, 619.]

107. Adom Getachew, *Worldmaking after Empire: The Rise and Fall of Self-Determination* (Princeton: Princeton University Press, 2019).

108. Deleuze and Guattari, *Anti-Oedipus*, 381.

Chapter 3

1. Oury discusses this in Jean Oury and Patrick Faugeras, *Préalables à toute clinique des psychoses* (Toulouse: Érès, 2012), 237–38.

2. Ibid., 234. See also Jean Oury, Félix Guattari, and François Tosquelles, *Pratique de l'institutionnel et politique* (Vigneux: Matrice, 1985), 41. As Gilles Deleuze put it in a text devoted to Guattari, "1936 was not only an event in the historical consciousness, but a complex of the unconscious." In "Préface de Gilles Deleuze: Trois problèmes de groupe," in Félix Guattari, *Psychanalyse et transversalité. Essais d'analyse institutionnelle* (Paris: La Découverte, 2003), ii.

174   NOTES TO PAGES 75–81

3. Oury and Faugeras, *Préalables à toute clinique des psychoses*, 239.

4. Félix Guattari, *De Leros à La Borde* (Paris: Lignes/Imec, 2011), 10.

5. Aïda Vasquez and Fernand Oury, *Vers une pédagogie institutionnelle* (Paris: François Maspero, 1967).

6. Deleuze and Guattari, *Anti-Oedipus*, xii.

7. For Julian Bourg, Deleuze and Guattari's notion of "ethics" was part of a broader "ethical turn" in French thought in the aftermath of May '68, a "transvaluation of May's contestatory energies." See Julian Bourg, *From Revolution to Ethics: May 1968 and Contemporary French Thought* (Montreal: McGill-Queen's University Press, 2007). Like Bourg, I am interested in the ethical dimension of institutional psychotherapy if we understand ethics as a practice of everyday life. Bourg, however, stresses the break between institutional psychotherapy and *Anti-Oedipus*, which he characterizes as Guattari's "definitive rupture" with the "ethically coherent thought and practice" of institutional psychotherapy (123). My own reading of *Anti-Oedipus* is much more in continuity with Guattari's clinical, political, and social activism. As I try to show here, many of the book's main concepts were first articulated in these other domains.

8. Oury and Faugeras, *Préalables à toute clinique des psychoses*, 83.

9. "La Constitution de l'an I," *Recherches: Histoires de la Borde: 10 ans de psychothérapie institutionnelle à Cour-Cheverny, 1953–1963*, no. 21 (Mar.–Apr. 1976): 19.

10. Ibid., 21. ["Prendre la responsabilité d'une tâche n'est pas simplement s'engager à l'assurer, c'est aussi la connecter à d'autres, la dénaturer, la réinventer."]

11. Ibid., 25.

12. Guattari, *De Leros à La Borde*, 64. See Guattari, "La Grille, 1987 (exposé fait au stage de formation de la Borde en janvier 1987)," in Archives IMEC, GTR2.Aa-10.27. See also Oury and Faugeras, *Préalables à toute clinique des psychoses*, 86; François Dosse, *Gilles Deleuze et Félix Guattari: Biographie croisée* (Paris: Découverte, 2007), 74–75; Susana Caló, *The Grid* (2016 [cited Apr. 10, 2020]); available from https://www.anthropocene-curriculum.org/contribution/the-grid.

13. *Recherches: Histoires de la Borde: 10 ans de psychothérapie institutionnelle à Cour-Cheverny, 1953–1963*, no. 21 (Mar.–Apr. 1976): 130–31.

14. Ibid., 61; Jean Oury and Marie Depussé, *À quelle heure passe le train . . . Conversations sur la folie* (Paris: Calmann-Lévy, 2003), 94.

15. Anne-Marie Norgeu, *La Borde: Le château des chercheurs de sens. La vie quotidienne à la clinique psychiatrique de La Borde* (Toulouse: Erès, 2006), 36. ["pièce maîtresse de la machinerie institutionnelle, machine à fomenter du désir, cycliquement révisée, interrogée par chacun dans sa construction paritaire."]

16. Jean Oury, *Séminaire de Sainte-Anne: Le Collectif* (Paris: Champs social, 2005), 163.

17. Guattari, *De Leros à La Borde*, 61. ["Il est vrai que je savais animer une réunion, structurer un débat, solliciter les personnes silencieuses à prendre la parole, faire se dégager des décisions pratiques, faire retour aux tâches précédemment décidées."]

18. *Recherches: Histoires de la Borde: 10 ans de psychothérapie institutionnelle à Cour-Cheverny, 1953–1963*, no. 21 (Mar.–Apr. 1976): 89. ["Les réunions prolifèrent. Nœuds, croisements, carrefours, elles vont brasser l'ensemble de la population de la clinique. Lieux de parole, elles accélèrent les échanges d'idées, d'informations. Elles permettent la mise à jour de questions nouvelles. Par leur dynamisme même, elles entraînent une remise en question du rôle de chacun, contribuant à modifier les habitudes des uns et des autres."]

19. Guattari, *De Leros à La Borde*, 17.

20. Archives of La Borde.

NOTES TO PAGES 81–85

21. Guattari, *De Leros à La Borde*, 67.

22. Nicolas Philibert, dir., *La moindre des choses*, Éditions Montparnasse, Paris, 1996.

23. In an interview, Oury recalled that Tosquelles told him upon his arrival at Saint-Alban in 1947: "Here, the first thing we do when we arrive is to read Lacan's thesis. It is the first step to approach the field of psychiatry." In Jean Oury and Danielle Roulot, *Dialogues à La Borde: Psychopathologie & structure institutionnelle* (Paris: Hermann, 2008), 102.

24. On Lacan's popularity during these years, see Sherry Turkle, *Psychoanalytic Politics: Freud's French Revolution* (New York: Basic Books, 1978).

25. This was apparently one of the reasons why Lacan never visited La Borde. According to Jean-Claude Polack, Lacan would say: "I won't go to a place where there are ten people in analysis with me." Private conversation with Polack on April 25, 2018.

26. Jean Oury, *Onze heures du soir à La Borde* (Paris: Gallilée, 1995), 316–17.

27. Oury and Roulot, *Dialogues à La Borde*, 101.

28. Jean Oury et al., "Entretien avec Jean Oury," *VST—Vie sociale et traitements* 88, no. 4 (2005): 18.

29. See Dylan Evans, *An Introductory Dictionary of Lacanian Psychoanalysis* (New York: Routledge, 1996); Silverman, *Subject of Semiotics*, 149–93; Bruce Fink, *The Lacanian Subject: Between Language and Jouissance* (Princeton: Princeton University Press, 1995); Franck Chaumon, *Lacan: La loi, le sujet et la jouissance* (Paris: Michalon, 2004); Jean-Pierre Cléro, *Le vocabulaire de Lacan* (Paris: Ellipses, 2012).

30. I refer to this as Lévi-Strauss's and Lacan's "structuralist social contract" in chapter 2 of Camille Robcis, *The Law of Kinship: Anthropology, Psychoanalysis, and the Family in France* (Ithaca: Cornell University Press, 2013).

31. Oury and Roulot, *Dialogues à La Borde*, 90. ["La forclusion du nom du père c'est ce qui invalide toute possibilité de rassemblement: autrement dit, c'est ce qui rend le désir impraticable. . . . Le nom du père, c'est ce qui va permettre la syntaxe. Dans l'existence schizophrénique, on peut dire que la syntaxe est foutue."]

32. Jean Oury, *Les symptômes primaires de la schizophrénie: Cours de psychopathologie, 1984–1986, suivi de Le corps et la psychose* (Paris: Éditions d'une, 2016), 409. ["un dépôt de signifiants purs, c'est-à-dire non articulés."]

33. Oury, *Onze heures du soir à La Borde*, 24. ["(Le schizophrène) pose, muet, la question impossible du référent."] On Saussure, see Jonathan D. Culler, *Ferdinand de Saussure* (Ithaca, NY: Cornell University Press, 1986).

34. Cited by Oury in Oury and Faugeras, *Préalables à toute clinique des psychoses*, 72.

35. Oury, *Séminaire de Sainte-Anne*, 197.

36. Oury, *Onze heures du soir à La Borde*, 161. ["Le psychotique est dans le réel; il vit dans un réseau troué; la symbolique est délabrée."]

37. Oury, *Séminaire de Sainte-Anne*, 43. ["La schizophrénie, la *Spaltung*, est une rupture d'un anneau. Toute la chaîne, à ce moment-là, se brise; et il n'y a pas d'objet *a*. Il faut bien 'fonctionner' quand même. Ce sont des bouts de corps, des bouts d'existence, de souvenirs, qui en arrivent à tenir lieu d'objet *a*, pour que ça tienne à peu près."] See also Oury, *Les symptômes primaires de la schizophrénie*, 194.

38. Oury and Roulot, *Dialogues à La Borde*, 90.

39. Préface by Pierre Delion in Oury, *Les symptômes primaires de la schizophrénie*, 18. ["La topique de ce vécu d'enfer schizophrénique est ce qu'il propose d'appeler le 'point d'horreur' situé derrière un miroir qui ne joue pas son rôle de rassemblement du corps éparpillé, dissocié, sous l'œil bienveillant de l'Autre."]

40. Ibid., 307.

176 NOTES TO PAGES 86-88

41. Ibid., 245.

42. See Gisela Pankow, *L'homme et sa psychose* (Paris: Flammarion, 2009). For an introduction to Pankow's life and thought, see Marie-Lise Lacas, *Gisela Pankow: Un humanisme au-delà de la psychose* (Paris: Campagne première, 2014).

43. Oury, *Séminaire de Sainte-Anne*, 202.

44. Oury, *Onze heures du soir à La Borde*, 244. ["L'astuce de la psychothérapie institutionnelle est peut-être d'avoir voulu métaboliser ces investissements massifs par la mise en place contrôlée de relations multiples, d'arborisations diverses, tenant compte ainsi de ce qui est particulièrement caractéristique dans l'existence schizophrénique: l'éparpillement, la dissociation du transfert, l'accolement des choses et des mots, si bien que l'organisation d'un groupe, la mise en place de systèmes de responsabilités partielles (bar, théâtre, bibliothèque, instances d'animation, etc.) arrivent à être 'représentatives' à un niveau inconscient."]

45. Ibid., 246.

46. Gilles Deleuze, *Pourparlers, 1972–1990* (Paris: Editions de Minuit, 1990), 28. See also Deleuze and Guattari, *Anti-Oedipus*, 333. [Gilles Deleuze and Félix Guattari, *L'Anti-Œdipe* (Paris: Éditions de Minuit, 1972), 398.] ["Freud made the most profound discovery of the abstract subjective essence of desire—Libido. But . . . he realienated this essence, reinvesting it in a subjective system of representation of the ego, and . . . he recorded this essence on the residual territory of Oedipus and under the despotic signifier of castration."]

47. See for example Guattari, *Psychanalyse et transversalité*, 93; Deleuze and Guattari, *Anti-Oedipus*, 46. Lacan's 1953 "The Function and Field of Speech and Language in Psychoanalysis," also known as the "Rome Discourse," marked Lacan's departure from the IPA (his "excommunication," to use his term) and also functioned as a theoretical manifesto for his new psychoanalytic association, the SFP (Société Française de Psychanalyse). The text began with Lacan's call for a "return to Freud," by which Lacan meant a return to the main two concepts of Freud, which, in Lacan's view, had been obliterated by ego psychology: the unconscious and sexuality. In Jacques Lacan, *Ecrits*, 31–104. [*Écrits*, 237–322.]

48. Guattari's relation to Lacan was complex and constantly wavered between admiration and condemnation. This is best evident, perhaps, in Guattari's diaries, in which Guattari recounted several of his dreams that focused on Lacan during the writing of *Anti-Oedipus*. For example: "Another dream about Lacan! This is insane! I can hear them, from here, saying: 'badly eliminated transfer,' etc. In a sense, it's true if transfer is oedipal reterritorialization artificially woven onto the space of the couch. I have oedipal rot sticking to my skin. Not passively, but with all the will to power of the death drive. The more I become disengaged—the more I try to become disengaged—from twenty years of Lacano-Labordian comfort, the more this familialist carcass enfolds me secretly. I would rather admit anything else." In Félix Guattari, *The Anti-Oedipus Papers* (New York: Semiotext(e), 2006), 305. See also 343–44.

49. Oury and Faugeras, *Préalables à toute clinique des psychoses*, 137.

50. Oury and Depussé, *À quelle heure passe le train*, 70.

51. For more on Guattari's political activism, see Dosse, *Gilles Deleuze et Félix Guattari*.

52. Cited in Valentin Schaepelynck, "Une critique en acte des institutions: Émergence et résidus de l'analyse institutionnelle dans les années 1960," Université Paris 8, 2013, 424.

53. Jacques Lacan, *L'envers de la psychanalyse: Le Séminaire, Livre XVII, 1969–1970*

NOTES TO PAGES 88–92

(Paris: Seuil, 1991), 239. See also Jacques Sédat, "Lacan et Mai 68," *Figures de la psychanalyse* 18, no. 2 (2009): 221–26.

54. For more on this meeting, see Dosse, *Gilles Deleuze et Félix Guattari*.

55. For more on Vincennes, see Jean-Michel Djian, ed., *Vincennes: Une aventure de la pensée critique* (Paris: Flammarion, 2009); Virginie Linhart, dir., *Vincennes, l'université perdue*, Blaq out, Paris, 2018. And on Deleuze's role in the university: Charles Soulié, "La pédagogie charismatique de Gilles Deleuze à Vincennes," *Actes de la recherche en sciences sociales* 216–17, no. 1 (2017): 42–63.

56. Robert Castel, "Les enfants de La Borde: review of Jean-Claude Polack and Danielle Sabourin, *La Borde ou le droit à la folie*." Archives of La Borde.

57. Gilles Deleuze, *Desert Islands and Other Texts, 1953–1974* (Los Angeles: Semiotext(e), 2004), 216.

58. Cited in Deleuze and Guattari, *Anti-Oedipus*, 29. [*L'Anti-Œdipe*, 36-37.] For an excellent overview of this intellectual moment, see Michel Feher, "Mai 68 dans la pensée," in *Histoire des gauches en France*, vol. 2, ed. Jean-Jacques Becker and Gilles Candar (Paris: La Découverte, 2004).

59. These were translated into English as Gilles Deleuze, *Spinoza, Practical Philosophy* (San Francisco: City Lights Books, 1988); Deleuze, *Expressionism in Philosophy: Spinoza* (New York: Zone Books, 1990). On Deleuze's philosophical formation, see Bourg, *From Revolution to Ethics*, 144–58.

60. Deleuze and Guattari, *Anti-Oedipus*, 4–5. [*L'Anti-Œdipe*, 9–10.]

61. Deleuze and Guattari, *Anti-Oedipus*, 29. [*L'Anti-Œdipe*, 36.]

62. Deleuze and Guattari, *Anti-Oedipus*, 26. [*L'Anti-Œdipe*, 34.]

63. Deleuze and Guattari, *Anti-Oedipus*, 121. [*L'Anti-Œdipe*, 144.]

64. Deleuze and Guattari, *Anti-Oedipus*, 67. [*L'Anti-Œdipe*, 80.] See also Ibid, 121. [*L'Anti-Œdipe*, 144.]

65. Deleuze and Guattari, *Anti-Oedipus*, 111. [*L'Anti-Œdipe*, 132.]

66. Deleuze and Guattari, *Anti-Oedipus*, 112. [*L'Anti-Œdipe*, 132–33.] See also Gilles Deleuze and Claire Parnet, *Dialogues* (Paris: Flammarion, 1977), 95; Gilles Deleuze and David Lapoujade, *L'île déserte et autres textes: Textes et entretiens, 1953–1974* (Paris: Editions de Minuit, 2002), 244. This vocabulary of flows and power as *puissance* is close to Nietzsche's, an author that Deleuze returned to regularly throughout his life. See chapter 2 in Gilles Deleuze, *Nietzsche et la philosophie* (Paris: Presses universitaires de France, 1962).

67. Deleuze and Guattari, *Anti-Oedipus*, 53. [*L'Anti-Œdipe*, 61.]

68. Deleuze and Guattari, *Anti-Oedipus*, 82. [*L'Anti-Œdipe*, 97–98.] See also Deleuze and Parnet, *Dialogues*, 100.

69. Deleuze and Guattari, *Anti-Oedipus*, 107. [*L'Anti-Œdipe*, 128.]

70. Deleuze and Guattari, *Anti-Oedipus*, 75. [*L'Anti-Œdipe*, 89.]

71. Deleuze and Guattari, *Anti-Oedipus*, 23. [*L'Anti-Œdipe*, 30.]

72. Deleuze and Guattari, *Anti-Oedipus*, 50, 92. [*L'Anti-Œdipe*, 58 and 110.]

73. Deleuze and Guattari, *Anti-Oedipus*, 57. [*L'Anti-Œdipe*, 67.]

74. Deleuze and Guattari, *Anti-Oedipus*, 297. [*L'Anti-Œdipe*, 353.] Eric L. Santner explored how taking into account this historical and political context might have led to a different reading of the Schreber case in *My Own Private Germany: Daniel Paul Schreber's Secret History of Modernity* (Princeton: Princeton University Press, 1996).

75. Deleuze and Guattari, *Anti-Oedipus*, 83. [*L'Anti-Œdipe*, 99.]

76. Deleuze and Guattari, *Anti-Oedipus*, 94. [*L'Anti-Œdipe*, 112.]

178 NOTES TO PAGES 92–96

77. Deleuze and Guattari, *Anti-Oedipus*, 130–37. [*L'Anti-Œdipe*, 155–62.]

78. Deleuze and Guattari, *Anti-Oedipus*, 103. [*L'Anti-Œdipe*, 123.]

79. Deleuze and Guattari, *Anti-Oedipus*, 103. [*L'Anti-Œdipe*, 124.] On this question of desire vs. ideology, see also Isabelle Garo, *Foucault, Deleuze, Althusser & Marx: La politique dans la philosophie* (Paris: Demopolis, 2011), 226; Herzog, *Cold War Freud*, 160–64.

80. Deleuze and Guattari, *Anti-Oedipus*, 104. [*L'Anti-Œdipe*, 124.]

81. Deleuze and Guattari, *Anti-Oedipus*, 105. [*L'Anti-Œdipe*, 124.]

82. Deleuze and Guattari, *Anti-Oedipus*, 30. [*L'Anti-Œdipe*, 38.]

83. Wilhelm Reich, *The Mass Psychology of Fascism* (New York: Farrar, Straus and Giroux, 1970).

84. Deleuze and Guattari, *Anti-Oedipus*, 118. [*L'Anti-Œdipe*, 140–41.]

85. Deleuze and Guattari, *Anti-Oedipus*, 29. [*L'Anti-Œdipe*, 37.]

86. Deleuze and Guattari, *Anti-Oedipus*, 29. [*L'Anti-Œdipe*, 37.] See also the preface by Gilles Deleuze in Guattari, *Psychanalyse et transversalité*, iii.

87. Deleuze and Guattari, *Anti-Oedipus*, xii.

88. Félix Guattari, *Chaosophy* (New York: Semiotext(e), 1995), 171.

89. For more on the intellectual crisis of French Marxism during these years, see Camille Robcis, "'China in Our Heads': Althusser, Maoism, and Structuralism," *Social Text* 30, no. 1 (110) (2012): 51–69. See also Herzog, *Cold War Freud*, especially chap. 5.

90. Deleuze and Guattari, *Anti-Oedipus*, xiii.

91. Ibid., 75. [*L'Anti-Œdipe*, 89.]

92. Gilles Deleuze, *Two Regimes of Madness: Texts and Interviews, 1975–1995* (Los Angeles: Semiotext(e), 2006), 238.

93. Deleuze says this explicitly in his letter to his Japanese translator and friend Kuniichi Uno, in ibid. In this sense, much of the speculation concerning the Deleuze and Guattari collaboration—who wrote what, when, whose ideas are they *really*, etc.—is somewhat misplaced. It is clear that Deleuze became aware of institutional psychotherapy through Guattari (even though, as many commentators have noted, Deleuze was supposedly "terrified of the mad" and never fully comfortable at La Borde). He was, however, already very interested in the question of desire and of institutions much prior to meeting Guattari, in his work on Hume and Sacher-Masoch, for instance. On this question, see Valentin Schaepelynck, "'Machines de guerre': Entre concepts, institutions et expérimentation sociale," in *Agencer les multiplicités avec Deleuze*, ed. Anne Querrien, Anne Sauvagnargues, and Arnaud Villani (Paris: Éditions Hermann, 2019).

94. Deleuze, *Two Regimes of Madness*, 307.

95. Ibid., 239. On the writing of *Anti-Oedipus*, see also Stéphane Nadaud's introduction to Guattari, *Anti-Oedipus Papers*, 11–22.

96. See also Guattari, *Chaosophy*, 73.

97. Deleuze and Guattari, *Anti-Oedipus*, 380. [*L'Anti-Œdipe*, 456.]

98. Deleuze and Guattari, *Anti-Oedipus*, 381. [*L'Anti-Œdipe*, 358.]

99. Deleuze and Guattari, *Anti-Oedipus*, 362. [*L'Anti-Œdipe*, 434.]

100. Deleuze and Guattari, *Anti-Oedipus*, 296. [*L'Anti-Œdipe*, 352.]

101. Deleuze and Guattari, *Anti-Oedipus*, 81–82. [*L'Anti-Œdipe*, 97.]

102. Deleuze and Guattari, *Anti-Oedipus*, 116. [*L'Anti-Œdipe*, 138.]

103. Deleuze and Guattari, *Anti-Oedipus*, 105. [*L'Anti-Œdipe*, 125.]

104. Deleuze and Guattari continued to theorize this notion of "minoritarian" practices in Gilles Deleuze and Félix Guattari, *Kafka, pour une littérature mineure* (Paris: Éditions de Minuit, 1975).

NOTES TO PAGES 96–99   179

105. Deleuze and Guattari, *Anti-Oedipus: Capitalism and Schizophrenia*, 98. [*L'Anti-Œdipe*, 116.]

106. Deleuze and Guattari, *Anti-Oedipus*, 105. [*L'Anti-Œdipe*, 125.]

107. Deleuze and Guattari, *Anti-Oedipus*, 64. [*L'Anti-Œdipe*, 75.] The distinction between *groupes-sujets* and *groupes-assujettis* could also be read as Deleuze and Guattari's take on Sartre's distinction between *collectif sériel* and *groupe en fusion* in his 1960 *Critique of Dialectical Reason*.

108. Deleuze and Guattari, *Anti-Oedipus*, 348. [*L'Anti-Œdipe*, 417.]

109. Deleuze, *Pourparlers*, 31. ["Comme beaucoup d'autres, nous annonçons le développement d'un fascisme généralisé. . . . il n'y a aucune raison pour que le fascisme ne se développe pas. Ou plutôt: ou bien une machine révolutionnaire se montrera, capable de prendre en charge le désir et les phénomènes de désir, ou bien le désir restera manipulé par les forces d'oppression, de répression, et menacera, même du dedans, les machines révolutionnaires."] See also chap. 9, "Everybody Wants to Be a Fascist," in Guattari, *Chaosophy*.

110. Deleuze, *Pourparlers*, 32. ["lignes de fuite actives et positives, parce que ces lignes conduisent au désir, aux machines du désir et à l'organisation d'un champ social de désir."]

111. Guattari, *De Leros à La Borde*, 68. ["Je ne proposais nullement de généraliser l'expérience de La Borde à l'ensemble de la société, aucun modèle en la matière n'étant transposable. Mais il m'apparaissait que la subjectivité, à tous les étages du socius où l'on voudra la considérer, n'allait pas de soi, qu'elle était produite dans certaines conditions et que ces conditions pouvaient être modifiées par de multiples procédures de façon à l'orienter dans un sens plus créatif."]

112. Ibid., 67. ["L'on se prend à rêver de ce que pourrait devenir la vie dans les ensembles urbains, les écoles, les hôpitaux, les prisons, etc., si, au lieu de les concevoir sur le mode de la répétition vide, on s'efforçait de réorienter leur finalité dans le sens d'une re-création permanente interne."] See also Oury, Guattari, and Tosquelles, *Pratique de l'institutionnel et politique*, 48.

113. Guattari, *Chaosophy*, 197.

114. Deleuze, preface to Guattari, *Psychanalyse et transversalité*, vi. In the English version of this book, Ames Hodges translates *groupes-sujets* as "group-subjects" and *groupes-assujettis* as "subjugated groups," and Rosemary Sheed as "dependent" and "independent" groups. I have consulted their translations, but I prefer to keep the terms "subject" and "subjected" groups to signal the continuities between institutional analysis, which began in the early 1960s, and *Anti-Oedipus* in 1972. See *Psychoanalysis and Transversality: Texts and Interviews, 1955–1971*, trans. Ames Hodges (South Pasadena, CA: Semiotext(e), 2015), 14, and Félix Guattari, *Molecular Revolutions: Psychiatry and Politics*, trans. Rosemary Sheed (New York: Penguin Books, 1984), 14. On Guattari and institutions, see Valentin Schaepelynck, *L'institution renversée: folie, analyse institutionnelle et champ social* (Paris: Editions Etérotopia, 2018).

115. Guattari, *Psychanalyse et transversalité*, 288–89.

116. Tosquelles cited in Olivier Apprill, *Une avant-garde psychiatrique: le moment GTPSI (1960–1966)* (Paris: Epel, 2013), 84. ["c'est 'l'Institution' qui est le lieu habituel de notre agir."]

117. Ibid., 33–34. The proceedings of the GTPSI meetings (currently archived at La Borde) have been published in recent years by the Éditions d'une. See http://www.gtpsi.fr.

180   NOTES TO PAGES 99–101

118. Oury cited in ibid., 64. ["L'analyse individuelle du praticien lui-même est utile, nécessaire, mais c'est insuffisant. Il est souhaitable que les groupes de travail ne soient pas vécus comme des réunions de simples confrontations de champs d'expérience divers, mais s'efforcent de faire apparaître ce qui est mis en jeu dans tout ce qui se passe. Cela nécessite une méthodologie qui doit être constamment à l'épreuve."]

119. One of the meetings of the GTPSI in July 1964 occurred one month after Lacan founded the École Française de Psychanalyse (which eventually became the École Freudienne de Paris) after he was expelled from the Société Française de Psychanalyse (SFP), the official psychoanalytic school recognized by the International Psychoanalytic Association (IPA). One of Lacan's goals was to create a section on "applied psychoanalysis" (along with a second section devoted to "pure psychoanalysis" and a third to "psychoanalysis and sciences"). In this context, the GTPSI decided to send him a delegation to convince him that "applied psychoanalysis" was exactly what was happening at Saint-Alban and at La Borde. Oury recounts that Lacan welcomed the idea enthusiastically but that some of his close associates eventually turned the group—and the idea—away. In Oury and Depussé, À quelle heure passe le train, 252.

120. Guattari, Psychanalyse et transversalité, 288.

121. Ibid., 79. [Psychoanalysis and Transversality, 112.]

122. Guattari, Psychanalyse et transversalité, 79. [Psychoanalysis and Transversality, 112.]

123. Guattari, Psychanalyse et transversalité, 80. [Psychoanalysis and Transversality, 113.] On groupes-sujets vs. groupes-assujettis, see also Psychanalyse et transversalité, 76. [Psychoanalysis and Transversality, 107.]

124. Guattari, Psychanalyse et transversalité, 84. [Psychoanalysis and Transversality, 118.] ["le lieu du sujet inconscient du groupe, l'au-delà des lois objectives qui le fondent, le support du désir de groupe."]

125. Guattari, Psychanalyse et transversalité, 82. [Psychoanalysis and Transversality, 116.] ["un dialogue d'un nouveau genre: le délire et toute autre manifestation inconsciente, au sein de laquelle le malade restait jusqu'alors muré et solitaire, pouvant parvenir à un mode d'expression collective."]

126. Guattari, Psychanalyse et transversalité, 83. [Psychoanalysis and Transversality, 117.] ["Un tel remaniement des idéaux du moi modifie les données d'accueil du surmoi et permet la mise en circuit d'un type de complexe de castration articulé avec des exigences sociales différentes de celles que les malades avaient connues précédemment dans leurs relations familiales, professionnelles, etc. L'acceptation d'être 'mis en cause,' d'être mis à nu par la parole de l'autre, un certain style de contestation réciproque, d'humour, l'élimination des prérogatives de la hiérarchie, etc., tout cela tendra à fonder une nouvelle loi du groupe . . ."]

127. Guattari, Psychanalyse et transversalité, 85. [Psychoanalysis and Transversality, 119–20.]

128. For more on this history, see Dosse, Gilles Deleuze et Félix Guattari, chap. 4. See also Hervé Hamon and Patrick Rotman, Génération, 2 vols. (Paris: Seuil, 1987 and 1988); Dominique Damamme et al., Mai-juin 68 (Ivry-sur-Seine: Les Éditions de l'Atelier, 2008).

129. Guattari, Psychanalyse et transversalité, 117. [Psychoanalysis and Transversality, 161.]

130. Guattari, Psychanalyse et transversalité, 126. [Psychoanalysis and Transversality, 174.]

131. Archives IMEC, Fonds Guattari, GTR 52.12. ["Le but du CERFI est de poursuivre les études et recherches concrètes dans l'esprit de synthèse des sciences humaines et de recherche interdisciplinaire qui caractérise les travaux de la FGERI. 1) réaliser les études

NOTES TO PAGES 101–104

relatives à la gestion et aux conditions de développement économique et social des collectivités locales, organismes d'animation culturelle, entreprises et institutions sociales, etc. 2) Promouvoir la recherche statistique, les enquêtes économiques, sociologiques et psychosociologiques, urbanistiques, concernant l'aménagement des villes et des régions. 3) développer ces recherches et études avec la participation des usagers à toutes les phases des investigations. 4) organiser la formation des éducateurs, instituteurs, animateurs culturels, infirmier(e)s, cadres administratifs, architectes, économistes, etc . . . dans l'esprit qui préside aux recherches elles-mêmes."]

132. Guattari, *De Leros à La Borde*, 69–70. On the genesis of the CERFI, see "CERFI: Four Remarks" and François Fourquet, "The History of CERFI" in the IMEC Archives, Fonds Guattari, IMEC GTR81.32. See also Schaepelynck, "Une critique en acte des institutions," and Meredith TenHoor, "State-Funded Militant Infrastructure? CERFI's *Équipements Collectifs* in the Intellectual History of Architecture," *Journal of Architecture* 24, no. 7 (2019): 999–1019.

133. All issues of *Recherches* are available online at http://www.editions-recherches.com/revue3.php (accessed April 13, 2020). See the presentation by Stéphane Nadaud: "Recherches (1966–1982: histoire d'une revue)," *La Revue des revues (Entr'revues)*, no. 34 (2004): 47–72.

134. Archives IMEC, Fonds Guattari, GTR 53.6: "La Borde: correspondence et documents administratifs." As Oury put it in a letter to the CERFI from November 14, 1967: "D'une façon générale, le CERFI prendrait en charge l'ensemble des activités regroupées sous la rubrique de thérapeutique institutionnelle: soit à l'intérieur de la Clinique ou de ses dépendances (ateliers d'ergothérapie, socialthérapie, psychothérapies de groupe, animation culturelle, éducation spécialisée, etc), soit hors de l'enceinte de la Clinique (réinsertion sociale des pensionnaires, sorties culturelles, excursions, visites d'expositions, etc . . .)."

135. For example, the double issue of *Recherches* no. 17 from March 1975 titled "Histoire de la psychiatrie de secteur ou le secteur impossible?" recounted the genesis of institutional psychotherapy at La Borde and traced its evolution through the 1970s. Bonnafé, Tosquelles, Oury, Daumézon, Guattari and others all contributed to this issue.

136. See also "Les barricades mystérieuses: La bande à Félix Guattari," Sur les docs, France Culture, Mar. 14, 2011, podcast, https://www.franceculture.fr/emissions/sur-les-docks/champ-libre-15-les-barricades-mysterieuses-la-bande-felix-guattari.

137. "Éditorial," *Recherches*, no. 1 (Jan. 1966): 1.

138. "Éditorial," *Recherches*, no. 1 (Jan. 1966): 2. ["La répétition, c'est la mort. Se servir de Marx ou de Freud sur le mode de la répétition, c'est se livrer à une sorte d'encensement mortifère."]

139. Félix Guattari, "Réflexions quelque peu philosophiques sur la psychothérapie institutionnelle" *Recherches*, no. 1 (Jan. 1966): 7. ["Comment un groupe peut-il se saisir de la parole, dans une institution donnée, à un moment donné de son histoire, sans renforcer les mécanismes sériels et aliénants qui caractérisent généralement les collectivités dans les sociétés industrielles?"]

140. "Éditorial," *Recherches*, no. 2 (Feb. 1966): 1. ["pas de comité de rédaction qui détermine la ligne, qui trie les articles, pas de théories ni de concepts à défendre."]

141. "Éditorial," *Recherches*, no. 2 (Feb. 1966): 1. ["La règle du jeu est la suivante: chacun parle son propre langage sans concession, sans honte, sans ces compromis de mondanité qui donnent l'illusion d'une compréhension mais replient chacun dans son système, sur sa 'vérité.'"]

142. Guy Hocquenghem, *Le désir homosexuel* (Paris: Fayard, 2000). For more on

182 NOTES TO PAGES 105–109

Hocquenghem's relationship to *Anti-Oedipus*, see Robcis, *Law of Kinship*, 205–9. On Hocquenghem more generally, see Antoine Idier, *Les vies de Guy Hocquenghem: politique, sexualité, culture* (Paris: Fayard, 2017); Todd Shepard, *Sex, France, and Arab Men, 1962–1979* (Chicago University of Chicago Press, 2017); Ron Haas, "Guy Hocquenghem and the Cultural Revolution in France after May 1968," in *After the Deluge: New Perspectives on the Intellectual and Cultural History of Postwar France*, ed. Julian Bourg (Lanham, MD: Lexington Books, 2004).

143. Dosse, *Gilles Deleuze et Félix Guattari*, 321. Some of this comes from my interview with Anne Querrien on June 17, 2019. See also Anne Querrien, "Le CERFI, l'expérimentation sociale et l'État: Témoignage d'une petite main," in *L'État à l'épreuve des sciences sociales. La fonction recherche dans les administrations sous la Ve République*, ed. Philippe Bezes, 72–87 (Paris: La Découverte, 2005); Liane Mozère, *Le printemps des crèches: Histoire et analyse d'un mouvement* (Paris: L'Harmattan, 1992).

144. This issue was republished as François Fourquet and Lion Murard, *Les équipements du pouvoir: Villes, territoires et équipements collectifs* (Paris: Union générale d'éditions, 1976). On the CERFI and urbanism, see Susana Caló and Godofredo Pereira, "CERFI: From the Hospital to the City," *London Journal of Critical Thought (LJCT)* 1, no. 2 (2017): 83–100.

145. See https://progressivegeographies.com/resources/foucault-resources/foucaults -collaborative-projects/ and Stuart Elden, *Foucault: The Birth of Power* (Malden, MA: Polity, 2017), 168–77. All of these research contracts are available at the IMEC Archives, Fonds Michel Foucault, FCL 4.14. See also Liane Mozère, "Foucault et le CERFI: Instantanés et actualité," *Le Portique* 13–14 (2004).

Chapter 4

1. Didier Eribon, *Michel Foucault: 1926–1984* (Paris: Flammarion, 1991), 60.

2. Michel Foucault, *Maladie mentale et personnalité* (Paris: Presses universitaires de France, 1954), 109.

3. Éliane Amado Lévy-Valensi, "Histoire et Psychologie?," *Annales. Histoire, Sciences Sociales*, no. 5 (Sept.–Oct. 1965): 923.

4. "La conception idéologique de 'L'Histoire de la Folie' de Michel Foucault (Journées annuelles de *L'Évolution Psychiatrique*, Toulouse, 6–7 Décembre 1969," *L'Évolution psychiatrique* 36, no. 2 (1971): 226. ["Il s'agit là d'une position 'psychiatricide' si lourde de conséquences pour l'idée même de l'Homme et de ses rapports constitutifs avec son corps et le corps social, que nous eussions beaucoup désiré la présence de Michel Foucault parmi nous. Tout à la fois pour lui rendre le juste hommage de notre admiration pour les démarches systématiques de sa pensée, et pour contester que la 'maladie mentale' puisse être considérée comme la merveilleuse manifestation de la divine Folie, ou plus exceptionnellement comme l'étincelle du génie poétique, car elle est 'autre chose' qu'un phénomène culturel."]

5. Oury and Faugeras, *Préalables à toute clinique des psychoses*, 110.

6. Ibid., 176–77.

7. See Saïd Chebili, "Foucault et l'antipsychiatrie," *L'Information psychiatrique* 92, no. 8 (2016): 671–76; Robert Castel, "Les aventures de la pratique," *Le Débat* 41, no. 4 (1986): 41–51. See also Foucault's own account in Michel Foucault, "Histoire de la folie et antipsychiatrie," *Cahier de L'Herne* 95 (2011): 95–102.

8. "Prisons et asiles dans le mécanisme du pouvoir" (no. 136, 1974) in Michel Foucault, *Dits et écrits, 1954–1988* (Paris: Gallimard Quarto, 2001), 1: 1392. ["La frontière po-

NOTES TO PAGES 109–113   183

litique a changé son tracé, et, maintenant, des sujets comme la psychiatrie, l'internement, la médicalisation d'une population sont devenus des problèmes politiques."]

9. "Le grand enfermement" (no. 105, 1972) in ibid., 1: 1169. ["Écrire aujourd'hui la suite de mon *Histoire de la folie* qui irait jusqu'à l'époque actuelle est pour moi dépourvu d'intérêt. En revanche, une action politique concrète en faveur des prisonniers me paraît chargée de sens."]

10. For a detailed chronology of these publications, see Stuart Elden's blog: https:// progressivegeographies.com/resources/foucault-resources/foucaults-collaborative -projects/

11. Deleuze and Guattari, *Anti-Oedipus*, xii.

12. Deleuze, *Pourparlers*, 36. See also Gilles Deleuze, *Foucault* (Paris: Editions de Minuit, 1986).

13. Michel Foucault, *Psychiatric Power: Lectures at the Collège de France, 1973–74* (Basingstoke, UK: Palgrave Macmillan, 2006), 39.

14. Eribon, *Michel Foucault*, 60; David Macey, *The Lives of Michel Foucault* (New York: Vintage Books, 1995), 36. Many of Foucault's notes on these lectures are available at the Bibliothèque Nationale de France (BNF).

15. Foucault even thought of writing his thesis on the birth of psychology in post-Cartesian philosophy. He lectured on these thinkers in his first seminars as a tutor at the École Normale Supérieure, as we know from the notes of his student Jacques Lagrange, held at the Archives IMEC, Fonds Michel Foucault, Côte FCL 3.8 (1ère chemise: Problèmes de l'Anthropologie).

16. Eribon, *Michel Foucault*, 48. See Maurice Merleau-Ponty, *Child Psychology and Pedagogy: The Sorbonne Lectures, 1949–1952* (Evanston, IL: Northwestern University Press, 2010).

17. On Lagache and this institutionalization of psychology in France, see Elisabeth Roudinesco, *Histoire de la psychanalyse en France: 1925–1985*, vol. 2 (Paris: Fayard, 1994); Ohayon, *Psychologie et psychanalyse en France.*

18. Bibliothèque Nationale de France, Fonds Michel Foucault, Côte NAF 28730 (38): Rue d'Ulm, circa 1944–1950. See especially pochettes 1 and 4.

19. Bibliothèque Nationale de France, Fonds Michel Foucault, Côte NAF 28730 (44a): Neurophysiologie Lagache EEG.

20. Bibliothèque Nationale de France, Fonds Michel Foucault, Côte NAF 28730 (44b): Neurophysiologie Lagache EEG. On Goldstein and Head, see Geroulanos and Meyers, *Human Body in the Age of Catastrophe.*

21. Bibliothèque Nationale de France, Fonds Michel Foucault, Côte NAF 28730 (37): Années de formation: Sorbonne, rue d'Ulm. Foucault briefly joined the Communist Party but quit it by October 1952.

22. In addition to the Eribon and Macey biographies, see Jean-François Bert, "Retour à Münsterlingen," in Jean-François Bert and Elisabetta Basso, *Foucault à Münsterlingen: À l'origine de l'Histoire de la folie* (Paris: Éditions EHESS, 2015). See also Philippe Artières and Jean-François Bert, *Un succès philosophique: L'histoire de la folie à l'âge classique de Michel Foucault* (Caen: Presses universitaires de Caen, 2011).

23. See for example in the Bibliothèque littéraire Jacques Doucet, Fonds Jean Delay, DLY MS 173, Delay's note on psychiatry: "Située par son objet même à la jointure des sciences biologiques et des sciences morales, qu'on appelle aujourd'hui sciences humaines, elle a largement bénéficié du développement des unes et des autres. C'est une erreur que d'opposer ces deux tendances, biologique et psychologique, qui sont complémentaires, et de vouloir séparer deux types de praticiens, le spécialiste des maladies du

184 NOTES TO PAGES 113–116

cerveau et le spécialiste de la pathologie des relations humaines, car c'est précisément la réunion de ces deux ordres de savoir qui caractérise le psychiatre."

24. Bibliothèque Nationale de France, Fonds Michel Foucault, Côte NAF 28730 (46), Cours à l'Université de Lille, 1952–1953: Connaissance de l'homme et réflexion transcendentale; Phénoménologie et psychologie; Binswanger et phénoménologie; Cours sur Freud et psychanalyse. On these courses, see Philippe Sabot, "Entre psychologie et philosophie: Foucault à Lille, 1952–1955," in Bert and Basso, *Foucault à Münsterlingen*, 103–20.

25. Philippe Sabot, "L'expérience, le savoir et l'histoire dans les premiers écrits de Michel Foucault," *Archives de Philosophie* 69 (2006): 292.

26. "Introduction to Binswanger, *Le Rêve et l'Existence* (trad. J. Verdeaux), Paris, Desclée de Brouwer, 1954, pp.9–128)" (1954, no. 1), Foucault, *Dits et écrits*, 1: 94. On Foucault's preface, see Elisabetta Basso, "Le rêve et l'existence, histoire d'une traduction," in Bert and Basso, *Foucault à Münsterlingen*, 143–66; Elisabetta Basso, *Michel Foucault e la daseinsanalyse: Un'indagine metodologica* (Milan: Mimesis, 2007). On Binswanger, see Caroline Gros, *Ludwig Binswanger: Entre phénoménologie et expérience psychiatrique* (Chatou: Les Éditions de la Transparence, 2009).

27. Jean-François Bert, "Retour à Münsterlingen," in Bert and Basso, *Foucault à Münsterlingen*, 36–37.

28. The photos are published in Bert and Basso, *Foucault à Münsterlingen*, 274–79.

29. Foucault, "La folie et la fête" (Jan. 7, 1963), cited in Jean-François Bert, "Retour à Münsterlingen" in ibid., 12. ["De nos jours . . . on essaye de reconstituer dans les hôpitaux psychiatriques des formes de vie voisines, autant qu'il est possible, de ce que, vous et moi, de ce que tout le monde appelle le 'normal.' Et par un étrange paradoxe, par un étrange retour, on organise pour eux, autour d'eux, avec eux, tout un défilé, avec danse et masque, tout un carnaval qui est au sens strict du terme une nouvelle fête des fous."]

30. Foucault, "Vérité, pouvoir et soi" (Oct. 25, 1982) cited in Jean-François Bert, "Retour à Münsterlingen," in ibid., 15. ["Dans un premier temps, j'ai accepté ces choses comme nécessaires, mais . . . au bout de trois mois, j'ai quitté cet emploi et je suis allé en Suède, avec un sentiment de grande malaise; là j'ai commencé à écrire une histoire de ces pratiques."]

31. "La psychologie de 1850 à 1950" (no. 2, 1957), in Foucault, *Dits et écrits*, 1: 148–65.

32. Ibid., 1: 156. ["c'est à l'intérieur du système freudien que s'est produit ce grand renversement de la psychologie; c'est au cours de la réflexion freudienne que l'analyse causale s'est transformée en genèse des significations, que l'évolution a fait place à l'histoire, et qu'au recours à la nature s'est substituée l'exigence d'analyser le milieu culturel."]

33. Ibid., 1: 165. ["L'avenir de la psychologie n'est-il pas dès lors dans la prise au sérieux de ces contradictions, dont l'expérience a justement fait naître la psychologie? Il n'y aurait dès lors de psychologie possible que par l'analyse des conditions d'existence de l'homme et par la reprise de ce qu'il y a de plus humain en l'homme, c'est-à-dire son histoire."] On this essay, see Jean-François Bert, "Un siècle de recherche psychologique revu et corrigé par Foucault," in Bert and Basso, *Foucault à Münsterlingen*, 228–32.

34. On the conditions of production of the text, see Luca Paltrinieri, "Philosophie, psychologie, histoire dans les années 1950. *Maladie mentale et personnalité* comme analyseur," in Giuseppe Bianco and Frédéric Fruteau de Laclos, *L'angle mort des années 1950: Philosophie et sciences humaines en France* (Paris: Publications de la Sorbonne, 2016), 169–91.

35. Luca Paltrinieri, "De quelques sources de *Maladie mentale et personnalité*: Ré-

NOTES TO PAGES 116–118   185

flexologie pavlovienne et critique sociale," in Bert and Basso, *Foucault à Münsterlingen*, 199–219.

36. Foucault, *Maladie mentale et personnalité*, 1. ["Sous quelles conditions peut-on parler de maladie mentale dans le domaine psychologique? Quels rapports peut-on définir entre les faits de la pathologie mentale et ceux de la pathologie organique?"]

37. Ibid., 10–12.

38. Ibid., 81.

39. Ibid., 91–92. ["La maladie relève donc de deux sortes de contradictions: les conditions sociales et historiques, qui fondent les conflits psychologiques sur les contradictions réelles du milieu; et les conditions psychologiques qui transforment le contenu conflictuel de l'expérience en forme conflictuelle de la réaction."]

40. On Foucault's reading of Pavlov, see Luca Paltrinieri "De quelques sources de *Maladie mentale et personnalité*," in Bert and Basso, *Foucault à Münsterlingen*, 199–219.

41. Foucault, *Maladie mentale et personnalité*, 102. ["Il y a maladie lorsque le conflit, au lieu d'amener une différenciation dans la réponse, provoque une réaction diffuse de défense; en d'autres termes, lorsque l'individu ne peut maîtriser, au niveau de ses réactions, les contradictions de son milieu, lorsque la dialectique psychologique de l'individu ne peut se retrouver dans la dialectique de ses conditions d'existence. C'est dire en d'autres termes qu'il est aliéné; non plus en ce sens classique qu'il serait devenu étranger à la nature humaine, comme le disaient médecins et juristes au XIXe siècle; mais en ce sens que le malade ne peut se reconnaître, en tant qu'homme dans des conditions d'existence que l'homme lui-même a constituées. L'aliénation, avec ce contenu nouveau, n'est plus une aberration psychologique, elle est définie par un moment historique: c'est en lui seulement qu'elle est rendue possible."]

42. Ibid., 103. ["La pathologie classique admet volontiers que le fait premier est dans *l'anormal* à l'état pur; que l'anormal cristallise autour de lui les conduites pathologiques dont l'ensemble forme la *maladie*; et que l'altération de la personnalité qui en résulte, constitue l'aliénation. Si ce que nous venons de dire est exact, il faudrait renverser l'ordre des termes, et en partant de l'aliénation comme situation originaire, découvrir ensuite le malade, pour définir en dernier lieu, l'anormal."]

43. Contrary to what is often said, Canguilhem was not Foucault's teacher. Canguilhem was on the *jury* (committee) of Foucault's *agrégation* in 1951, but he barely knew Foucault when he agreed to sponsor the *History of Madness*. From these early texts, however, it is obvious that *The Normal and the Pathological* became a crucial reference for Foucault. Foucault recognized this intellectual debt clearly, not only in his dedication in *History of Madness*, but also in his 1978 preface to the English translation of *The Normal and the Pathological* in which he celebrated Canguilhem's "philosophy of concepts" (Georges Canguilhem, *The Normal and the Pathological* [New York: Zone Books, 1989]). Similarly, Canguilhem's influence is striking in Michel Foucault, *The Birth of the Clinic: An Archaeology of Medical Perception* (New York: Vintage Books, 1994). Canguilhem himself noted the confluence of his argument in *The Normal and the Pathological* with institutional psychotherapy when he wrote in 1943, right after his stay at Saint-Alban: "It is interesting to note that in their own discipline contemporary psychiatrists have brought about a rectification and restatement of the concepts of *normal* and *pathological* from which physicians and physiologists apparently have not cared to draw a lesson concerning themselves." In Canguilhem, *Normal and the Pathological*, 115.

44. Foucault, *Maladie mentale et personnalité*, 106. ["Le matérialisme, en psychopathologie, doit donc éviter deux erreurs: celle qui consisterait à identifier le conflit psy-

186 NOTES TO PAGES 118–120

chologique et morbide avec les contradictions historiques du milieu, et à confondre ainsi l'aliénation sociale et l'aliénation mentale; et celle, d'autre part, qui consisterait à vouloir réduire toute maladie à une perturbation du fonctionnement nerveux, dont les mécanismes, encore inconnus, pourraient, en droit, être analysés d'un point de vue purement physiologique."]

45. Ibid., 108. ["que la condition première de la maladie est à trouver dans un conflit du milieu humain, et que le propre de la maladie est d'être réaction généralisée de défense devant ce conflit; alors, la thérapeutique doit prendre une allure nouvelle."]

46. Ibid., 109. ["La psychanalyse psychologise le réel, pour l'irréaliser: elle contraint le sujet à reconnaître dans ses conflits la loi déréglée de son cœur, pour lui éviter d'y lire les contradictions du monde. A ces sortes de psychothérapies, il faut préférer les thérapeutiques qui offrent au malade des moyens concrets de dépasser sa situation de conflit, de modifier son milieu, ou de répondre d'une manière différenciée, c'est-à-dire adaptée, aux contradictions de ses conditions d'existence. Il n'y a pas de guérison possible quand on irréalise les rapports de l'individu et de son milieu; il n'y a, en fait, de guérison que celle qui réalise des rapports nouveaux avec le milieu."]

47. Ibid., 110. ["L'erreur est la même qui veut épuiser l'essence de la maladie dans ses manifestations psychologiques et trouver dans l'explication psychologique le chemin de la guérison. Vouloir détacher le malade de ses conditions d'existence, et vouloir séparer la maladie de ses conditions d'apparition, c'est s'enfermer dans la même abstraction; c'est impliquer la théorie psychologique et la pratique sociale de l'internement dans la même complicité: c'est vouloir maintenir le malade dans son existence d'aliéné. La vraie psychologie doit se délivrer de ces abstractions qui obscurcissent la vérité de la maladie et aliènent la réalité du malade; car, quand il s'agit de l'homme, l'abstraction n'est pas simplement une erreur intellectuelle; la vraie psychologie doit se débarrasser de ce psychologisme, s'il est vrai que, comme toute science de l'homme, elle doit avoir pour but de le désaliéner."]

48. Michel Foucault, *Maladie mentale et psychologie* (Paris: Presses universitaires de France, 1962), 89. ["Jamais la psychologie ne pourra dire sur la folie la vérité, puisque c'est la folie qui détient la vérité de la psychologie. . . . Poussée jusqu'à sa racine, la psychologie de la folie, ce serait non pas la maîtrise de la maladie mentale et par là la possibilité de sa disparition, mais la destruction de la psychologie elle-même et la remise à jour de ce rapport essentiel, non psychologique parce que non moralisable, qui est le rapport de la raison à la déraison."]

49. Eribon, *Michel Foucault*, 92. For a close analysis of the differences between the 1954 and 1962 texts, see Pierre Macherey, "Aux sources de *L'Histoire de la folie*: Une rectification et ses limites," *Critique* 46, no. 471 (1986): 753–74.

50. "La folie n'existe que dans une société" (1961), no. 5 in Foucault, *Dits et écrits*, 1: 195. ["La bonne conscience des psychiatres m'a déçu."]

51. Jean Hyppolite, "Pathologie mentale et organisation" (1955), cited in Eribon, *Michel Foucault*, 93. ["J'ai été confirmé dans l'idée que l'étude de la folie—l'aliénation au sens profond du terme—était au centre d'une anthropologie, d'une étude de l'homme. L'asile est le refuge de ceux qu'on ne peut plus faire vivre dans notre milieu interhumain. C'est donc un moyen de comprendre indirectement ce milieu et les problèmes qu'il pose incessamment à l'homme normal."]

52. Georges Canguilhem, "Qu'est-ce que la psychologie," *Revue de Métaphysique et de Morale*, no. 1 (1958): 12–25. This text was originally delivered at the Collège philosophique on December 18, 1956. Canguilhem recounts the conditions of production of Foucault's

NOTES TO PAGES 121–123   187

thesis in Georges Canguilhem, "Sur *l'Histoire de la folie* en tant qu'évènement," *Le Débat* 41, no. 4 (1986): 37–40.

53. See for example Castel, "Les aventures de la pratique"; Chebili, "Foucault et l'antipsychiatrie."

54. "Michel Foucault, l'illégalisme et l'art de punir" (1976), no. 175 in Foucault, *Dits et écrits*, 2: 88–89. ["Personne ne s'est intéressé au départ à mon premier livre, sauf des littéraires comme Barthes et Blanchot. Mais aucun psychiatre, aucun sociologue, aucun homme de gauche. Avec la *Naissance de la clinique*, ce fut encore pis: silence total. La folie, la santé, ce n'était pas encore un problème théorique et politique noble, à cette époque. Ce qui était noble, c'était la relecture de Marx, la psychanalyse, la sémiologie. De sorte que j'ai été fort déçu de cet inintérêt, je ne m'en cache pas. . . . Et puis, en 1968, brusquement, ces problèmes de santé, de folie, de sexualité, de corps sont entrés directement dans le champ des préoccupations politiques. Le statut des fous intéressait tout à coup toute la population. Ces livres-là, soudain, furent donc sur-consommés, alors qu'ils avaient été sous-consommés pendant la période précédente. J'ai donc repris mon sillon après cette date, avec plus de sérénité d'esprit et avec plus de certitude sur le fait que je ne m'étais pas trompé."] See also "Radioscopie de Michel Foucault" (1975), no. 161, in ibid., 1: 1668, in which Foucault recounts a radio show in which the psychiatrist Henri Baruk got up and told Foucault he had no right to speak because he was not a doctor.

55. Many of these reviews can be found in the excellent collection edited by Philippe Artières, Jean-François Bert, Philippe Chevallier, et al., *Histoire de la folie à l'âge classique de Michel Foucault: Regards critiques, 1961–2011* (Caen: Presses universitaires de Caen, 2011). Two notable exceptions to this lack of interest from the psyche disciplines were the reviews by the psychoanalyst Octave Mannoni, "Histoire de la folie," *Les Temps Modernes*, no. 187 (Dec. 1961): 802–5, and by the psychiatrist Pierre Mondoloni, "Folie et Déraison. Histoire de la folie à l'âge classique, par Michel Foucault, Plon éd.," *L'information psychiatrique* 38, no. 3 (1962): 317–19.

56. Macey, *Lives of Michel Foucault*, 61.

57. Préface (1961), no. 4 in Foucault, *Dits et écrits*, 1: 192. ["Faire l'histoire de la folie voudra donc dire: faire une étude structurale de l'ensemble historique—notions, mesures juridiques et policières, concepts scientifiques—qui tient captive une folie dont l'état sauvage ne peut jamais être restitué en lui-même."] I consulted the English translation of the Jean Khalfa edition: Michel Foucault, *History of Madness*, trans. Jonathan Murphy and Jean Khalfa (London: Routledge, 2006).

58. "Préface" (1961), no. 4 in Foucault, *Dits et écrits*, 1: 188. ["La folie et non-folie, raison et non-raison sont confusément impliquées, inséparables du moment qu'elles n'existent pas encore, et existant l'une pour l'autre, l'une par rapport à l'autre dans l'échange qui les sépare."]

59. Ibid., 187. ["aucun des concepts de psychopathologie ne devra . . . exercer de rôle organisateur."]

60. Michel Foucault, *Histoire de la folie à l'âge classique* (Paris: Gallimard, 1972), 212. [*History of Madness*, 159.]

61. Foucault, *Histoire de la folie à l'âge classique*, 626–27. [*History of Madness*, 505–7.]

62. Lucien Bonnafé, "Le personnage du psychiatre III: ou les métamorphoses," *L'Évolution psychiatrique* 37 (Jan.–Mar. 1967): 8.

63. Ibid., 32.

64. On the Ey/Foucault relation, see Saïd Chebili, *Foucault et la psychologie* (Paris: L'Harmattan, 2005).

188   NOTES TO PAGES 124–128

65. Eribon, *Michel Foucault*, 150.

66. "La conception idéologique de 'L'Histoire de la Folie' de Michel Foucault," 225. ["On peut s'étonner que son 'Histoire de la Folie à l'âge classique' qui entend remettre en cause le concept même de 'maladie mentale' et la raison d'être de notre fonction thérapeutique, que cet ouvrage si radicalement contestataire du bien-fondé de la Psychiatrie, n'ait pas suscité de plus violentes réactions parmi les Psychiatres."]

67. Ibid., 223. ["délivrer l'homme de la société qui l'aliène ou, au contraire, tout en tenant compte évidemment des facteurs socio-culturels qui diversifient la maladie mentale, de reconnaître d'abord l'originalité du fait psychiatrique en tant que maladie mentale."]

68. Ibid., 243. ["L'enjeu d'un débat comme celui qui nous rassemble ici est très clair: celui de la nature morale du concept de maladie mentale. Ou bien celle-ci est une réalité pathologique naturelle, malheureuse atténuation de la responsabilité de l'homme—ou bien elle est un artéfact culturel, scandaleux effet de la répression sociale."]

69. Ibid., 227.

70. Ibid., 228. ["J'ai été très tôt embarrassé par la constante confusion entre la Folie, catégorie du langage trivial, je veux dire banal et quotidien, et les troubles mentaux que nous sommes chargés de traiter, qui sont l'objet de notre fonction, de notre petit savoir, de notre pratique."]

71. Ibid., 234. ["ne peut-on, avec plus de rigueur, aborder le problème épistémologique de façon différente: considérer plutôt ce qui bloquait le regard médical devant le trouble mental pour les prédécesseurs des Médecins de la fin du 18e siècle, et enregistrer comment s'est opérée la mise en place de l'appareil conceptuel qui pouvait embrasser le désordre mental?"]

72. Ibid., 239. ["mais la thèse propagée a été reprise et amplifiée par maints lecteurs et plus encore par des non-lecteurs. Certains jeunes psychiatres sont imprégnés de cette vue déformée, leur pratique quotidienne est infléchie par le tourment qu'elle leur inflige, leur conduite en face du malade est dictée par la crainte d'être pour lui le geôlier médical campé par Foucault."]

73. Ibid., 267. ["La médecine bourgeoise ne soigne pas, elle répare les travailleurs."]

74. Ibid., 282.

75. "Prisons et asiles dans le mécanisme du pouvoir" (1974), no. 136 in Foucault, *Dits et écrits*, 1: 1391. [*L'Histoire de la folie* "a servi de tool-box à des personnes différentes les unes des autres, comme les psychiatres de l'antipsychiatrie britannique, comme Szasz aux États-Unis, comme les sociologues en France: ils l'ont fouillé, ont trouvé un chapitre, une forme d'analyse, quelque chose qui leur a servi ultérieurement."]

76. "Entretien avec Michel Foucault" (1980), no. 281 in Foucault, *Dits et écrits*, 2: 864.

77. Ibid., 2: 879.

78. "Ibid., 2:879–80. Foucault also expressed this idea in "Enfermement. Prison. Psychiatrie" (1977), no. 209 in ibid., 2: 337.

79. For a detailed history of the publication of *History of Madness*, see Artières and Bert, *Un succès philosophique*, 106–27.

80. David Cooper, *Psychiatry and Anti-Psychiatry* (London: Tavistock, 1967).

81. Reader's report reproduced in Jean Khalfa's edition of Foucault, *History of Madness*, ii.

82. R. D. Laing, "The Invention of Madness," *New Statesman*, June 16, 1967, 843.

83. Ibid.

84. R. D. Laing, *The Divided Self: An Existential Study in Sanity and Madness* (London: Penguin Books, 1990), 12. On Laing's life, see Gavin Miller, *R. D. Laing* (Edin-

NOTES TO PAGES 129–131   189

burgh: Edinburgh Review in association with Edinburgh University Press, 2004). See also Staub, *Madness Is Civilization*.

85. See "L'antipsychiatrie britannique," in Hochmann, *Les antipsychiatries*, 169–94.

86. Republished as Stokely Carmichael et al., *The Dialectics of Liberation* (London: Verso, 2015).

87. Basaglia, Laing, and Cooper had all visited La Borde during the 1960s according to Guattari, but their perspectives fundamentally differed from those of institutional psychotherapy. See Jean-Jacques Brochier, "'Antipsychiatrie, antipsychanalyse': entretien avec Felix Guattari," *Magazine littéraire*, nos. 112–13 (May 1976): 28.

88. The proceedings of the colloquium were published in a special issue of *Recherches* in December 1968 titled "Enfance aliénée (II): L'enfant, la psychose et l'institution." ["La maladie mentale, comme le rappelle Foucault, est devenue 'folie aliénée,' aliénée dans cette psychologie qu'elle-même a rendu possible."]

89. Maud Mannoni, *Ce qui manque à la vérité pour être dite* (Paris: Denoël, 1988), 79. ["mise en question continue du cadre institutionnel."] See also Maud Mannoni, Robert Lefort, and Roger Gentis, *Un lieu pour vivre: Les enfants de Bonneuil, leurs parents et l'équipe des soignants* (Paris: Seuil, 1976); Timothy Scott Johnson and Sophie Wustefeld, "Maud Mannoni and Piera Aulagnier on Mental Illness and Disability: Parents at the Boundary between Society and Childhood (France, 1960–80)," *Psychoanalysis and History* 21, no. 2 (August 2019).

90. Maud Mannoni, *Le psychiatre, son "fou" et la psychanalyse* (Paris: Seuil, 1990), 175. ["Pour l'anti-psychiatrie, la guérison est un processus normal qui ne demande aucune thérapeutique. Il suffit de laisser à ce processus la liberté de se développer."]

91. Ibid., 172. ["C'est pourquoi toute idée de réforme institutionnelle est rejetée par l'anti-psychiatrie: elle revendique une mise en question radicale des structures économiques et politiques qui ont amené la naissance des institutions aliénantes."]

92. David Cooper, *Psychiatrie et anti-psychiatrie*, trans. Michel Braudeau (Paris: Seuil, 1970); Erving Goffman, *Asiles: Études sur la condition sociale des malades mentaux et autres reclus*, trans. Liliane Lainé and Claude Lainé (Paris: Éditions de Minuit, 1968); Thomas Stephen Szasz, *Le mythe de la maladie mentale*, trans. Denise Berger (Paris: Payot, 1975).

93. Republished as "Enfermement. Prison. Psychiatrie" (1977), no. 209 in Foucault, *Dits et écrits*, 2: 332–60.

94. John Foot, *The Man Who Closed the Asylums: Franco Basaglia and the Revolution in Mental Health Care* (London: Verso, 2015), 23.

95. Castel, "Les aventures de la pratique," 6.

96. Castel recounts this in Marc Bessin, Bernard Doray, and Jean-Paul Gaudillière, "De la psychiatrie à la société salariale: Une socio-histoire du présent: Entretien avec Robert Castel," *Mouvements* 27–28, no. 3 (2003): 179.

97. Castel, "Présentation," in Goffman, *Asiles*.

98. Ibid., 15. ["L'*asilation* exemplifie ce processus spécial d'adaptation à un univers claustral où le compromis de l'homme et de l'institution dans un temps immobile réalise la symbiose passive de l'initiative et de la répétition."]

99. Ibid., 30. ["L'institution totalitaire est en effet à la fois un modèle réduit, une épure et une caricature de la société globale."]

100. Ibid., 27. ["Il s'agit bien évidemment d'une filiation logique et non d'une influence directe."]

101. Ibid., 26–27. ["Il serait essentiel pour notre propos de distinguer deux moments dans l'histoire de la 'psychothérapie institutionnelle.' Les positions des fondateurs sont

190 NOTES TO PAGES 131–133

très proches de la formulation sociologique du problème, à cette réserve près que leurs analyses demeurent commandées par le souci thérapeutique. On peut se demander si certains des théoriciens les plus récents de ce courant, surtout influencés par les hypothèses de la psychanalyse, de la psychosociologie des groupes, voire de la linguistique structurale, n'ont pas tendance à réinterpréter les déterminismes institutionnels dans une perspective plus étroitement psychosociologique, illustrant ainsi la variante la plus moderne de ce que j'ai appelé ici le 'discours psychiatrique.'"]

102. Ibid., 16. ["La prolifération actuelle des réunions dans les services ne fait qu'institutionnaliser cette perception de l'hôpital comme milieu thérapeutique par le verbe."]

103. Robert Castel, *Le psychanalysme* (Paris: Maspero, 1973); Robert Castel, *L'ordre psychiatrique: L'âge d'or de l'aliénisme* (Paris: Éditions de Minuit, 1976).

104. Robert Castel, *The Regulation of Madness: The Origins of Incarceration in France* (Cambridge, UK: Polity Press, 1988), 8. This is an English translation (by W. D. Halls) of *L'ordre psychiatrique*.

105. Castel, *Le psychanalysme*, 161.

106. "L'asile illimité" (1977), no. 202 in Foucault, *Dits et écrits*, 2: 271–75.

107. Castel, *Regulation of Madness*, 6–7.

108. "L'asile illimité," in Foucault, *Dits et écrits*, 2: 274. ["Le secteur n'est-il pas une autre façon, plus souple, de faire fonctionner la médecine mentale comme hygiène publique, présente partout et toujours prête à intervenir?"]

109. "Enfermement. Prison. Psychiatrie" (1977), no. 209 in Foucault, *Dits et écrits*, 2: 333. ["dès le départ, la psychiatrie a eu pour projet d'être une fonction d'ordre social."]

110. Bessin, Doray, and Gaudillière, "De la psychiatrie à la société salariale," 180; Castel, "Les aventures de la pratique," 6.

111. See "Manifeste du GIP" (1971), no. 86 in Foucault, *Dits et écrits*, 1: 1042–43. Much has been written on the GIP, but for a selective bibliography, see Groupe d'information sur les prisons, *Intolérable*, ed. Philippe Artières (Paris: Verticales, 2013); Philippe Artières, Michelle Zancarini-Fournel, and Laurent Quéro, eds., *Le Groupe d'information sur les prisons: Archives d'une lutte, 1970–1972* (Paris: Éditions de l'IMEC, 2003); François Boullant, *Michel Foucault et les prisons* (Paris: Presses Universitaires de France, 2003); Elden, *Foucault*, chap. 5; Daniel Defert, *Une vie politique* (Paris: Seuil, 2014); Bourg, *From Revolution to Ethics*, 79–95.

112. Liane Mozère develops this comparison in "Foucault et le CERFI."

113. Published in the group's newsletter *Psychiatrisés en lutte* and reproduced in Philippe Bernardet, *Les Dossiers noirs de l'internement psychiatrique (avec la participation du Groupe Information Asiles)* (Paris: Fayard, 1989), 362. ["Cette charte ne vise pas à l'amélioration de la psychiatrie, mais vise à la destruction complète de l'appareil médico-policier. Cette charte s'inscrit dans le combat pour conquérir, dans un premier temps, les droits démocratiques les plus élémentaires qui sont enlevés à tout travailleur que la psychiatrie parvient à isoler."]

114. Ibid., 363. ["1) détruisant l'institution carcérale; 2) en brisant l'isolement de l'interné dans son statut d'assisté, d'irresponsable et de fou; 3) en brisant l'isolement dû au silence."]

115. Archives Bibliothèque Nationale de France, fol. JO. 18236.

116. Groupe Information Asiles, *Psychiatrie: La peur change de camp* (1973), 52–54. ["même les anti-psychiatres ne sortent pas de cette logique et conçoivent la guérison comme une affaire individuelle."] ["L'asile" et le "secteur" ne sont que les deux faces, les deux aspects d'un même ennemi: l'appareil psychiatrique dans son ensemble."]

NOTES TO PAGES 133–138   191

117. Ibid., 47. ["contre le terrorisme de la loi; le comité de défense des internés; contre le terrorisme du savoir; dépsychiatriser la folie; sortir la folie de son statut privé."]

118. *Psychiatrisés en lutte* (Feb.–Apr. 1975).

119. For more on these different groups, see Artières and Bert, *Un succès philosophique*, 225–39. See also Jacques Lagrange, "Course Context," in Foucault, *Psychiatric Power*, 353. On the GIS and Foucault, see the transcription of their roundtable, published as "Médecine et lutte de classes" in *La Nef*. 49 (1972).

120. François Gantheret and Jean-Marie Brohm, *Garde-fous, arrêtez de vous serrer les coudes* (Paris: Maspero, 1975), 5. ["Il n'y a pas si longtemps encore les fous étaient enfermés pêle-mêle avec les prostituées, les chômeurs, les truands, la pègre, en un mot avec tous ceux qui n'étaient pas 'normaux' face aux valeurs consacrées par la société de classe; avec tous ceux qui dérangeaient les normes de la propriété privée et l'institution de la conformité des mœurs."]

121. *Gardes-fous*, no. 10 (Winter 1976): 23.

122. "Table ronde sur l'expertise psychiatrique" (1974), no. 142 in Foucault, *Dits et écrits*, 1: 1532–43.

123. Ibid., 1: 1539–40. [Hassoun: "Toute la psychiatrie manie les concepts de réadaptabilité, de dangerosité, de responsabilité." Foucault: "Elles ne sont ni dans le droit ni dans la médecine. Ce sont des notions ni juridiques, ni psychiatriques, ni médicales, mais disciplinaires. Ce sont toutes ces petites disciplines de l'école, de la caserne, de la maison de correction, de l'usine, qui ont pris plus d'ampleur."]

124. "Asiles, Sexualité, Prisons" (1975), no. 160 in ibid., 1: 1641. ["D'une façon générale, je dirais que l'antipsychiatrie de Laing et de Cooper, entre 1955 et 1960, marque le début de cette analyse critique et politique des phénomènes de pouvoir. Je pense que, jusqu'à 1970–1975, des analyses du pouvoir, des analyses critiques, en même temps théoriques et pratiques, ont tourné essentiellement autour de la notion de répression. Dénoncer le pouvoir répressif, le rendre visible, lutter contre lui. Mais, à la suite des changements opérés en 1968, il faut l'aborder dans un autre registre; nous n'avancerions pas si nous continuions à poser le problème dans ces termes: il nous faut poursuivre cette analyse théorique et politique du pouvoir, mais d'une autre manière."]

125. Eribon, *Michel Foucault*, 170.

126. Foucault, *Histoire de la folie à l'âge classique*, 9. [*History of Madness*, xxxvii.]

127. "Le grand enfermement," no. 105 (1972), in Foucault, *Dits et écrits*, 1: 1169. See chap. 4, n. 9, above.

128. Defert, *Une vie politique*. When Defert asked Foucault to participate in the GIP, "Foucault me confia qu'il était enchanté, que c'était dans le droit-fil de l'*Histoire de la folie*."

129. "Entretien avec Michel Foucault" (1977), no. 192 in Foucault, *Dits et écrits*, 2: 146. ["On n'a pu commencer à faire ce travail qu'après 1968, c'est-à-dire à partir de luttes quotidiennes et menées à la base, avec ceux qui avaient à se débattre dans les maillons les plus fins du réseau du pouvoir. C'est là où le concret du pouvoir est apparu et en même temps la fécondité vraisemblable de ces analyses du pouvoir pour se rendre compte de ces choses qui étaient restées jusque-là hors du champ de l'analyse politique. Pour dire les choses très simplement, l'internement psychiatrique, la normalisation mentale des individus, les institutions pénales ont sans doute une importance assez limitée si on en cherche seulement la signification économique. En revanche, dans le fonctionnement général des rouages du pouvoir, ils sont sans doute essentiels."]

130. See for example "Par-delà le bien et le mal" (1971), no. 98 in ibid., 1: 1099. ["Notre

action . . . ne cherche pas l'âme ou l'homme derrière le condamné, mais à effacer cette frontière profonde entre l'innocence et la culpabilité."]

131. "Un problème m'intéresse depuis longtemps, c'est celui du système penal" (1971), no. 95 in ibid., 1: 1077. ["Depuis quelques années s'est développé en Italie, autour de Basaglia, et en Angleterre un mouvement qu'on appelle antipsychiatrie. Ces gens-là ont, bien sûr, développé leur mouvement à partir de leurs idées et de leurs expériences de psychiatres, mais ils ont vu dans le livre que j'avais écrit une sorte de justification historique et ils l'ont, d'une certaine façon, réassumé, repris en compte, ils s'y sont, jusqu'à un certain point, retrouvés, et voilà que ce livre historique est en train d'avoir une sorte d'aboutissement pratique. Alors, disons que je suis un peu jaloux et que, maintenant, je voudrais faire les choses moi-même. Au lieu d'écrire un livre sur l'histoire de la justice, qui serait ensuite repris par des gens qui remettraient pratiquement en question la justice, je voudrais commencer par la remise en question pratique de la justice et puis, ma foi! si je vis encore et si je n'ai pas été mis en prison, eh bien, j'écrirai le livre . . ."]

132. Michel Foucault, *Discipline and Punish: The Birth of the Prison* (New York: Vintage Books, 1995), 31. [Michel Foucault, *Surveiller et punir: Naissance de la prison* (Paris: Gallimard, 1975), 35.] For how the book was written in conversation with the GIP experience, see Philippe Artières, Jean-François Bert, Pierre Lascoumes, et al., eds., *Surveiller et punir de Michel Foucault: Regards critiques, 1975–1979* (Caen: Presses universitaires de Caen, 2010).

133. Foucault, *Psychiatric Power*, 12–13.

134. Ibid., 4.

135. Ibid., 13.

136. Ibid., 14.

137. Ibid., 15.

138. Ibid., 16.

139. Ibid., 39.

140. Ibid., 59.

141. Ibid., 41.

142. Ibid., 189.

143. Barnes and Berke, *Mary Barnes*. Foucault cites the French translation in his course.

144. Foucault, *Psychiatric Power*, 254.

145. Michel Foucault, "Histoire de la folie et antipsychiatrie," 95.

146. Ibid., 96.

147. Ibid., 98. ["l'hôpital comme lieu d'affrontement entre la passion et la volonté perturbée du malade, la passion, la volonté orthodoxe du médecin et du personnel hospitalier."]

148. Ibid., 99.

149. Ibid., 100. ["tout ce qui remet en question le rôle d'un psychiatre chargé autrefois de produire la vérité de la maladie dans l'espace hospitalier."]

150. Ibid., 102. ["Enfin, quatrième type de psychiatrie, celle qui consisterait non pas exactement à supposer, comme le font Laing et Cooper, que le rapport de pouvoir peut être éludé, peut être mis entre parenthèses, peut être en quelque sort anéanti d'un coup; c'est une antipsychiatrie au contraire qui considère que les rapports de pouvoir ne surprennent pas la folie de l'extérieur sous le seul visage du médecin ou de l'administrateur, mais qu'au fond les rapports de pouvoir ont tramé toute l'existence du malade et ont tramé sa folie et que, par conséquent, c'est bien la mise au jour et en même temps

NOTES TO PAGES 143–148   193

la destruction, et la destruction politique de tous ces rapports de pouvoir, qu'ils soient ceux qui ont rendu possible la folie ou que ce soit ceux qui s'exercent contre la folie; c'est cette destruction de tous les rapports de pouvoir qui doit être la tâche de l'antipsychiatrie, et c'est cela, si vous voulez, qui permet—je crois—de situer dans ce très large panorama les recherches de Basaglia ou celles qui sont actuellement menées en France par des gens comme Guattari."]

Epilogue

1. See for example Judith Butler, *Notes toward a Performative Theory of Assembly* (Cambridge: Harvard University Press, 2015).

2. Michel Feher, *Rated Agency: Investee Politics in a Speculative Age* (New York: Zone Books, 2018); Wendy Brown, *Undoing the Demos: Neoliberalism's Stealth Revolution* (New York: Zone Books, 2015); Michel Foucault, *The Birth of Biopolitics: Lectures at the Collège de France, 1978–79* (New York: Palgrave Macmillan, 2008).

3. Pierre Dardot and Christian Laval, *Commun: Essai sur la révolution au XXIe siècle* (Paris: La Découverte, 2014). [Pierre Dardot and Christian Laval, *Common: On Revolution in the 21st Century*, trans. Matthew MacLellan (London: Bloomsbury Academic, 2019).]

4. Dardot and Laval, *Commun*, 583.

5. On this point, Dardot and Laval targeted in particular the second volume of Michael Hardt and Antonio Negri's trilogy, *Commonwealth*, published between *Empire* in 2000 and *Assembly* in 2017: Michael Hardt and Antonio Negri, *Commonwealth* (Cambridge: Belknap Press of Harvard University Press, 2009).

6. Dardot and Laval, *Commun*, 451.

7. Ibid., 445. ["la praxis instituante est donc tout à la fois l'activité qui établit un nouveau système de règles *et* l'activité qui cherche à relancer en permanence cet établissement de manière à éviter l'enlisement de l'instituant dans l'institué."]

8. Ibid. ["la praxis anticipe consciemment dès le début la nécessité d'avoir à modifier et à réinventer l'institué qu'elle n'a posé que pour mieux le faire vivre dans la durée."]

9. Ibid. ["La praxis instituante produit son propre sujet dans la continuité d'un exercice qui est toujours à renouveler au-delà de l'acte créateur. Plus exactement, elle est autoproduction d'un sujet collectif dans et par la coproduction continuée de règles de droit."]

10. Ibid., 446. ["Terme d'"institutionnalisation' désigne ici non pas la création de nouvelles institutions par la loi . . . ou encore moins l'officialisation de ce qui existait déjà sans être reconnu, mais très précisément la réinvention permanente de l'institution par laquelle le groupe qui l'a créée peut contrecarrer son inertie. Tout le dispositif du Collectif est ordonné à cette exigence de la relance de l'activité instituante."]

11. See for example, Miriam Ticktin, "No Borders in the Time of COVID-19," in *American Anthropologist*, July 2, 2020: http://www.americananthropologist.org/2020/07/02/no-borders-in-the-time-of-covid-19/.

12. Thomas Frank, *What's the Matter with Kansas?: How Conservatives Won the Heart of America* (New York: Metropolitan Books, 2004).

13. Wilder, *Freedom Time*, 12.

14. Ibid., 13. LaCapra develops this notion throughout much of his work, but see, for example, Dominick LaCapra, *History & Criticism* (Ithaca: Cornell University Press, 1985); Dominick LaCapra, *Rethinking Intellectual History: Texts, Contexts, Language* (Ithaca: Cornell University Press, 1983).

BIBLIOGRAPHY

Archives

Archives de l'Association des amis de Septfonds
Archives de La Borde
Archives départementales de Tarn-et-Garonne: Camp de Septfonds
Archives Pere Mata in Reus, Spain
Archives Saint-Alban, Centre hospitalier François Tosquelles, Lozère
Bibliothèque littéraire Jacques Doucet: Fonds Jean Delay
Bibliothèque Nationale de France: Fonds Michel Foucault
IMEC (Institut mémoires de l'édition contemporaine)
  Fonds Lucien Bonnafé
  Fonds Fernand Deligny
  Fonds Frantz Fanon
  Fonds Michel Foucault
  Fonds Groupe d'information sur les prisons (GIP)
  Fonds Félix Guattari
  Fonds Gisela Pankow
POUM / Fundación Andreu Nin (Barcelona)

Published Sources

Abadie, Daniel, ed. *Dubuffet: Catalogue de l'exposition "Jean Dubuffet" présentée à l'occasion du centenaire de la naissance de l'artiste, Centre Pompidou, 2001.* Paris: Centre Pompidou, 2001.

Alba, Víctor, and Stephen Schwartz. *Spanish Marxism versus Soviet Communism: A History of the P.O.U.M.* New Brunswick, NJ: Transaction Books, 1988.

Anderson, Warwick, Deborah Jenson, and Richard C. Keller. *Unconscious Dominions: Psychoanalysis, Colonial Trauma, and Global Sovereignties.* Durham, NC: Duke University Press, 2011.

Apprill, Olivier. *Une avant-garde psychiatrique: Le moment GTPSI (1960–1966).* Paris: Epel, 2013.

Arnall, Gavin. *Subterranean Fanon: An Underground Theory of Radical Change.* New York: Columbia University Press, 2020.

BIBLIOGRAPHY

Arrighi, Paul. *Silvio Trentin: Un Européen en résistance, 1919–1943.* Portet-sur-Garonne: Loubatières, 2007.

Arthur, Paige. *Unfinished Projects: Decolonization and the Philosophy of Jean-Paul Sartre.* London: Verso, 2010.

Artières, Philippe, Jean-François Bert, Philippe Chevallier, et al., eds. *Histoire de la folie à l'âge classique de Michel Foucault: Regards critiques, 1961–2011.* Caen: Presses universitaires de Caen, 2011.

Artières, Philippe, and Jean-François Bert. *Un succès philosophique: L'histoire de la folie à l'âge classique de Michel Foucault.* Caen: Presses universitaires de Caen, 2011.

Artières, Philippe, Jean-François Bert, Pierre Lascoumes, et al., eds. *Surveiller et punir de Michel Foucault: Regards critiques, 1975–1979.* Caen: Presses universitaires de Caen, 2010.

Artières, Philippe, Michelle Zancarini-Fournel, and Laurent Quéro, eds. *Le Groupe d'information sur les prisons: Archives d'une lutte, 1970–1972.* Paris: Éditions de l'IMEC, 2003.

Ayme, Jean. "Essai sur l'histoire de la psychothérapie institutionnelle." *Actualités de la psychothérapie institutionnelle* (1985).

Bailly-Salin, Pierre. "The Mentally Ill under Nazi Occupation in France." *International Journal of Mental Health* 35, no. 4 (2006–7): 11–25.

Balvet, Paul. "L'ambre du musée." *L'Information psychiatrique* 54, no. 8 (1978): 861–64.

Barnes, Mary, and Joseph H. Berke. *Mary Barnes: Two Accounts of a Journey through Madness.* New York: Harcourt Brace Jovanovich, 1972.

Basso, Elisabetta. *Michel Foucault e la daseinsanalyse: Un'indagine metodologica.* Milan: Mimesis, 2007.

Bégué, Jean-Michel. "French Psychiatry in Algeria (1830–1962): From Colonial to Transcultural." *History of Psychiatry* 7 (1996): 533–48.

Bellahsen, Mathieu. *La santé mentale vers un bonheur sous contrôle.* Paris: La Fabrique, 2014.

Benjamin, Walter. *The Origin of German Tragic Drama.* London: Verso, 2003.

Bentouhami, Hourya. "L'emprise du corps: Fanon à l'aune de la phénoménologie de Merleau-Ponty." *Cahiers Philosophiques* 3, no. 138 (2014): 34–46.

Bernardet, Philippe. *Les Dossiers noirs de l'internement psychiatrique (avec la participation du Groupe Information Asiles).* Paris: Fayard, 1989.

Bert, Jean-François, and Elisabetta Basso. *Foucault à Münsterlingen: À l'origine de l'Histoire de la folie.* Paris: Éditions EHESS, 2015.

Berthelier, Robert. *L'homme maghrébin dans la littérature psychiatrique.* Paris: L'Harmattan, 1994.

Bessin, Marc, Bernard Doray, and Jean-Paul Gaudillière. "De la psychiatrie à la société salariale: Une socio-histoire du présent: Entretien avec Robert Castel." *Mouvements* 27–28, no. 3 (2003): 177–85.

Bianco, Giuseppe. "La réaction au bergsonisme: Transformations de la philosophie française de Politzer à Deleuze." Université Charles de Gaulle—Lille 3, 2009.

Bianco, Giuseppe, and Frédéric Fruteau de Laclos. *L'angle mort des années 1950: Philosophie et sciences humaines en France.* Paris: Publications de la Sorbonne, 2016.

Bonnafé, Lucien. *Désaliéner?: Folie(s) et société(s).* Toulouse: Presses universitaires du Mirail, 1991.

———. "Le personnage du psychiatre III: Ou les métamorphoses." *L'Évolution psychiatrique* 37 (Jan.–Mar. 1967): 1–36.

Bonnet, Marius. "Le témoignage d'un infirmier." *Esprit* 197, no. 12 (1952): 815–20.

BIBLIOGRAPHY

Boulanger, Christophe. "La conation esthétique de Jean Oury." In *Le Collectif à venir*, 101–14. Toulouse: ERES, 2018.

Boulanger, Christophe, Sabine Faupin, Mireille Gauzy, and Madeleine Lommel. *Trait d'union: Les chemins de l'art brut à Saint-Alban-sur-Limagnole*. Lille: Musée d'art moderne Lille, 2007.

Boullant, François. *Michel Foucault et les prisons*. Paris: Presses Universitaires de France, 2003.

Bourg, Julian. *From Revolution to Ethics: May 1968 and Contemporary French Thought*. Montreal: McGill-Queen's University Press, 2007.

Brochier, Jean-Jacques. "'Antipsychiatrie, antipsychanalyse': Entretien avec Félix Guattari." *Magazine littéraire*, nos. 112–13 (May 1976): 28–30.

Brown, Wendy. *Undoing the Demos: Neoliberalism's Stealth Revolution*. New York: Zone Books, 2015.

Buck-Morss, Susan. *Hegel, Haiti, and Universal History*. Pittsburgh: University of Pittsburgh Press, 2009.

Bueltzingsloewen, Isabelle von. *L'hécatombe des fous: La famine dans les hôpitaux psychiatriques français sous l'Occupation*. Paris: Aubier, 2007.

Bulhan, Hussein Abdilahi. *Frantz Fanon and the Psychology of Oppression*. New York: Plenum Press, 1985.

Butler, Judith. *Notes toward a Performative Theory of Assembly*. Cambridge: Harvard University Press, 2015.

Caló, Susana. *The Grid* 2016. https://www.anthropocene-curriculum.org/contribution /the-grid. Accessed April 10, 2020.

Caló, Susana, and Godofredo Pereira. "CERFI: From the Hospital to the City." *London Journal of Critical Thought (LJCT)* 1, no. 2 (2017): 83–100.

Canguilhem, Georges. *Le normal et le pathologique*. Paris: Quadrige/PUF, 2005.

———. *The Normal and the Pathological*. New York: Zone Books, 1989.

———. *Résistance, philosophie biologique et histoire des sciences, 1940–1965*. Ed. Camille Limoges. Paris: Librairie philosophique J. Vrin, 2015.

———. "Sur *l'Histoire de la folie* en tant qu'événement." *Le Débat* 41, no. 4 (1986): 37–40.

Carmichael, Stokely, David Cooper, R. D. Laing, and Herbert Marcuse. *The Dialectics of Liberation*. London: Verso, 2015.

Castel, Robert. *L'ordre psychiatrique: L'âge d'or de l'aliénisme*. Paris: Éditions de Minuit, 1976.

———. *Le psychanalysme*. Paris: Maspero, 1973.

———. "Les aventures de la pratique." *Le Débat* 41, no. 4 (1986): 41–51.

———. *The Regulation of Madness: The Origins of Incarceration in France*. Cambridge, UK: Polity Press, 1988.

Chanoit, Pierre. *La psychothérapie institutionnelle*. Paris: Presses Universitaires de France, 1995.

Chaumon, Franck. *Lacan: La loi, le sujet et la jouissance*. Paris: Michalon, 2004.

Chebili, Saïd. "Foucault et l'antipsychiatrie." *L'Information psychiatrique* 92, no. 8 (2016): 671–76.

———. *Foucault et la psychologie*. Paris: L'Harmattan, 2005.

Cherki, Alice. *Frantz Fanon: Portrait*. Paris: Seuil, 2000.

Chettiar, Teri. "Democratizing Mental Health: Motherhood, Therapeutic Community and the Emergence of the Psychiatric Family at the Cassel Hospital in Post–Second World War Britain." *History of the Human Sciences* 25, no. 5 (2012): 107–22.

BIBLIOGRAPHY

Christ, Michel. *Le POUM: Histoire d'un parti révolutionnaire espagnol (1935–1952)*. Paris: Harmattan, 2005.

Cléro, Jean-Pierre. *Le vocabulaire de Lacan*. Paris: Ellipses, 2012.

Cole, Jennifer. *Forget Colonialism?: Sacrifice and the Art of Memory in Madagascar*. Berkeley: University of California Press, 2001.

Comelles, Josep M. "Forgotten Paths: Culture and Ethnicity in Catalan Mental Health Policies (1900–39)." *History of Psychiatry* 21, no. 4 (2010): 406–23.

"La conception idéologique de 'L'Histoire de la Folie' de Michel Foucault (Journées annuelles de *l'Évolution Psychiatrique*, Toulouse, 6–7 Décembre 1969)." *L'Évolution Psychiatrique* 36, no. 2 (1971): 223–98.

"La Constitution de l'an I." *Recherches: Histoires de la Borde: 10 ans de psychothérapie institutionnelle à Cour-Cheverny, 1953–1963*, no. 21 (Mar.–Apr. 1976).

Cooper, David. *Psychiatrie et anti-psychiatrie*. Trans. Michel Braudeau. Paris: Seuil, 1970.

———. *Psychiatry and Anti-Psychiatry*. London: Tavistock, 1967.

Cooper, Frederick. *Citizenship between Empire and Nation: Remaking France and French Africa, 1945–1960*. Princeton: Princeton University Press, 2014.

Cottias, Myriam, and Madeleine Dobie. *Relire Mayotte Capécia: Une femme des Antilles dans l'espace colonial français*. Paris: Armand Colin, 2012.

Courtois, Stéphane. *Le PCF dans la guerre: De Gaulle, la Résistance, Staline*. Paris: Ramsay, 1980.

Culler, Jonathan D. *Ferdinand de Saussure*. Ithaca, NY: Cornell University Press, 1986.

Daeninckx, Didier. *Caché dans la maison des fous*. Paris: Gallimard, 2017.

Dalzell, Thomas G. *Freud's Schreber between Psychiatry and Psychoanalysis: On Subjective Disposition to Psychosis*. London: Karnac Books, 2011.

Damamme, Dominique, Boris Gobille, Frédérique Matonti, and Bernard Pudal. *Mai–juin 68*. Ivry-sur-Seine: Les Éditions de l'Atelier, 2008.

Damousi, Joy, and Mariano Ben Plotkin. *Psychoanalysis and Politics: Histories of Psychoanalysis under Conditions of Restricted Political Freedom*. New York: Oxford University Press, 2012.

Dardot, Pierre, and Christian Laval. *Common: On Revolution in the 21st Century*. Trans. Matthew MacLellan. London: Bloomsbury Academic, 2019.

———. *Commun: Essai sur la révolution au XXIe siècle*. Paris: La Découverte, 2014.

Daumézon, Georges. "Le poids des structures." *Esprit* 197 (Dec. 1952): 935–44.

Dean, Carolyn J. *The Self and Its Pleasures: Bataille, Lacan, and the History of the Decentered Subject*. Ithaca: Cornell University Press, 1992.

de Felipe-Redondo, Jesus. "Worker Resistance to 'Social' Reform and the Rise of Anarchism in Spain, 1880–1920." *Critical Historical Studies* 1, no. 2 (2014): 255–84.

Defert, Daniel. *Une vie politique*. Paris: Seuil, 2014.

Deleuze, Gilles. *Desert Islands and Other Texts, 1953–1974*. Los Angeles: Semiotext(e), 2004.

———. *Expressionism in Philosophy: Spinoza*. New York: Zone Books, 1990.

———. *Foucault*. Paris: Editions de Minuit, 1986.

———. *Nietzsche et la philosophie*. Paris: Presses universitaires de France, 1962.

———. *Pourparlers, 1972–1990*. Paris: Editions de Minuit, 1990.

———. *Spinoza, Practical Philosophy*. San Francisco: City Lights Books, 1988.

———. *Two Regimes of Madness: Texts and Interviews, 1975–1995*. Los Angeles: Semiotext(e), 2006.

Deleuze, Gilles, and Félix Guattari. *Anti-Oedipus: Capitalism and Schizophrenia*. Minneapolis: University of Minnesota Press, 1983.

BIBLIOGRAPHY 199

———. *L'Anti-Œdipe*. Paris: Éditions de Minuit, 1972.

———. *Kafka, pour une littérature mineure*. Paris: Éditions de Minuit, 1975.

Deleuze, Gilles, and David Lapoujade. *L'île déserte et autres textes: Textes et entretiens, 1953–1974*. Paris: Editions de Minuit, 2002.

Deleuze, Gilles, and Claire Parnet. *Dialogues*. Paris: Flammarion, 1977.

Deligny, Fernand. *Œuvres*. Ed. Sandra Alvarez de Toledo. Paris: L'Arachnéen, 2007.

Deyres, Martine. *Les heures heureuses*. Marseille: Les Films du tambour de soie, 2019.

Diagne, Souleymane Bachir. "La Négritude comme mouvement et comme devenir." *Rue Descartes* 83, no. 4 (2014): 50–61.

Di Capua, Yoav. *No Exit: Arab Existentialism, Jean-Paul Sartre, and Decolonization*. Chicago: The University of Chicago Press, 2018.

Dicks, Henry Victor. *Fifty Years of the Tavistock Clinic*. London: Routledge, 1970.

Dieudonné, Julien, and Marianne Jakobi. *Dubuffet*. Paris: Perrin, 2007.

Djian, Jean-Michel, ed. *Vincennes: Une aventure de la pensée critique*. Paris: Flammarion, 2009.

Dosse, François. "François Maspero: La joie de lire, 1932–." In *Les hommes de l'ombre: Portraits d'éditeurs*. Paris: Perrin, 2014.

———. *Gilles Deleuze et Félix Guattari: Biographie croisée*. Paris: Découverte, 2007.

Dreyfus-Armand, Geneviève. *L'exil des républicains espagnols en France: De la Guerre civile à la mort de Franco*. Paris: Albin Michel, 1999.

———. *Septfonds, 1939–1944 dans l'archipel des camps français*. Perpignan: Le Revenant, 2019.

Dreyfus-Armand, Geneviève, and Émile Temime. *Les camps sur la plage: Un exil espagnol*. Paris: Autrement, 1995.

Druet, Anne-Cécile. "La psychiatrie espagnole et la psychanalyse des années 1910 à la guerre civile. De la presse médicale au discours social." *El Argonauta Español* 8 (2001).

Dubuffet, Jean. *L'art brut préféré aux arts culturels*. Paris: Galerie René Drouin, 1949.

Duong, Kevin. *The Virtues of Violence: Democracy against Disintegration in Modern France*. New York: Oxford University Press, 2020.

Dutrenit, Jean-Marc. *Sociologie, travail social et psychiatrie: Le berceau lozérien de la psychothérapie institutionnelle*. Paris: Études vivantes, 1981.

Ealham, Chris. *Class, Culture, and Conflict in Barcelona, 1898–1937*. London: Routledge, 2005.

Elden, Stuart. *Canguilhem*. Cambridge, UK: Polity, 2019.

———. *Foucault: The Birth of Power*. Malden, MA: Polity, 2017.

Eribon, Didier. *Michel Foucault: 1926–1984*. Paris: Flammarion, 1991.

Evans, Dylan. *An Introductory Dictionary of Lacanian Psychoanalysis*. New York: Routledge, 1996.

Fanon, Frantz. *Alienation and Freedom*. Ed. Jean Khalfa and Robert Young. Trans. Steve Corcoran. London: Bloomsbury, 2018.

———. *Black Skin, White Masks*. Trans. Richard Philcox. New York: Grove Press, 2008.

———. *Écrits sur l'aliénation et la liberté*. Ed. Jean Khalfa and Robert Young. Paris: La Découverte, 2015.

———. *Frantz Fanon par les textes de l'époque*. Paris: Les Petits Matins, 2012.

———. *Œuvres*. Paris: La Découverte, 2011.

———. *Toward the African Revolution: Political Essays*. Trans. Haakon Chevalier. New York: Grove Press, 1967.

———. *The Wretched of the Earth*. Trans. Richard Philcox. New York: Grove Press, 2004.

Fau, Jean-Claude. "Le camp des réfugiés espagnols de Septfonds (Tarn-et-Garonne)

1939–1940." In *Les camps du Sud-Ouest de la France 1939–1944: Exclusion, internement et déportation*, ed. Monique-Lise Cohen and Éric Malo. Toulouse: Privat, 1994.

Faugeras, Patrick, ed. *L'ombre portée de François Tosquelles*. Ramonville Saint-Agne: Érès, 2007.

Feher, Michel. "Mai 68 dans la pensée." In *Histoire des gauches en France*, vol. 2. Ed. Jean-Jacques Becker and Gilles Candar. Paris: La Découverte, 2004.

———. *Rated Agency: Investee Politics in a Speculative Age*. New York: Zone Books, 2018.

Fink, Bruce. *The Lacanian Subject: Between Language and Jouissance*. Princeton: Princeton University Press, 1995.

Foot, John. *The Man Who Closed the Asylums: Franco Basaglia and the Revolution in Mental Health Care*. London: Verso, 2015.

Foucault, Michel. *The Birth of Biopolitics: Lectures at the Collège de France, 1978–79*. New York: Palgrave Macmillan, 2008.

———. *The Birth of the Clinic: An Archaeology of Medical Perception*. New York: Vintage Books, 1994.

———. *Discipline and Punish: The Birth of the Prison*. New York: Vintage Books, 1995.

———. *Dits et écrits, 1954–1988*. 2 vols. Collection Quarto, ed. Daniel Defet and François Ewald. Paris: Gallimard, 2001.

———. *Histoire de la folie à l'âge classique*. Paris: Gallimard, 1972.

———. "Histoire de la folie et antipsychiatrie." *Cahier de L'Herne* 95 (2011): 95–102.

———. *History of Madness*. Ed. by Jean Khalfa. Trans. Jean Khalfa and Jonathan Murphy. London: Routledge, 2006.

———. *Maladie mentale et personnalité*. Paris: Presses universitaires de France, 1954.

———. *Maladie mentale et psychologie*. Paris: Presses universitaires de France, 1962.

———. *Psychiatric Power: Lectures at the Collège de France, 1973–74*. Basingstoke, UK: Palgrave Macmillan, 2006.

———. *Surveiller et punir: Naissance de la prison*. Paris: Gallimard, 1975.

Fourquet, François, and Lion Murard. *Les équipements du pouvoir: Villes, territoires et équipements collectifs*. Paris: Union générale d'éditions, 1976.

Frank, Thomas. *What's the Matter with Kansas?: How Conservatives Won the Heart of America*. New York: Metropolitan Books, 2004.

Freud, Sigmund. *The Schreber Case*. Trans. Andrew Webber. New York: Penguin Books, 2003.

Gantheret, François, and Jean-Marie Brohm. *Garde-fous, arrêtez de vous serrer les coudes*. Paris: Maspero, 1975.

Garo, Isabelle. *Foucault, Deleuze, Althusser & Marx: La politique dans la philosophie*. Paris: Demopolis, 2011.

Gateau, Jean-Charles. *Paul Éluard ou le frère voyant, 1895–1952*. Paris: Robert Laffont, 1988.

Geroulanos, Stefanos, and Todd Meyers. *The Human Body in the Age of Catastrophe: Brittleness, Integration, Science, and the Great War*. Chicago: University of Chicago Press, 2018.

Getachew, Adom. *Worldmaking after Empire: The Rise and Fall of Self-Determination*. Princeton: Princeton University Press, 2019.

Gibson, Nigel C., and Roberto Beneduce. *Decolonizing Madness: The Psychiatric Writings of Frantz Fanon*. New York: Palgrave Macmillan, 2014.

Glick, Thomas F. "The Naked Science: Psychoanalysis in Spain, 1914–1948." *Comparative Studies in Society and History of European Ideas* 24 (1982): 533–71.

Goffman, Erving. *Asiles: Études sur la condition sociale des malades mentaux et autres reclus.* Trans. Liliane Lainé and Claude Lainé. Paris: Éditions de Minuit, 1968.

Goldstein, Jan. *Console and Classify: The French Psychiatric Profession in the Nineteenth Century.* Chicago: University of Chicago Press, 2001.

———. *The Post-Revolutionary Self: Politics and Psyche in France, 1750–1850.* Cambridge: Harvard University Press, 2005.

Gougoulis, Nicolas. "Freud et les psychiatres." *Topique* 88, no. 3 (2004): 17–35.

Gros, Caroline. *Ludwig Binswanger: Entre phénoménologie et expérience psychiatrique.* Chatou: Les Éditions de la Transparence, 2009.

Groupe d'information sur les prisons. *Intolérable.* Ed. Philippe Artières. Paris: Verticales, 2013.

Grütter, Angela. *Hermann Simon: Die Entwicklung der Arbeits- und Beschäftigungstherapie in der Anstaltspsychiatrie: Eine biographische Betrachtung.* Herzogenrath: Murken-Altrogge, 1995.

Grynberg, Anne. *Les camps de la honte: Les internés juifs des camps français, 1939–1944.* Paris: La Découverte, 1999.

Guattari, Félix. *The Anti-Oedipus Papers.* New York: Semiotext(e), 2006.

———. *Chaosophy.* New York: Semiotext(e), 1995.

———. *De Leros à La Borde.* Paris: Lignes/IMEC, 2011.

———. *Molecular Revolutions: Psychiatry and Politics.* Trans. Rosemary Sheed. New York: Penguin Books, 1984.

———. *Psychanalyse et transversalité. Essais d'analyse institutionnelle.* Paris: La Découverte, 2003.

———. *Psychoanalysis and Transversality: Texts and Interviews, 1955–1971.* Trans. Ames Hodges. South Pasadena, CA: Semiotext(e), 2015.

Guenther, Katja. *Localization and Its Discontents: A Genealogy of Psychoanalysis and the Neuro Disciplines.* Chicago: University of Chicago Press, 2015.

Guichard, Bruno, Julien Hage, and Alain Léger. *François Maspero et les paysages humains.* Lyon: La fosse aux ours, 2009.

Guillemain, Hervé. "Les effets secondaires de la technique. Patients et institutions psychiatriques au temps de l'électrochoc, de la psychochirurgie et des neuroleptiques retard (années 1940–1970)." *Revue d'histoire moderne & contemporaine* 67-1, no. 1 (2020): 72–98.

Haas, Ron. "Guy Hocquenghem and the Cultural Revolution in France after May 1968." In *After the Deluge: New Perspectives on the Intellectual and Cultural History of Postwar France,* ed. Julian Bourg, 175–99. Lanham, MD: Lexington Books, 2004.

Hage, Julien. "François Maspero: Éditeur partisan." *Contretemps* 13 (2005): 100–107.

Hamon, Hervé, and Patrick Rotman. *Génération.* 2 vols. Paris: Seuil, 1987 and 1988.

Hardt, Michael, and Antonio Negri. *Commonwealth.* Cambridge: Belknap Press of Harvard University Press, 2009.

Harrington, Anne. *Mind Fixers: Psychiatry's Troubled Search for the Biology of Mental Illness.* New York: W. W. Norton, 2019.

Heaton, Matthew M. *Black Skin, White Coats: Nigerian Psychiatrists, Decolonization, and the Globalization of Psychiatry.* Athens: Ohio University Press, 2013.

Herzog, Dagmar. *Cold War Freud: Psychoanalysis in an Age of Catastrophes.* Cambridge, UK: Cambridge University Press, 2017.

———. *Unlearning Eugenics: Sexuality, Reproduction, and Disability in Post-Nazi Europe.* Madison: University of Wisconsin Press, 2018.

Hochmann, Jacques. *Histoire de la psychiatrie*. Paris: Presses Universitaires de France, 2015.

———. *Les antipsychiatries: Une histoire*. Paris: Odile Jacob, 2015.

Hocquenghem, Guy. *Le désir homosexuel*. Paris: Fayard, 2000.

Idier, Antoine. *Les vies de Guy Hocquenghem: Politique, sexualité, culture*. Paris: Fayard, 2017.

Jay, Martin. *The Dialectical Imagination: A History of the Frankfurt School and the Institute of Social Research, 1923–1950*. Boston: Little Brown, 1973.

Johnes, Lucile. "Désaliénisme à l'hôpital psychiatrique de Saint-Alban-sur-Limagnole: L'accueil de la folie dans un hôpital public de Lozère de la fin de la deuxième guerre mondiale au début des années 1970." Université de Lettres Paul Valéry, 2010.

Johnson, Timothy Scott, and Sophie Wustefeld. "Maud Mannoni and Piera Aulagnier on Mental Illness and Disability: Parents at the Boundary between Society and Childhood (France, 1960–80)." *Psychoanalysis and History* 21, no. 2 (August 2019).

Jones, Edgar. "War and the Practice of Psychotherapy: The UK Experience, 1939–1960." *Medical History* 48 (2004): 493–510.

Jones, Maxwell. *Social Psychiatry: A Study of Therapeutic Communities*. London: Tavistock, 1952.

Judaken, Jonathan. *Jean-Paul Sartre and the Jewish Question: Anti-Antisemitism and the Politics of the French Intellectual*. Lincoln: University of Nebraska Press, 2006.

Kazanjian, David. *The Brink of Freedom: Improvising Life in the Nineteenth-Century Atlantic World*. Durham, NC: Duke University Press, 2016.

Keller, Richard C. "Clinician and Revolutionary: Frantz Fanon, Biography, and the History of Colonial Medicine." *Bulletin of the History of Medicine* 81 (2007): 823–41.

———. *Colonial Madness: Psychiatry in French North Africa*. Chicago: University of Chicago Press, 2007.

Khalfa, Jean. "Fanon and Psychiatry." *Nottingham French Studies* 54, no. 1 (2015): 52–71.

Khanna, Ranjana. *Dark Continents: Psychoanalysis and Colonialism*. Durham, NC: Duke University Press, 2003.

Krtolica, Igor. "La 'tentative' des Cévennes: Deligny et la question de l'institution." *Chimères* 72, no. 1 (2010): 73–97.

Kuby, Emma. "'Our Actions Never Cease to Haunt Us': Frantz Fanon, Jean-Paul Sartre, and the Violence of the Algerian War." *Historical Reflections* 41, no. 3 (2015): 59–78.

Lacan, Jacques. *De la psychose paranoïaque dans ses rapports avec la personnalité*. Paris: Seuil, 1975.

———. *Ecrits: The First Complete Edition in English*. Trans. Bruce Fink. New York: W. W. Norton, 2006.

———. *L'envers de la psychanalyse: Le Séminaire, Livre XVII, 1969–1970*. Paris: Seuil, 1991.

LaCapra, Dominick. *History & Criticism*. Ithaca: Cornell University Press, 1985.

———. "History, Language, and Reading: Waiting for Crillon." *American Historical Review* 100, no. 3 (1995): 799–828.

———. *Rethinking Intellectual History: Texts, Contexts, Language*. Ithaca: Cornell University Press, 1983.

Lacas, Marie-Lise. *Gisela Pankow: Un humanisme au-delà de la psychose*. Paris: Campagne première, 2014.

Lafont, Max. *L'extermination douce: La mort de 40,000 malades mentaux dans les hôpitaux psychiatriques en France sous le Régime de Vichy*. Ligné: Editions de l'Arefppi, 1987.

Laing, R. D. *The Divided Self: An Existential Study in Sanity and Madness*. London: Penguin Books, 1990.

———. "The Invention of Madness." *New Statesman*, June 16, 1967, 843.

Lane, Christopher. "Psychoanalysis and Colonialism Redux: Why Mannoni's 'Prospero Complex' Still Haunts Us." *Journal of Modern Literature* 25, nos. 3/4 (2002): 127–50.

Lecourt, Dominique. *Georges Canguilhem*. Paris: PUF, 2016.

Le Guillant, Louis, and Lucien Bonnafé. "Le condition du malade à l'hôpital psychiatrique." *Esprit* 197 (Dec. 1952): 843–69.

Lévy-Valensi, Éliane Amado. "Histoire et Psychologie?" *Annales. Histoire, Sciences Sociales*, no. 5 (Sept.–Oct. 1965): 923–38.

Lieb, Peter, and Robert O. Paxton. "Maintenir l'ordre en France occupée. Combien de divisions?" *Vingtième Siècle. Revue d'histoire* 112, no. 4 (2011): 115–26.

Linhart, Virginie, dir. *Vincennes, l'université perdue*. Blaq out, Paris, 2018.

Linstrum, Erik. *Ruling Minds: Psychology in the British Empire*. Cambridge: Harvard University Press, 2016.

Mabin, Dominique, and Renée Mabin. "Art, folie et surréalisme à l'hôpital psychiatrique de Saint-Alban-sur-Limagnole pendant la guerre de 1939–1945." *ASTU* (2015). https://melusine-surrealisme.fr/wp/?p=1775#_ftn12

Macey, David. "Fanon, Phenomenology, Race." *Radical Philosophy* 95, no. (May/June 1999): 8–14.

———. *Frantz Fanon: A Biography*. London: Verso Books, 2012.

———. *The Lives of Michel Foucault*. New York: Vintage Books, 1995.

Macherey, Pierre. "Aux sources de *L'Histoire de la folie*: Une rectification et ses limites." *Critique* 46, no. 471 (1986): 753–74.

Mahone, Sloan, and Megan Vaughan. *Psychiatry and Empire*. Basingstoke, UK: Palgrave Macmillan, 2007.

Makari, George. *Soul Machine: The Invention of the Modern Mind*. New York: W. W. Norton, 2015.

Mannoni, Maud. *Ce qui manque à la vérité pour être dite*. Paris: Denoël, 1988.

———. *Le psychiatre, son "fou" et la psychanalyse*. Paris: Seuil, 1990.

Mannoni, Maud, Robert Lefort, and Roger Gentis. *Un lieu pour vivre: Les enfants de Bonneuil, leurs parents et l'équipe des soignants*. Paris: Seuil, 1976.

Mannoni, Octave. *Prospero and Caliban: The Psychology of Colonization*. Ann Arbor: University of Michigan Press, 1990.

———. *Psychologie de la colonisation*. Paris: Seuil, 1950.

Manuellan, Marie-Jeanne. *Sous la dictée de Fanon*. Paris: L'Amourier, 2017.

Marriott, David S. *Whither Fanon? Studies in the Blackness of Being*. Stanford: Stanford University Press, 2018.

Mbembe, Achille. *Politiques de l'inimitié*. Paris: La Découverte, 2016.

McCulloch, Jock. *Colonial Psychiatry and "the African Mind."* Cambridge, UK: Cambridge University Press, 1995.

Melas, Natalie. "Untimeliness, or Négritude and the Poetics of Contramodernity." *South Atlantic Quarterly* 108, no. 3 (2009): 563–80.

Merleau-Ponty, Maurice. *Child Psychology and Pedagogy: The Sorbonne Lectures, 1949–1952*. Evanston, IL: Northwestern University Press, 2010.

Mestre, Claire, and Marie-Rose Moro. "L'intime et le politique: Projet pour une ethnopsychanalyse critique." *L'Autre* 13, no. 3 (2012/13): 263–72.

Micale, Mark S., and Roy Porter. *Discovering the History of Psychiatry*. New York: Oxford University Press, 1994.

Miller, Gavin. *R. D. Laing*. Edinburgh: Edinburgh Review in association with Edinburgh University Press, 2004.

BIBLIOGRAPHY

Mintz, Frank. *Anarchism and Workers' Self-Management in Revolutionary Spain*. Oakland, CA: AK Press, 2013.

Mira y López, Emilio. *Psychiatry in War*. New York: Norton, 1943.

Mornet, Joseph. *Psychothérapie institutionnelle: Histoire & actualité*. Nîmes: Champ Social Editions, 2007.

Mozère, Liane. "Foucault et le CERFI: Instantanés et actualité." *Le Portique* 13–14 (2004).

———. *Le printemps des crèches: Histoire et analyse d'un mouvement*. Paris: L'Harmattan, 1992.

Mülberger, Annette, and Ana Maria Jacó-Vilela. "Es mejor morir de pie que vivir de rodillas: Emilio Mira y López y la revolucion nacional." *Dynamis* 27 (2006): 309–32.

Murard, Numa. "Psychothérapie institutionnelle à Blida." *Tumultes* 31, no. 2 (2008): 31–45.

Nadaud, Stéphane. "Recherches (1966–1982: histoire d'une revue)." *La Revue des revues (Entr'revues)*, no. 34 (2004): 47–72.

Norgeu, Anne-Marie. *La Borde: Le château des chercheurs de sens. La vie quotidienne à la clinique psychiatrique de La Borde*. Toulouse: Erès, 2006.

Ohayon, Annick. *Psychologie et psychanalyse en France: L'impossible rencontre, 1919–1969*. Paris: La Découverte, 2006.

Ophir, Orna. *Psychosis, Psychoanalysis and Psychiatry in Postwar USA: On the Borderland of Madness*. London: Routledge, 2015.

Orwell, George. *Homage to Catalonia*. London: Secker and Warburg, 1938.

Ourabah, Marie-Rose. *À l'ombre des poiriers: Hélène et François Tosquelles, un secret de famille*. Saint-Denis: Édilivre, 2014.

Oury, Jean. *Essai sur la création esthétique*. Paris: Hermann, 2008.

———. *Onze heures du soir à La Borde*. Paris: Gallilée, 1995.

———. *La psychothérapie institutionnelle de Saint-Alban à la Borde*. Paris: Éditions d'une, 2016.

———. *Séminaire de Sainte-Anne: Le Collectif*. Paris: Champs social, 2005.

———. *Les symptômes primaires de la schizophrénie: Cours de psychopathologie, 1984–1986, suivi de Le corps et la psychose*. Paris: Éditions d'une, 2016.

Oury, Jean, and Marie Depussé. *À quelle heure passe le train . . . Conversations sur la folie*. Paris: Calmann-Lévy, 2003.

Oury, Jean, and Patrick Faugeras. *Préalables à toute clinique des psychoses*. Toulouse: Érès, 2012.

Oury, Jean, Thierry Goguel d'Allondans, Jean-François Gomez, and Lise Gaignard. "Entretien avec Jean Oury." *VST—Vie sociale et traitements* 88, no. 4 (2005): 18–22.

Oury, Jean, Félix Guattari, and François Tosquelles. *Pratique de l'institutionnel et politique*. Vigneux: Matrice, 1985.

Oury, Jean, and Danielle Roulot. *Dialogues à La Borde: Psychopathologie & structure institutionnelle*. Paris: Hermann, 2008.

Pagès i Blanch, Pelai. *War and Revolution in Catalonia, 1936–1939*. Leiden: Brill, 2013.

Pain, François, Jean-Claude Polack, and Danielle Sivadon, dirs. *Francesc Tosquelles: Une politique de la folie*. 1989.

Palem, Robert Michel. *Henri Ey et la philosophie: Les racines et référents philosophiques et anthropologiques d'Henri Ey*. Paris: L'Harmattan, 2013.

Pankow, Gisela. *L'homme et sa psychose*. Paris: Flammarion, 2009.

Peschanski, Denis. *La France des camps: L'internement, 1938–1946*. Paris: Gallimard, 2002.

Philibert, Nicolas, dir. *La moindre des choses*. Éditions Montparnasse, Paris, 1996.

BIBLIOGRAPHY

Preston, Paul. *The Spanish Civil War: Reaction, Revolution and Revenge*. New York: W. W. Norton, 2007.

Proctor, Robert N. *Racial Hygiene: Medicine under the Nazis*. Cambridge: Harvard University Press, 1988.

Querrien, Anne. "Le CERFI, l'expérimentation sociale et l'État: Témoignage d'une petite main." In *L'État à l'épreuve des sciences sociales. La fonction recherche dans les administrations sous la Ve République*, ed. Philippe Bezes, 72–87. Paris: La Découverte, 2005.

Ranzanajao, Claudine, and Jacques Postel. "La vie et l'œuvre psychiatrique de Frantz Fanon." *Sud/Nord* 22, no. 1 (2007): 147–74.

Reich, Wilhelm. *The Mass Psychology of Fascism*. New York: Farrar, Straus and Giroux, 1970.

Rioux, Jean-Pierre, Antoine Prost, and Jean-Pierre Azéma. *Le Parti communiste français des années sombres 1938–1941*. Paris: Seuil, 1986.

Robcis, Camille. "'China in Our Heads': Althusser, Maoism, and Structuralism." *Social Text* 30, no. 1 (110) (2012): 51–69.

———. *The Law of Kinship: Anthropology, Psychoanalysis, and the Family in France*. Ithaca: Cornell University Press, 2013.

Rose, Nikolas S. *Inventing Our Selves: Psychology, Power, and Personhood*. Cambridge, UK: Cambridge University Press, 1996.

Roth, Michael S. *Knowing and History: Appropriations of Hegel in Twentieth-Century France*. Ithaca: Cornell University Press, 1988.

Roudinesco, Elisabeth. *La bataille de cent ans: Histoire de la psychanalyse en France*. Vol. 1. Paris: Ramsay, 1982.

———. *Histoire de la psychanalyse en France: 1925–1985*. Vol. 2. Paris: Fayard, 1994.

———. *Jacques Lacan: Esquisse d'une vie, histoire d'un système de pensée*. Paris: Fayard, 1993.

———. *Philosophes dans la tourmente*. Paris: Points, 2011.

Sabot, Philippe. "L'expérience, le savoir et l'histoire dans les premiers écrits de Michel Foucault." *Archives de Philosophie* 69 (2006): 285–303.

Sadowsky, Jonathan. *Imperial Bedlam: Institutions of Madness in Colonial Southwest Nigeria*. Berkeley: University of California Press, 1999.

Salamon, Gayle. "'The Place Where Life Hides Away': Merleau-Ponty, Fanon, and the Location of Bodily Being." *differences* 17, no. 2 (2006): 96–112.

Santner, Eric L. *My Own Private Germany: Daniel Paul Schreber's Secret History of Modernity*. Princeton: Princeton University Press, 1996.

Schaepelynck, Valentin. "Une critique en acte des institutions: Émergence et résidus de l'analyse institutionnelle dans les années 1960." Université Paris 8, 2013.

———. *L'institution renversée: Folie, analyse institutionnelle et champ social*. Paris: Editions Etérotopia, 2018.

———. "'Machines de guerre': Entre concepts, institutions et expérimentation sociale." In *Agencer les multiplicités avec Deleuze*, ed. Anne Querrien, Anne Sauvagnargues, and Arnaud Villani, 365–76. Paris: Éditions Hermann, 2019.

Schmidgen, Henning. "Jean Oury et la conation esthétique: Un parcours entre Sartre, Goldstein et Lacan." *Revue germanique internationale* 30 (2019).

Scull, Andrew. *Madness in Civilization: A Cultural History of Insanity, from the Bible to Freud, from the Madhouse to Modern Medicine*. Princeton: Princeton University Press, 2015.

BIBLIOGRAPHY

Sédat, Jacques. "Lacan et la psychiatrie." *Topique* 88, no. 3 (2004): 37–46.

———. "Lacan et Mai 68." *Figures de la psychanalyse* 18, no. 2 (2009): 221–26.

Seigel, Jerrold E. *The Idea of the Self: Thought and Experience in Western Europe since the Seventeenth Century*. New York: Cambridge University Press, 2005.

Shepard, Todd. *Sex, France, and Arab Men, 1962–1979*. Chicago: University of Chicago Press, 2017.

Shorter, Edward. *A History of Psychiatry: From the Era of the Asylum to the Age of Prozac*. New York: John Wiley, 1997.

Silverman, Kaja. *The Subject of Semiotics*. New York: Oxford University Press, 1983.

Simon, Hermann. *Une thérapeutique plus active à l'hôpital*. Translated from German by Jacques Tosquelles and André Chaurand. Berlin: Walter de Gruyter, 1929.

Solano, Wilebaldo. *El POUM en la historia: Andreu Nin y la revolución española*. Madrid: Los Libros de Catarata, 1999.

Soo, Scott. *The Routes to Exile: France and the Spanish Civil War Refugees, 1939–2009*. Manchester: Manchester University Press, 2013.

Soulié, Charles. "La pédagogie charismatique de Gilles Deleuze à Vincennes." *Actes de la recherche en sciences sociales* 216–17, no. 1 (2017): 42–63.

Staub, Michael E. *Madness Is Civilization: When the Diagnosis Was Social, 1948–1980*. Chicago: University of Chicago Press, 2011.

Szasz, Thomas Stephen. *Le mythe de la maladie mentale*. Trans. Denise Berger. Paris: Payot, 1975.

Termes, Josep. *Història del moviment anarquista a Espanya (1870–1980)*. Barcelona: Avenç, 2011.

Terranti, Idriss. "Fanon vu de Blida." *Sud/Nord* 22, no. 1 (2007): 89–95.

Tosquellas, Jacques. "Courriers Tosquelles-Balvet." *Sud/Nord* 19, no. 1 (2003): 171–84.

Tosquelles, François. "L'effervescence saint-albanaise." *L'Information psychiatrique* 63, no. 8 (1987): 957–63.

———. *L'enseignement de la folie*. Paris: Dunod, 2014.

———. *Fonction poétique et psychothérapie: Une lecture de "In memoriam" de Gabriel Ferrater*. Ramonville Saint-Agne: Érès, 2003.

———. "Francesc Tosquelles." *Primera Plana* (1984): 18–23.

———. "François Tosquelles par lui-même." *L'âne: Le magazine freudien*, no. 13 (Nov.–Dec. 1983): 3–5.

———. "Frantz Fanon à Saint-Alban." *Sud/Nord* 22, no. 1 (2007): 9–14.

———. "Frantz Fanon et la psychothérapie institutionnelle." *Sud/Nord* 22, no. 1 (2007): 71–78.

———. "La guerre d'Espagne." *VST—Vie sociale et traitements* (1987): 35–38.

———. "La société vécue par les malades psychiques." *Esprit* 197 (Dec. 1952): 897–904.

———. *"Trait-d'union" journal de Saint-Alban: Éditoriaux, articles, notes (1950–1962)*. Paris: Éditions d'une, 2015.

———. *Le travail thérapeutique à l'hôpital psychiatrique*. Paris: Editions du Scarabée, 1967.

———. *Le vécu de la fin du monde dans la folie: Le témoignage de Gérard de Nerval*. Grenoble: Jérôme Millon, 2012.

Tosquelles, François, Lucien Bonnafé, and André Chaurand. "Note sur l'originalité du pathologique d'après la psychanalyse et sur la valeur du complexe comme perspective structurale dans l'existence pathologique." *Annales médico-psychologiques* 2 (1946): 96–101.

Tristram, Didier. "Frantz Fanon, le 'chaînon manquant' de la psychiatrie martiniquaise." *Sud/Nord* 22, no. 1 (2007): 39–43.

Turkle, Sherry. *Psychoanalytic Politics: Freud's French Revolution.* New York: Basic Books, 1978.

Vasquez, Aïda, and Fernand Oury. *Vers une pédagogie institutionnelle.* Paris: François Maspéro, 1967.

Vaughan, Megan. *Curing Their Ills: Colonial Power and African Illness.* Stanford: Stanford University Press, 1991.

Vergès, Françoise. "Chains of Madness, Chains of Colonialism." In *The Fact of Blackness: Fanon and Visual Representation,* ed. Alan Read, 47–75. London: Institute of Contemporary Arts, 1996.

———. "Creole Skin, Black Mask: Fanon and Disavowal." *Critical Inquiry* 23, no. 3 (1997): 578–95.

Vialette, Aurélie. *Intellectual Philanthropy: The Seduction of the Masses.* West Lafayette, IN: Purdue University Press, 2018.

Vidal, Fernando. *The Sciences of the Soul: The Early Modern Origins of Psychology.* Chicago: University of Chicago Press, 2011.

von Platen, Alice Ricardi. *L'extermination des malades mentaux dans l'Allemagne nazie.* Toulouse: Erès, 2001.

Walter, B. "Hermann Simon—Psychiatriereformer, Sozialdarwinist, Nationalsozialist?" *Der Nervenarzt* 73, no. 11 (2002): 1047–54.

Widlöcher, Daniel. "Psychanalyse et psychiatrie française. 50 ans d'histoire." *Topique* 88, no. 3 (2004): 7–16.

Wilder, Gary. *Freedom Time: Negritude, Decolonization, and the Future of the World.* Durham, NC: Duke University Press, 2015.

———. "Race, Reason, Impasse: Césaire, Fanon, and the Legacy of Emancipation." *Radical History Review* 90 (Fall 2004): 31–61.

Zahzah, Abdenour, and Bachir Ridouh, dirs. *Frantz Fanon, mémoire d'asile.* Centre national de la cinématographie, Paris, 2008.

Zaretsky, Eli. *Political Freud: A History.* New York: Columbia University Press, 2015.

INDEX

Abraham, Karl, 111

Adler, Alfred, 111

AERLIP (Association pour l'étude et la rédaction du livre des institutions psychiatriques), 133

Aichhorn group, 21

Aimée (Lacan's patient), 23

Ajuriaguerra, Julian de, 74, 111

Algeria, 7, 13, 48–50, 61–63, 67–70, 72–73

Algiers School, 54, 63, 67

alienation: childhood, 129; Daumézon on, 39–40; double, 10, 131; Fanon on, 48, 50; Foucault on, 111–13, 117–22, 127; Guattari on, 83; Lacan on, 83–84; linguistic, 22; Marx on, 58, 112; Oury on, 82–83, 85; racial, 56; social and psychic, 8, 17, 73, 78, 82, 101, 116, 131; and subjectivity, 89; theory of, 9–12, 82, 143, 148; Tosquelles on, 8, 38, 101. *See also* disalienation

Alienation and Freedom (Fanon), 50

Almodovar del Campo, Spain, 26

alterity, 4, 51, 56, 84

Althusser, Louis, 89, 115–16

anarchism, 2–3, 17, 19, 28, 47, 74, 128

Angelergues, René, 74

Annales médico-psychologiques, 25, 35–36, 108

anthropology, 9, 52, 59, 77, 82, 90, 101, 113, 115, 120, 122

anti-austerity movements, 143, 145

anti-authoritarianism, 8–9, 18, 41, 46, 87–88, 121, 129

anticolonialism, 7, 13, 58–59, 63, 69, 101

anti-oedipal politics, 8, 78, 94, 104

Anti-Oedipus (Guattari and Deleuze), 8, 11, 78, 86–98, 104–5, 110, 118, 174n7, 176n48

antipsychiatry: in Britain, 12, 47, 83, 128–29; and Foucault, 9, 107–9, 125–37, 139–42; and Guattari, 82–83, 87–88, 92, 106; vs. institutional psychotherapy, 6, 12, 78, 82–83, 106, 130–31

antiracism, 59. *See also* racism

Anti-Semite and Jew (Sartre), 56

anti-Semitism, 23, 28, 56

anti-Stalinism, 2, 18, 88

Apprill, Olivier, 99

Ariès, Philippe, 120

Army Psychiatric Services (UK), 26

art and therapy, 30, 44–46, 81–82. *See also* ergotherapy; theater, in hospitals

Artaud, Antonin, 45

art brut, 3, 44–45. *See also* Dubuffet, Jean

assemblages (Deleuze and Guattari), 47, 95–96

assujettissement, 89

asylums. *See individual institutions*

Asylums (Goffman), 130–31

asylum-village, 39

auberges de jeunesse. See youth hostels

authoritarianism, 1, 11–12, 18, 73, 78–79, 90, 93–94, 96, 143, 145–46

210 INDEX

autism, 7, 112, 129
Ayme, Jean, 98, 129
Azoulay, Jacques, 64, 66–68

Bachelard, Gaston, 35, 111, 121
Badiou, Alain, 88
Balvet, Paul, 15, 31–34, 37, 39, 60
Barcelona, Spain, 17, 20–21, 27
Barnes, Mary, 140. *See also* Kingsley Hall clinic
Barthes, Roland, 121
Basaglia, Franco, 6, 83, 130, 138, 141, 189n87. *See also* Gorizia asylum; *psichiatria democratica*
behaviorism, 5, 87, 115, 158n5
Bellevue Sanatorium, 114
Benjamin, Walter, 13
Bergson, Henri, 88, 111
Binswanger, Ludwig, 108, 114; *Dream and Existence*, 107, 113
biological determinism, 51, 60
biological essentialism, 3, 16, 51, 56–57, 60, 72–73, 111, 118
biopolitics, 33–34
Birth of the Clinic, The (Foucault), 107, 121, 130, 185n43
Black Skin, White Masks (Fanon), 6, 51, 53, 55–58, 116
Blanchot, Maurice, 121
Bleuler, Eugen, 86, 111
Blida-Joinville hospital, 7, 13, 48, 61–63, 65–67, 69–72
BOC (Bloque Obrero y Campesino), 17
Bonnafé, Lucien, 15, 25, 33–40, 43, 55, 78, 108, 116–18, 123–26, 128
Bonnet, Marius, 15, 34, 36, 39, 41
Bonneuil, école expérimentale de, 129
Borisov, Vladimir, 130
Bourdieu, Pierre, 89, 130–31
Bourg, Julian, 174n7
Braudel, Fernand, 108
Brohm, Jean-Marie, 133
Brown, Wendy, 143
Brunschvicg, Léon, 111, 121
Burghölzli hospital, 23

Café maure (Blida), 68
Cahiers de psychopathologie, 112, 116
Cahiers pour la folie, 133

Camp de Judes, 27–32, 60. *See also* Septfonds, France
Canguilhem, Georges, 3, 15, 37, 116, 120–21, 186n52; *The Normal and the Pathological*, 34–36, 118, 185n43
Capécia, Mayotte, 57
capitalism, 10, 58, 71, 101, 144
Capitalism and Schizophrenia (Guattari and Deleuze), 8, 87. See also *Anti-Oedipus* (Guattari and Deleuze); *Thousand Plateaus, A* (Guattari and Deleuze)
Carmichael, Stokely, 129
Castel, Robert, 83, 88–89, 130, 134; *Le psychanalysme*, 131; *L'ordre psychiatrique*, 131–32
Castoriadis, Cornelius, 144–45
castration, 85–87, 91, 95, 100, 176n46
Catalan-Balearic Communist Federation, 20
Catalonia, 2, 13, 16–21, 26, 47
Catholicism, 32, 55, 74, 116
Centre de sociologie européenne, 130
Centre hospitalier François Tosquelles. *See* Saint-Alban Hospital
CERFI (Centre d'étude, de recherche et de formation institutionnelles), 8, 101–5, 109, 129, 132, 134–35, 142, 145–46. See also *Recherches* (journal)
Césaire, Aimé, 49, 54, 57
Chaban-Delmas, Jacques, 105
Chaos (Surrealist group), 34
Charcot, Jean-Martin, 30, 141
Charles-Nicolle day center, 7, 69
Châtelet, François, 88
Chaurand, André, 25, 31, 35–37
Cherki, Alice, 64
Claude, Henri, 23
Cluboscope (La Borde), 81
Club Paul Balvet (Saint-Alban), 41–44, 46, 60, 64, 74, 80
CNT (Confederación Nacional del Trabajo), 17
cognitive behavior therapies, 148
Cold War, 10, 70, 78, 94, 97, 106
collectif soignant. See healing collectives
collective infrastructures, 105, 109, 146
Collège de France, 109, 130, 137–38, 142
colonialism/imperialism, 2, 13, 18, 67,

149; psychic effects of, 7, 48–51, 54–60, 62–64, 70–73, 171n62. *See also* decolonization

comarcas, 19, 26

Comelles, Josep, 19

Comintern, 18

Commun (Dardot and Laval), 144

communism, 3, 17–18, 34, 55, 144, 161n32. *See also individual parties*

Compagnie de l'art brut, 45

complex (psychoanalytic concept), 25, 56, 59, 91, 100. *See also* Oedipus complex

Conan, Michel, 105

concentration camps, 2, 16, 31, 36, 39, 47; camp psychosis, 30. *See also* Camp de Judes

concentrationism, 2, 8, 12, 30, 36–37, 50, 73, 78, 103, 143, 146

Congress of Psychiatry and Neurology (1942), 38–39

Congress of the UEC (1965), 101

Cooper, David, 6, 83, 128–29, 136, 140–41, 189n87; *Psychiatry and Anti-Psychiatry*, 127, 130

Cotard delusion, 32

countertransference, 148. *See also* transference

COVID-19 pandemic, 143, 145

Crimini di pace (manifesto), 130

Daladier, Édouard, 28

Dardot, Pierre, 145; *Commun*, 144

Daseinanalyse, 113–14

Daumézon, Georges, 34, 39, 55, 74, 107–8, 111, 116–17, 123–25, 131

day hospitalization, 68–70

Dechaume, Jean, 51–52, 55

decolonization, 48–49, 51, 57, 70–73, 78. *See also* colonialism/imperialism

Defert, Daniel, 137

Delay, Jean, 112–13, 120

Deleuze, Gilles: *Anti-Oedipus*, 8, 11, 78, 86–98, 104–5, 110, 118, 174n7, 176n48; on assemblages, 47, 95–96; *Capitalism and Schizophrenia*, 8, 87; and CERFI, 103; on fascism, 11, 93–94, 97; and Foucault, 108–10, 118; and Guattari, 8, 11, 73, 78, 86–97, 105, 107–10, 149,

178n93; on oedipalization, 8, 11, 78, 86–97, 105, 110, 118; on psychosis, 91–92, 98–99; *Spinoza et le problème de l'expression*, 90; *Spinoza: Philosophie pratique*, 90; *A Thousand Plateaus*, 8; on the unconscious, 91, 93–94, 96, 98, 100

Deligny, Fernand, 7

Der Gestaltkreis (Weizsäcker), 107–8, 123

Derrida, Jacques, 121

desire, 10, 13, 75, 79–80, 144–45, 176n46; for authoritarianism, 11–12, 78, 94, 146; Deleuze and Guattari on, 86–101, 110, 178n93; Fanon on, 70; Foucault on, 110; Hocquenghem on, 104; Lacan on, 53, 83–84; and oedipalization, 8; Oury on, 85; and projection, 5. *See also* fantasy; lack (Lacan)

desiring machines (Deleuze and Guattari), 90, 95

Despinoy, Maurice, 64, 171n59

deterritorialization, 8, 13, 73, 78, 92, 94–96, 106

Dewey, John, 75

"Dialectics of Liberation" conference, 129

dialogic history, 13, 148

Dide, Maurice, 20–21, 31

disalienation: Fanon on, 50, 55, 57–58, 68, 71, 73; Foucault on, 119; of the hospital, 39, 47, 74, 80; Oury and Guattari on, 78, 98; theory of, 9–11, 148; Tosquelles on, 16, 80. *See also* alienation

disciplinary power, 9, 110, 136, 138–40

Discipline and Punish (Foucault), 137–38

Divided Self, The (Laing), 128

Dolto, Françoise, 129

Domenach, Jean-Marie, 55, 116

Dream and Existence (Binswanger), 107, 113

Dubuffet, Jean, 3, 44–46

Duhamel, Colette, 121

École Française de Psychanalyse, 180n119

École Normale Supérieure, 74, 104, 107–8, 110–12, 116, 120, 183n15

Écrits (Lacan), 23

Éditions de la Table Ronde (Gallimard), 121

Éditions de Minuit, 130–31

212   INDEX

Éditions du Seuil, 51, 55
Éditions Flammarion, 136–37
Éditions Gallimard, 121, 127, 137
Éditions Julliard, 136
Éditions Plon, 120, 127
ego, 83–84, 95, 103, 176n46; ego ideal, 53, 100
ego psychology, 5, 87, 176n47
Eiminder, Sandor, 21
electroencephalograms, 112
electroshock therapy, 6, 61, 70, 82, 136
Elementary Structures of Kinship (Lévi-Strauss), 83–84
Ellenberger, Henri, 141
El Moudjahid, 69
Éluard, Paul, 2, 34–36, 46
ERC (Esquerra Republicana de Catalunya), 17
ergotherapy, 5, 41, 44, 60, 64, 66–68, 74, 81, 133, 145
Eribon, Didier, 119, 130
Erlebnis, 53, 56, 113
Esprit (journal), 13, 39–40, 51, 55–56, 108, 116, 119
Esquirol, Jean-Étienne Dominique, 117, 125
ethics, 22, 47, 72–73, 105, 122, 149, 174n7; Foucauldian, 3, 8, 78, 94–95, 110
ethnopsychiatry, 51, 67
eugenics, 1, 11, 33, 161n32
Évolution psychiatrique, 23–24, 52, 108, 123–25
existentialism, 6, 11, 52, 107, 127–28, 147
Ey, Henri, 23–24, 52–53, 108, 111–12, 116, 123–24

familialism, 90, 92, 99, 104, 176n48
Fanon, Frantz: on alienation, 48, 50; *Alienation and Freedom*, 50; and Azoulay, 66–68; "Black Orpheus," 58; *Black Skin, White Masks*, 6, 51, 53, 55–58, 116; at Blida-Joinville, 48, 61–70, 72; on colonialism, 48–50, 54–56, 64, 70–73; on disalienation, 50, 55, 57–58, 68, 71, 73; and Freud, 52, 56; and institutional psychotherapy, 6–8, 13, 50–51, 64, 68–70, 73, 106, 145, 147, 149; and Lacan, 52–53, 61; and Lacroix, 116; "Letter to a Frenchman," 63; "The Lived Expe-

rience of the Black Man," 55, 116; on madness, 69–70; and Octave Mannoni, 58–60; "Mental Alterations, Character Modifications, Psychic Disorders, and Intellectual Deficit," 51; and Merleau-Ponty, 111; on national culture, 71–72; "The North African Syndrome," 6, 51, 54–56; "Notes on Muslim Psychiatry," 63; on psychiatry, 48–54, 61, 68–69; and racism, 7, 48, 50, 54–60, 72; at Saint-Alban, 6–7, 13, 43, 50–51, 53, 55, 60–62, 64, 70, 73; on subjectivity, 51, 56–60, 73; and Tosquelles, 7, 50, 60–61, 64; *Toward the African Revolution*, 63, 69; on the unconscious, 51, 56; *The Wretched of the Earth*, 7, 50, 69–72; *The Year Five of the Algerian Revolution*, 69–70
fantasy, 10–13, 46, 78, 98–99, 145–46; and Deleuze and Guattari, 93, 95; and Fanon, 70–71; and Freud, 4–5. *See also* desire
fascism: Deleuze and Guattari on, 11, 78, 90, 93–94, 97, 146; Foucault on, 8, 11, 78, 93–94, 146; and institutional psychotherapy, 1, 10–12, 34, 93, 146, 148; and POUM, 18, 27; and Tosquelles, 2, 16, 21, 33, 78, 93. *See also* Franco, Francisco; Hitler, Adolf; Mussolini, Benito; Nazism; Pétain, Philippe; Third Reich; Trump, Donald; Vichy France
Faye, Jean-Pierre, 130
Feher, Michel, 143
Ferenczi, Sándor, 111
FFI (Forces françaises de l'intérieur), 35
FFL (Forces françaises libres), 35
FGERI (Fédération des groupes d'études et de recherches institutionnelles), 8, 101–2, 103, 105, 129
FHAR (Front homosexuel d'action révolutionnaire), 104
Fifth Republic, 135
Fleury-les-Aubrais hospital, 111
FLN (Front de libération nationale), 7, 49, 68–69
Forestier, Auguste, 45–46
Foucault, Michel: on alienation, 111–13, 117–22, 127; and antipsychiatry, 9, 107–

9, 125–37, 139–42; on *assujettissement*,
89; on biopolitics, 33; *The Birth of the
Clinic*, 107, 121, 130, 185n43; and Canguilhem, 120, 185n43; and Castel, 130–
32; and CERFI, 8, 103, 105, 142; and
Deleuze, 108–10, 118; on disalienation,
119; *Discipline and Punish*, 137–38;
on ethics, 3, 8, 78, 94–95, 110; on fascism, 8, 11, 78, 93–94, 146; and Freud,
107, 111–13, 118; and Guattari, 108–10,
118; *History of Madness*, 91, 107–11,
114–17, 119–27, 130–31, 136–39, 185n43;
The History of Sexuality, 109–10; "The
Hospital Institution in the Eighteenth Century," 109; and institutional
psychotherapy, 9, 12, 109–10, 116–17,
123, 125, 132, 147; and La Borde, 107–
9; and Lacan, 107, 111–12; on madness,
107, 112, 114–15, 117, 119–23, 129, 139–41;
Madness and Civilization, 127–29; *Maladie mentale et personnalité*, 107–8, 111,
115–20, 122, 130; and Marxism, 112–13,
117; on mental illness, 108, 116–19, 123–
25, 129; and neoliberalism, 143; and
the normal, 112, 114–15; and Oury, 83,
108; on power, 136–42; and psychiatry, 9, 13, 107–14, 116–24, 127, 139–40;
and psychoanalysis, 107, 116, 118, 121;
and psychology, 107, 116–20, 129–30;
on psychosis, 112; and Saint-Alban,
107, 114–15, 140; thesis by, 120, 183n15;
on the unconscious, 110, 112–13; at Vincennes, 88, 130
Fourquet, François, 102–3, 105, 109, 134
Fourth Republic, 54, 57
France: antipsychiatry in, 108, 126–31;
and colonialism, 48–49, 54–55, 58, 60,
62–63; "French theory," 13, 73, 147; gay
liberation movement in, 104; intellectual life in, 7, 13, 55, 73, 77, 103; Marxism in, 94; postwar thought in, 2, 13;
psychiatric institutions in, 1, 23, 33, 60,
63, 113, 123; psychiatry in, 16, 19–20,
23–24, 50–52, 61–62, 69, 74, 121, 123,
148; psychology in, 111–12; and racism, 56–57, 60; and Spanish Civil War,
16, 27–31; Vichy, 1–3, 16, 33–34, 93, 146,
163n80. *See also* Fifth Republic; Fourth
Republic

Franco, Francisco, 2, 18, 26–27, 146
Frank, Thomas, 146
Frankfurt School, 11
Freinet, Célestin, 75
French Communist Party (PCF), 34, 74,
97, 101, 183n21
French Popular Front, 34, 74
French Resistance, 2–3, 34–36, 146
Fresnes prison, 107, 113
Freud, Sigmund: and CERFI, 102–3; and
Deleuze, 87, 91–92, 96; and Fanon, 52,
56; and Foucault, 107, 111–13, 118; and
Guattari, 87, 91–92, 96, 102; and insti-
tutional psychotherapy, 6, 10–11; and
Lacan, 23–25, 84, 87; and Mira, 20–
21; on Oedipus complex, 90–91; and
Oury, 84–86; and psychiatry, 4, 16, 23–
24; and psychoanalysis, 4–6, 16–17, 23,
56, 86, 96, 106, 115, 118; on psychosis,
40, 86, 91, 159n5; on subjectivity, 5, 24;
on talking cure, 4; and Tosquelles, 10,
16–17; on transference, 4–5; on the unconscious, 4–5, 24
Friedreich's ataxia, 52–53, 55
Fromm, Erich, 11

Galerie René Drouin, 45
Gantheret, François, 133
Garde-fous (journal), 133–34, 136
généalogie des équipements collectifs,
105
*Généalogie des équipements de normalisa-
tion*, 109
Genet, Jean, 103
Gentis, Roger, 98
geopsychiatry, 27, 37
George III (king of the United King-
dom), 140
Germany, 1, 4, 18, 21, 27–28, 33–34, 36, 93,
112–13, 163n80. *See also* Weimar Re-
public
Géronimi, Charles, 64
Gestalt theory, 22, 52
Getachew, Adom, 72
GIA (Groupe information asiles), 132–33
GIP (Groupe d'information sur les pris-
ons), 109, 132–33, 137–38, 142
GIS (Groupe information santé), 133–34
Goffman, Erving, *Asylums*, 130–31

Goldstein, Kurt, 52–53, 112, 116

Gombrowicz, Witold, 81–82

Gorizia asylum, 130. *See also* Basaglia, Franco

Great Britain, 6, 12, 22, 26, 108, 127–29, 138, 140

Grenelle Agreements (1968), 89

groupes-sujets vs. *groupes-assujettis*, 96–97, 98–101, 109, 142, 179n107, 179n114

GTPSI (Group de travail de psychothérapie et sociothérapie institutionnelle), 98–100, 108, 180n119

Guattari, Félix: and activism, 81, 105, 146, 174n7; on alienation, 78, 83; *Anti-Oedipus*, 8, 11, 78, 86–98, 104–5, 110, 118, 174n7, 176n48; and antipsychiatry, 82–83, 87–88, 92, 106; on assemblages, 47, 95–96; *Capitalism and Schizophrenia*, 8, 87; and CERFI, 8, 101–5, 129; and Deleuze, 8, 11, 73, 78, 86–97, 105, 107–10, 149, 178n93; on desire, 86–87, 89–97; on disalienation, 78, 98; on fascism, 11, 78, 90, 93–94, 97, 146; and FGERI, 8, 101, 103, 105, 129; and Foucault, 108–10, 118; and Freud, 87, 91–92, 96, 102; and the GTPSI, 98–100; on institutional analysis, 86–87, 98–100, 101, 105; and institutional psychotherapy, 6–9, 105–6, 145, 147; at La Borde, 7–8, 77–78, 87, 97–98, 100, 105–6, 189n87; and Lacan, 6–7, 82, 86–88, 90–92, 96, 102, 176n48; on madness, 82–83; and oedipalization, 8, 11, 78, 86–97, 104–5, 110, 118; and Oury, 8–9, 22, 75, 77–79, 82–83, 87–88, 146; on psychosis, 91–92, 98–99; at Saint-Alban, 105–6; and schizoanalysis, 95–98, 104–5, 109, 118; "Somewhat Philosophical Reflections on Institutional Psychotherapy," 103; on subjectivity, 91, 93–94, 96, 98, 100; *A Thousand Plateaus*, 8; on transversality, 5, 99–100; on the unconscious, 91, 93–94, 96, 98, 100

Gusdorf, Georges, 108, 111, 115

Gütersloh asylum, 21. *See also* Simon, Hermann

Hassoun, Jacques, 136

Head, Henry, 112

healing collectives, 40, 66

Hegel, Georg Wilhelm Friedrich, 24, 52

Heidegger, Martin, 52, 113

Herzog, Dagmar, 11

History of Madness (Foucault), 91, 107–11, 114–17, 119–27, 130–31, 136–39, 185n43

History of Sexuality, The (Foucault), 109–10

Hitler, Adolf, 11, 33, 78, 93, 161n32. *See also* Nazism; Third Reich

Hocquenghem, Guy, 8, 103, 149; *Le désir homosexuel*, 104

homosexuality, 104, 112, 149

Horney, Karen, 111

humanism, 50, 57, 70

Hume, David, 88, 178n93

Hyppolite, Jean, 52, 120

hysteria, 4–5, 63, 112, 136, 140–41

Ibáñez, Félix Martí, 19

Iberian Union of Socialist Republics, 18

ICE (Izquierda Comunista de España), 17

identification, 5–6, 25–26, 83–84

ideological state apparatuses, 89

Imaginary (Lacan), 83–84, 92, 100

incest taboo, 83–84

Institut de psychologie de Paris, 111–12

institutional analysis, 8, 87, 97–106

institutional psychotherapy: vs. antipsychiatry, 6, 12, 78, 82–83, 106, 130–31; decolonizing, 70–73; deterritorialization of, 8, 13, 73, 78, 92, 94–96, 106; diffusion of, 103; ethics of, 174n7; and Fanon, 6–8, 13, 50–51, 64, 68–70, 73, 106, 145, 147, 149; and fascism, 1, 10–12, 34, 93, 146, 148; first generation of, 93, 131; and Foucault, 9, 12, 109–10, 116–17, 123, 125, 132, 147; founding fathers of, 10, 25, 36, 39, 78, 143, 146; and Freud, 6, 10–11; future of, 148; goals of, 2–3, 6, 9, 36–37, 47, 73, 145; and Guattari, 6–9, 105–6, 145, 147; at La Borde, 7–9, 13, 101, 129; and madness, 21, 35, 37–38, 40; and mental illness, 22, 37–39, 47; and Oury, 2, 7, 12–13, 36–37, 86, 145, 147–48; at Saint-Alban, 1–3, 5–8, 13, 20, 36–47, 53, 78–80, 82, 146, 148; second generation of, 6, 9, 82, 109, 129, 131; theory

INDEX 215

and practice, 3, 22, 37, 78, 88, 98, 145; and Tosquelles, 2, 13, 37, 47, 78, 117–18, 131, 145, 147
institutions, 8, 22, 27, 37, 46, 100, 139–40, 144
Institut Pere Mata, 20, 160n24
insulin cures, 6, 61
International Psychoanalytic Association (IPA), 83
Irigaray, Luce, 103
Italy, 6, 12, 35, 68, 83, 93, 108, 114, 130, 138

Janet, Pierre, 111
Jeanson, Francis, 55
Jones, Maxwell, 26, 128
Jussieu campus, 132

Kant, Immanuel, 88
Keller, Richard, 62–63
Kingsley Hall clinic, 128–29, 140. *See also* Barnes, Mary; Laing, R. D.
Klein, Melanie, 111
Kojève, Alexandre, 24, 52
Kuhn, Roland, 114

La Borde, Clinic of: and CERFI, 101–2; Club at, 80–81, 86; critiques of, 134–36; daily life at, 77–82; Deleuze at, 178n93; and Foucault, 107–9; Fourquet at, 109; and the grid, 79–81, 100, 104; Guattari at, 7–8, 77–78, 87, 97–98, 100, 105–6, 189n87; and institutional psychotherapy, 7–9, 13, 101, 129; and Lacan, 82; Oury at, 77–79, 82, 102, 108, 131; and Saint-Alban, 7, 79–82; and University of Vincennes, 88–89; Vasquez at, 75
La Borde Éclair, 81
Laboucarié, Jean, 124
Lacan, Jacques: on alienation, 83–84; "Beyond the 'Reality Principle,'" 23–25; and CERFI, 102; and Deleuze, 91–92; *Écrits*, 23; and Fanon, 52–53, 61; and Foucault, 107, 111–12; and Freud, 23–25, 84, 87; "The Function and Field of Speech and Language in Psychoanalysis," 83–84, 87, 176n47; and GT-PSI, 180n119; and Guattari, 6–7, 82, 86–88, 90–92, 96, 102, 176n48; and La Borde, 82, 175n25; on madness, 22–24,

26–27, 38, 53; and Octave Mannoni, 58, 129; and mirror stage, 83–85, 112; "The Mirror Stage as Formative of the I Function," 25; *On Paranoid Psychosis and Its Relations to the Personality*, 5, 23–24, 53; and Oury, 74, 82–85; and psychiatry, 13, 16, 22–24, 111; psychoanalysis (Lacanian), 6–7, 87, 96, 106, 128, 180n119; on psychosis, 4–5, 22–24, 82–84, 175n23; on the Real, Imaginary, and Symbolic, 83–85, 92; Rome Discourse, 83–84, 87, 187n47; Saint-Alban (influence on), 23, 25; on subjectivity, 25, 86–87; thesis on psychosis, 5, 21, 23–24, 38, 82, 160n24, 160n26, 175n23; and Tosquelles, 16, 21–27, 61, 160n24, 160n26, 175n23; on the unconscious, 24, 83, 87
Lacano-Labordian complex, 87, 176n48
LaCapra, Dominick, 13, 148
Lacaton, Raymond, 63–64, 171n66
lack (Lacan), 84, 87, 90. *See also* desire
Lacoste, Robert, 48–49, 68
Lacroix, Jean, 116
Lagache, Daniel, 111–12, 116, 120
Laing, R. D., 6, 83, 127, 129, 131, 136, 140–41, 189n87; *The Divided Self*, 128. *See also* Kingsley Hall clinic
La Manouba hospital, 68–69
La moindre des choses (documentary), 81–82
Lapassade, Georges, 88
Laval, Christian, 145; *Commun*, 144
Law (Lacan), 22, 83–86, 90–91
Le désir homosexuel (Hocquenghem), 104
Le Goff, Jacques, 108
Le Guillant, Louis, 40, 55, 131
Lenin, Vladimir, 52
Le nouvel observateur (journal), 132
Le psychanalysme (Castel), 131
Leroi-Gouran, André, 52
Lévi-Strauss, Claude, 52, 84, 98; *Elementary Structures of Kinship*, 83–84
liberalism, 10, 12, 49, 51, 55, 58, 70–71, 146–47
libidinal economy, 78, 93, 96
libidinal investments, 92, 96–97
Lindroth, Stirn, 120
L'Information psychiatrique (journal), 66
L'ordre psychiatrique (Castel), 131–32

216 INDEX

Lozère, France, 1, 15, 37, 45
Lycée Henri IV, 120
Lycée Schoelcher, 57
Lyon, France, 6, 51–54, 60–61, 73, 116
Lyotard, Jean-François, 88

Macey, David, 50, 55, 60
madness: and antipsychiatry, 129, 133, 141;
Fanon on, 69–70; Foucault on, 107, 112,
114–15, 117, 119–23, 129, 139–41; and in-
stitutional psychotherapy, 21, 35, 37–
38, 40; Lacan on, 22–24, 26–27, 38, 53;
Oury and Guattari on, 82–83; politics
of, 3, 17, 47; and Surrealism, 2, 21, 35–
36, 45. *See also* mental illness
Madness and Civilization (Foucault),
127–29
Maladie mentale et personnalité (Foucault), 107–8, 111, 115–20, 122, 130
Mannoni, Maud, 8, 129–30
Mannoni, Octave, 57, 60; *Psychologie de
la colonisation*, 58–59
Manuellan, Marie-Jeanne, 69
Maoism, 88, 101, 104, 132
Marcuse, Herbert, 11, 125, 129
Martinique, 49, 57–58, 60, 64
Marx, Karl, 10–11, 16–17, 52, 58, 103, 112,
121
Marxism, 52, 103, 125–26, 146; critiques
of, 71, 109–10, 112–13, 117; existential,
11; fascism and, 12, 93–94, 146; revolu-
tionary, 78; state, 10. *See also individ-
ual parties*
Mary, Bertrand, 134–36
Maspero, François, 13, 69, 75, 131, 133
materialism, 25, 94, 96, 117–18, 126–27
Maurín, Joaquín, 17
Maury, Hervé, 103
Mauss, Marcel, 52, 67
May '68, 87–88, 97, 104, 105, 129, 174n7;
and Deleuze and Guattari, 88–89, 94,
110; and Foucault, 108, 110, 121, 125–27,
133, 136–38; Mouvement du 22 mars,
88
Memoirs of My Nervous Illness
(Schreber), 91
mental illness: causes of, 51, 56, 116, 123–
24; Foucault on, 108, 116–19, 123–25,

129; and institutional psychotherapy,
22, 37–39, 47; and the Third Reich, 33.
See also madness
Merleau-Ponty, Maurice, 52, 111, 113, 116,
168n10
Ministry of Health (France), 20, 61
Ministry of Infrastructure (France), 105
Mira y López, Emilio, 20–21, 26–27,
160n24
MLF (Mouvement de libération des
femmes), 104
moral treatment, 21–22, 24, 160n23
Moreno, Jacob, 46, 69
Mounier, Emmanuel, 55, 116
Mouvement de l'École moderne, 75
Mouvement du 22 mars, 88. *See also*
May '68
Mozère, Liane, 103
Münsterlingen asylum, 114–15
Murard, Lion, 103, 105, 134
Mussolini, Benito, 11, 78
Myth of Mental Illness, The (Szasz), 130

name-of-the-father (Lacan), 84–85, 91
national culture (Fanon), 50, 67, 70–72
Nazism, 1, 11, 33, 36, 93, 146, 161n32. *See
also* Hitler, Adolf; Third Reich
Negri, Antonio, 8, 103
négritude, 57–58, 60, 72
neoliberalism, 143–44, 146
neuroleptics, 6, 82, 113
neurological automatism, 24
neurological essentialism, 16, 118
neurological objectivism, 111
neurology, 3–5, 9, 23–24, 51–53, 61–62, 83
neuropsychiatry, 51, 107
neurosciences, 10, 24, 148
neurosis, 54; vs. psychosis, 5, 16, 82–87,
92, 98; war, 26–27, 29
Nietzsche, Friedrich, 88, 120
Nin, Andreu, 17
nom-du-père. See name-of-the-father
(Lacan)
Normal and the Pathological, The (Canguilhem), 34–36, 118, 185n43
"North African Syndrome, The" (Fanon),
6, 51, 54–56, 116
Notre journal (Blida), 66

INDEX

Nouvelles labordiennes (La Borde), 81
Nouvel observateur, 104, 132
Nuit Debout, 143
nurses, 15, 22, 39, 46, 61–62, 64, 72, 79

occupational therapy, 22
oedipalization, 8, 90–92, 95, 98. *See also* anti-oedipal politics
Oedipus complex, 84, 87, 90–92, 94–97, 99
On Paranoid Psychosis and Its Relations to the Personality (Lacan), 5, 23–24, 53
ontogeny, 52, 56
Opposition de gauche, 88, 100–101
organicism, 23, 51, 61
Ortigues, Edmond, 129
Oury, Fernand, 74–75
Oury, Jean: on alienation, 82–83, 85; and antipsychiatry, 82–83, 129; and CERFI, 102; and the collective, 12, 99; on disalienation, 78, 98; and Foucault, 83, 108; and Freud, 84–86; and the GTPSI, 98, 108; and Guattari, 8–9, 22, 75, 77–79, 82–83, 87–88, 146; and institutional pedagogy, 75; and institutional psychotherapy, 2, 7, 12–13, 36–37, 86, 145, 147–48; at La Borde, 77–79, 82, 102, 108, 131; and Lacan, 74, 82–85; on madness, 82–83; on psychosis, 46, 82–87; at Saint-Alban, 45–46, 74–75, 175n23; on schizophrenia, 85, 87; and Tosquelles, 8, 15, 22, 74–75, 175n23; *Toward an Institutional Pedagogy*, 75; on transference, 5, 81, 86, 99, 129; on transferential constellation, 5, 99, 129; on the unconscious, 75, 86; and youth hostels, 74–75, 145

Pankow, Gisela, 86, 98
pathogenesis, 53
Paumelle, Philippe, 69, 131
Pavlov, Ivan, 112, 117, 126–27
PCE (Partido Comunista Español), 17–18
PCF. *See* French Communist Party (PCF)
Perec, Georges, 103
personality (psychoanalytic concept), 5, 23–26, 38, 53, 59, 61, 118

Pétain, Philippe, 32. *See also* Vichy France
pharmacology, 113, 115, 148
phenomenology, 3, 91, 147; and Basaglia, 6; and Fanon, 51–53, 56; and Foucault, 107, 111, 113, 119, 122, 137; and Lacan, 23, 53; and Laing, 6, 127; and Mira, 20; and Tosquelles, 32
phylogeny, 52, 56
Pinel, Philippe, 21–22, 24, 40, 63, 117, 122–23
Polack, Jean-Claude, 98
politique de secteur, 19–20, 26, 69, 132, 134, 140, 148
Porot, Antoine, 62–63, 67
positivism, 20, 113, 115, 122
POUM (Partido Obrero de Unificación Marxista), 2, 17–19, 26–27, 41, 47, 146
Présence africaine (journal), 57
Presses Universitaires de France (PUF), 116
psichiatria democratica, 6, 130. *See also* Basaglia, Franco
psychiatric hospitals. *See* Bellevue Sanatorium; Blida-Joinville hospital; Burghölzli hospital; Charles-Nicolle day center; Fleury-les-Aubrais hospital; Gorizia asylum; Gütersloh asylum; Institut Pere Mata; Kingsley Hall clinic; La Borde, Clinic of; La Manouba hospital; Münsterlingen asylum; Rodez hospital; Rouffach hospital; Saint-Alban Hospital; Sainte-Anne hospital; Saint Elizabeth hospital; Tavistock
Psychiatrisés en lutte (newsletter), 133, 135
Psychiatrist, His "Mad," and Psychoanalysis, The (Mannoni), 129–30
psychiatry: colonial, 53, 59, 73; and criminology, 113, 136; disalienating, 50, 68; Fanon on, 48–54, 61, 68–69; Foucault on, 9, 13, 107–14, 116–24, 127, 139–40; in France, 16, 19–20, 23–24, 50–52, 61–62, 69, 74, 121, 123, 148; Freud on, 4, 16, 23–24; future of, 148; Lacan on, 13, 16, 22–24, 111; mainstream, 3–4, 36, 38, 50, 61, 147; and Marxism, 17, 125–26; materialist, 117–18, 126–27; as political practice, 3, 7, 10, 148; and psychoanalysis,

psychiatry (*continued*)
3, 6, 16, 21, 23–24, 52, 82, 97, 102, 105, 116, 131–32; radical, 6, 13, 51, 77; social, 27; Tosquelles on, 2, 16, 27, 30–31, 52, 55, 108, 123, 128–29; and war, 1, 26–33; Western, 13, 50. *See also* antipsychiatry; institutional psychotherapy

Psychiatry and Anti-Psychiatry (Cooper), 127, 130

psychic causality, 4, 51, 56, 111–12, 115

psychoanalysis: and alienation, 10; and antipsychiatry, 92, 141; applied, 180n119; Deleuze and Guattari on, 90–92, 95–97; and familialism, 90, 92, 96, 99, 104; and Foucault, 107, 116, 118, 121; Freudian, 4–6, 16–17, 23, 56, 86, 96, 106, 115, 118; Lacanian, 6–7, 87, 96, 106, 128, 180n119; and neurosis, 98; and Oedipus complex, 90–91, 95–97; and paranoia, 23; and psychiatry, 3, 6, 16, 21, 23–24, 51–52, 82, 97, 102, 105, 116, 131–32; and psychosis, 4–5; and race, 57–59; subjectivity in, 24; and Tosquelles, 16, 32; and transference, 99. *See also* talking cure

psychodramas, 46, 99

Psychologie de la colonisation (Mannoni), 58–59

psychology: clinical, 107, 111, 113; and colonialism, 58–59; degrees in, 107, 111–13; ego, 5, 87; and fascism, 93; and Foucault, 107, 116–20, 129–30; history of, 25, 107, 115, 119; profession of, 23, 111–13; and race, 57–58, 60, 63; social, 52

psychopathology, 17, 37, 107, 111, 122

psychopharmacology, 141

psychosis: and alienation, 10; camp, 32; Deleuze and Guattari on, 91–92, 98–99; and fascism, 148; Foucault on, 112; Lacan on, 4–5, 22–24, 83–85, 175n23; Laing and Cooper on, 128; Oury on, 46, 82–87; and psychoanalysis, 4–5; treatment of, 3, 6, 9, 46–47, 61

psychosurgery, 51, 141

psychotherapy. *See* institutional psychotherapy

Querrien, Anne, 102–3

racism, 12, 92; and colonialism, 51, 70–73; and Fanon, 7, 48, 50, 54–60, 72; in France, 54, 60–61; in medicine, 62–63, 68. *See also* anti-Semitism; eugenics

radical psychiatry, 6, 13, 51, 77

Ramée, Dr., 63

Real (Lacan), 83–85, 92

Recherches (journal), 8, 101–2, 103–5, 109, 129, 134–35, 181n135

reflexology, 126

refugees, 2, 16, 28–31, 60, 68

Regard sur la folie (Ruspoli), 114

Reich, Wilhelm, 93

Resistance (against Vichy France). *See* French Resistance

Retirada, 27

Reus, Spain, 17, 20–21

Revue de psychanalyse (journal), 112

rhizome (Deleuze and Guattari), 95–96

Rodez hospital, 45

Rome Discourse (Lacan), 83–84, 87, 187n47

Rorschach test, 112

Rouffach hospital, 33

Ruspoli, Mario, 114

Russia, 17–18, 101, 112, 117

Sacher-Masoch, Leopold von, 88, 178n93

Saint-Alban Hospital: and *art brut*, 44–46; Bonnafé at, 34–36; Canguilhem at, 35–36, 185n43; Club Paul Balvet at, 41–44, 46, 64, 80; early history of, 15; Fanon at, 6–7, 13, 43, 50–51, 53, 55, 60–62, 64, 70, 73; and Foucault, 107, 114–15, 140; Guattari at, 105–6; influence on La Borde, 7, 79–82; institutional psychotherapy at, 1–3, 5–8, 13, 20, 36–47, 53, 78–80, 82, 146, 148; Lacan's influence on, 23, 25; Oury at, 45–46, 74–75, 175n23; Tosquelles at, 5, 7, 20–22, 25–27, 33–34, 37–40, 47, 64, 114

Sainte-Anne hospital, 23, 86, 107–8, 111–12, 123, 140

Saint Elizabeth hospital, 130

Saint-Ylie of Dole hospital, 60

Salpêtrière, 122, 141

Sanchez, François, 64

Sarraut, Albert, 28

Sarró, Ramón, 21
Sartre, Jean-Paul, 11, 52, 57–58, 70; *Anti-Semite and Jew*, 56
Saumery clinic, 75
Sauret, Jaime, 30–31
Saussure, Ferdinand de, 85
Schérer, René, 88, 103
schizoanalysis, 78, 95–97, 104–5, 109, 118
schizoanalytic unconscious, 98
schizophrenia, 4–5, 21, 85–87, 128
Schreber, Daniel Paul, 4–5, 91–92. See also *Memoirs of My Nervous Illness* (Schreber)
self, 9–12, 48, 61, 83, 111, 113, 115–16, 144; and alterity, 24, 51–52, 56
Sellier, Henri, 34
Senghor, Léopold, 54, 57–58
Septfonds, France, 28–32. *See also* Camp de Judes
Service du travail obligatoire (STO), 36
shell shock, 27
signifier, 84–85, 87, 90–91
Simon, Hermann, 21–22, 27, 39, 44, 64, 161n32. *See also* Gütersloh asylum
Sivadon, Paul, 131
socialism, 11, 17–19, 71, 78, 159n9. *See also individual organizations and parties*
social psychiatry, 27
socialthérapie. See institutional psychotherapy
Société du Gévaudan, 37–38
sociodrames, 69
sociogeny, 52, 56
Sorbonne, 111–12, 120
Spain, 13, 143; Civil War in, 2, 16, 18, 26–28, 34, 146; fascism in, 21, 78, 93; refugees from, 17, 27, 28–31. *See also individual cities*
Spanish Popular Front, 18, 26, 28
Spinoza, Baruch, 88–90
Spinoza et le problème de l'expression (Deleuze), 90
Spinoza: Philosophie pratique (Deleuze), 90
Stalinism, 1, 16, 18, 26–27, 33, 74, 88, 101
storytellers, 68, 72
structuralism, 124, 147, 175; and Lacan, 6, 25, 83–85, 87, 90–92; structural anal-ysis, 7, 39, 50–51, 56, 58–60, 67, 69–70;
structural linguistics, 6, 131
subject-groups. See *groupes-sujets* vs. *groupes-assujettis*
subjectivity: Bourdieu on, 89, 97, 143; Fanon on, 51, 56–60, 73; Freud on, 5, 24; Guattari on, 78, 86, 90, 97–98, 103; Lacan on, 25, 86–87; theory of, 9–10, 12, 143; Tosquelles on, 19
Surrealism, 2, 20–21, 23–24, 34–36, 45, 47, 60
Svedberg laboratory, 120
Sweden, 115, 119–20
Switzerland, 23, 45–46, 68, 86, 113–14
Symbolic (Lacan), 4, 22, 75, 81, 83–85, 91–92, 100, 129, 131
Szasz, Thomas, 6, 83, 135; *The Myth of Mental Illness*, 130
Sztulman, Henri, 125

talking cure, 4
Tankonalasanté (Aslongaswehavehealth), 133–34
Tavistock, 26, 127, 129
theater, in hospitals, 5, 30, 41–42, 67, 81–82, 114–15
Thiers Foundation, 113
Third Reich, 1, 33, 146. *See also* Hitler, Adolf
Third World, 70–71, 101, 173n97
thirdworldism, 69, 88, 101
Thousand Plateaus, A (Guattari and Deleuze), 8
Tiselius, Arne, 120
Tosquelles, François: and alienation, 8, 38, 101, 118; and art, 45–46; and Canguilhem, 35–36; and Club Paul Balvet, 41–44, 46; on disalienation, 16, 80; on ergotherapy, 44; and Fanon, 7, 50, 60–61, 64; and fascism, 2, 16, 21, 33, 78, 93; and Freud, 10, 16–17; and GTPSI, 98; on healing collectives, 40, 46–47; and institutional psychotherapy, 2, 13, 37, 47, 78, 117–18, 131, 145, 147; and Lacan, 16, 21–27, 61, 160n24, 160n26, 175n23; and Marx, 10, 16–17; on May '68, 88; and Mira, 20–21, 27; and Oury, 8, 15, 22, 74–75, 175n23; and POUM, 18–19,

220 INDEX

Tosquelles, François (*continued*)
26, 146; and psychiatry, 2, 16, 27, 30–
31, 52, 55, 108, 123, 128–29; and psychoanalysis, 16, 32; at Saint-Alban, 5,
7, 20–22, 25–27, 33–34, 37–40, 47, 64,
114; on schizophrenia, 85; at Septfonds
camp, 28–32, 60; and Simon, 21–22, 44,
161n32; and subjectivity, 19; on transference, 5, 86, 99, 129; and the unconscious, 46
totalitarianism, 36–37, 78, 93, 131
Toulouse, Édouard, 23
tout-pouvoir, 2, 18, 146
Toward an Institutional Pedagogy
(F. Oury and Vasquez), 75
Toward the African Revolution (Fanon),
63, 69
Trait d'union (newsletter), 41–44, 61
transference, 6–7, 39–41, 75, 78, 98, 103,
145, 148; burst, 5, 99, 129; collective, 13;
dissociated, 81, 86; and Fanon, 60; and
Freud, 4, 16; and Mira, 20; transferential constellation, 5, 46, 99, 129. *See also*
countertransference
transversality, 5, 99–101
Trentin, Silvio, 35
Trotskyism, 18, 74, 88, 101
Trump, Donald, 143, 146–47
Tuke, William, 91, 122–23
Tunisia, 7, 13, 50, 68–70

unconscious (psychoanalytic concept):
and alienation, 78, 89; and CERFI,
102–3; Deleuze and Guattari on, 91,
93–94, 96, 98, 100; Fanon on, 51, 56;
Foucault on, 110, 112–13; Freud on, 4–
5, 24; Lacan on, 24, 83, 87; Oury on,
75, 86; and politics, 10–11, 146, 149;
schizoanalytic, 98; and the self, 9, 13;
Tosquelles on, 46; and transference,
7, 145
Union des Étudiants Communistes
(UEC), 101
Union fédérale des étudiants, 34

United Kingdom. *See* Great Britain
United States, 6, 12, 22, 45, 69–70, 83, 108,
130, 143
universalism, 54, 57, 70
University of Barcelona, 20
University of Lille, 107, 113
University of Paris VIII. *See* University of
Vincennes
University of Uppsala, 120
University of Vincennes, 88, 130

Vasquez, Aïda, *Toward an Institutional
Pedagogy*, 75
Verdeaux, Georges, 112–14
Verdeaux, Jacqueline, 112–14
Vichy France, 1–3, 16, 33–34, 93, 146,
163n80. *See also* French Resistance;
Pétain, Philippe
Vienna, Austria, 21
Vigouroux, Lieutenant Colonel, 30
Voie communiste, 88

war neuroses, 27, 29
Weber, Alfred, 115
Weimar Republic, 161n32
Weizsäcker, Viktor von, *Der Gestaltkreis*,
107–8, 123
Wilder, Gary, 147–48
Winnicott, Donald, 129
Wölfli, Adolf, 45
World Psychiatric Congress, 112
World War I, 27
World War II, 26, 28, 33, 38, 59, 78, 107,
123, 146; and institutional psycho-
therapy, 10, 15–16, 47, 146; and psycho-
analysis, 5. *See also* Third Reich; Vichy
France
Wretched of the Earth, The (Fanon), 7, 50,
69–72

Year Five of the Algerian Revolution, The
(Fanon), 69–70
York Retreat, 122
youth hostels, 74–75, 81, 146

Printed and bound by CPI Group (UK) Ltd, Croydon, CR0 4YY
15/10/2024

14574334-0002